Trials of an

ORDINARY
DOCTOR

To carry the mind in writing back into the past . . . is a task of great labor and judgment—the rather because in ancient transactions the truth is difficult to ascertain, and in modern it is dangerous to tell.

—Sir Francis Bacon, *De Dignitate et Augmentis Scientiarum* (1623)

HAROLD J. COOK

_Trials of an
ORDINARY
DOCTOR

*Joannes Groenevelt in
Seventeenth-Century
London*

The Johns Hopkins University Press

BALTIMORE AND LONDON

© 1994 The Johns Hopkins University Press
All rights reserved
Printed in the United States of America on acid-free paper
03 02 01 00 99 98 97 96 95 94   5 4 3 2 1

The Johns Hopkins University Press
2715 North Charles Street
Baltimore, Maryland 21218-4319
The Johns Hopkins Press Ltd., London

ISBN 0-8018-4778-8
Library of Congress Cataloging-in-Publication Data will be found
at the end of this book.
A catalog record for this book is available from the British Library.

Dedicated to
Faye
mijn echtgenoot

Contents

Illustrations

Acknowledgments

I WOULD LIKE to acknowledge the generous support of many people and agencies over the years who made this book possible. The Clark and Milton funds of Harvard University made possible summer travel to London, and the Graduate School of the University of Wisconsin–Madison helped make possible a semester in the Netherlands learning Dutch and beginning to trace Groenevelt through the archives there. During the 1989–90 year, I was able to live in the Netherlands and carry on research—part of which went into this book—thanks to the combined support of the Fulbright Commission and the Netherlands America Foundation for Educational Exchange, the National Endowment for the Humanities, the National Library of Medicine (NIH Grant LM 05066), and the Graduate School of the University of Wisconsin–Madison. At a time when this project was not quite formed, I had the encouragement of Simon Schama to tackle the Dutch language, and the very generous help of Francis Gouda and Dirk Struik in making rough initial translations of some of Groenevelt's letters. Brad Holtman later made a more complete translation of them for me, while Rob Howell introduced me to the modern tongue. My colleagues in the departments of the History of Medicine and the History of Science tolerated my crazy project, and Judy Leavitt and Ron Numbers even encouraged me in it. I also received support from Marten van Lieburg and from Daniel de Moulin, Wim Mulder, Godelieve van Heteren, and Hilary Marland. Thanks, too, to the archivists of many places, especially of the municipal archives in Amsterdam, Delft, Deventer, Grave, Haarlem, and Leiden, and to the librarians of the Koningklijk Bibliotheeck, the Leiden University Library, the Museum Boerhaave library, the London Guildhall, the Corporation of London Records Office, the Worshipful Company of Barbers, the Royal Society of London, the British Library, the Bodleian Library, the National Library of Medicine, the

University of Wisconsin–Madison special collections, the Middleton Library rare book collection, the Institute for Historical Research, and the Wellcome Institute for the History of Medicine, especially John Symons. Geoffrey Davenport, the librarian of the Royal College of Physicians, has been unfailingly helpful over the years, while the Fellows of the Royal College of Physicians generously allowed me to quote from their documents; Phyllis Kauffman organized facilities in Madison for photographing rare medical books. Mark Derez of the University Archives and Geert Vanpaemel, both of the Katholieke Universiteit Leuven, helped me sort out some leads regarding François Zypeaus; Francis McKee and Cathy Crawford both pointed out some connections to Groenevelt they had come across in their own research; Shigehisa Kuriyama helped with references to early European accounts of acupuncture; and Doctors Reginald Bruskewitz and David Bloom, urologists, read chapter 4 and verified that the surgical descriptions there were correct. An earlier version of Groenevelt's story appeared in the 1990 issue of *Tractrix*. Susan Lawrence generously offered comments on large parts of the work in an earlier draft, and David Sacks astutely suggested ways to streamline the last chapters.

But this study of Groenevelt and his world truly would have been impossible without the help of my Dutch friends. Antonie Luyendijk-Elshout's kindness to a stranger opened the doors through which Groenevelt walked. She graciously invited me to stay in Leiden when I first traveled to the Netherlands, took an interest in my work, and arranged many things for me. Over many years, too, Toon Kerkhoff patiently listened to my stories, helped with my Dutch, and introduced me to sailing on Dutch waters; without this experience my perception of his country would have been very different. Equally important, Gemma Beukers and Gabrielle Kerkhoff made me, and later Faye, feel quite at home in their lovely land. My deepest debt of gratitude is owed to my host in Leiden on many occasions since my first visit: Harm Beukers, who gave me a desk at which to work, encouraged me to speak in his tongue even when I butchered it badly, taught me an enormous amount about the medical history of his country, and even carefully read parts of the manuscript. Needless to say, all remaining errors are my own. Without the help and friendship of all these many people, Groenevelt would not have had his day. Above all, however, the wit, insight, and support of Faye made this study possible, even when she had to live with ghosts.

Introduction

The Importance of an Ordinary Doctor

JOANNES GROENEVELT, or John Greenfield, as his English friends sometimes called him, walked in the worlds on both sides of the North Sea. On the one side, the earth washed down from the Alpine mountains ended in a flat and often soggy land cut by a maze of rivers, inhabited by the people among whom Joannes Groenevelt was born: the Dutch. Neighborly and clannish, well educated and industrious, led as often by the interests of their merchants as by the dynastic policies of their nobles, and seeking a working consensus despite a welter of diverse regions, dialects, and religions, they peopled the northwestern corner of the continent more densely than anyone else anywhere else in Europe save the Italians. Near the coast they had already reclaimed considerable arable land from the water. From behind their rivers, dikes, and massive urban fortifications they had beaten off recent attempts at conquest from the south and east; in the bottoms of their ships traveled the goods of northern Europe and, increasingly, the wealth of Asia, Africa, and North America.

On the other side, sheltered by the rough sea, were the English, among whom Groenevelt died. A wealthy kingdom with a powerful aristocracy, committed to the defense of honor as much as to the pursuit of wealth, the more thinly settled people of England were never entirely comfortable with strangers from across the water, although the pressures of religious struggle, trade, and war had caused them to tolerate many of those fleeing war on the Continent and even to invite over some to teach them new industries. The capital city of London, strategically situated on the lower reaches of the Thames, within easy reach of both the North Sea and the Atlantic, was growing at a tremendous pace that would soon make it the largest city in Europe; and English merchants and English ships competed increasingly successfully with the Dutch for trade in Asia, Europe, the Levant, and America.

Within this militant, acquisitive, cool, and damp world on both sides of the North Sea, new ideas were flourishing. Much new information and many new ways of looking at the world flowed in from elsewhere: from France, Italy, Iberia, the Baltic, central Europe, and the Balkans, from the Middle East, Asia, Africa, and the Americas. Other ideas of a more local flavor bubbled to the surface in the cities and villages, universities and print shops. No one, most especially a person of education, could remain unaffected by the rapid changes. At least Groenevelt was not; and his life and ideas clearly show us that world of the northwest at the moment between "the scientific revolution" and the Enlightenment.

Like many of his peers, Groenevelt entered upon a life in which he made a living through the exercise of a particular kind of knowledge and skill. Like many of the most highly educated of the age, he joined those who ministered to the body rather than join those who ministered to the soul. He and his boyhood friends obtained one of the best medical educations available in Europe, let alone in the north. One of Groenevelt's boyhood friends, Herbert Dapper, went on to a distinguished career in his hometown of Deventer as a physician and burgomaster; another, Caspar Sibellius, became well known in medical circles from Amsterdam to the upper reaches of the Rhine, and for a time in England and Ireland as well. In a country overpopulated with learned physicians, however, many Dutch medical practitioners, like Dutchmen of so many other ways of life, were forced to look elsewhere and set out on what has been termed the Dutch diaspora. Willem ten Rhijne, for example, another boyhood friend of Groenevelt's, took service with the Dutch East India Company, where he not only became a man of importance but wrote the first detailed report to Europeans about the Japanese practice of acupuncture.

Groenevelt, too, had to leave his country for an uncertain future abroad, in his case England. Because of his education, interests, and friends, he soon became known among the members of the Royal Society for the Advancement of Natural Knowledge of London. He associated with an influential group of medical dissenters, innovators, and translators, including Edward Tyson, John Pechey, and Thomas Sydenham. His own publications earned a good, if modest, reputation in Europe for furthering surgical techniques and medical treatments. In London, he became a noted physician and lithotomist, surgically removing bladder stones. But the "Glorious Revolution" that brought a Dutchman to the English throne in 1688 soon brought Groenevelt grief:

the London medical establishment, fed up with Groenevelt and his friends, supported by new Dutch immigrants attempting to displace the old, tried to extinguish his livelihood. His notorious trial for malpractice in the mid-1690s became a cause célèbre, and his eventual vindication in the English courts established an important legal precedent. Only similarly antiestablishment medical practitioners and English regard for legal niceties came to his rescue. But not even professional allies and the law could save him from an impoverished old age and death in a country that was never his own. Despite defending himself successfully, his reputation never recovered and his practice declined, as did his health. When he died just a couple of months short of his sixty-eighth birthday, in London, he was virtually without means.

The medical interests of Groenevelt and his Dutch and English friends were closely connected to their enthusiasm for the new, experimental philosophy. They knew perfectly the new ideas of Descartes and Boyle; saw the hand of God in nature, although not always in the ways taught by orthodox doctrine; thought of their task as developing new and effective remedies for forceful diseases; and grasped eclectically at experimentally founded treatments. They campaigned for a new medical order. They had no patience for divisions between science and medicine, nor for those between medicine, surgery, and pharmacy. While they were on the front line fighting the diseases of humankind, however, the old guard tried to undermine them—or so they thought. The unsettled Dutch and the English dissenters became allies. In the end, perhaps Groenevelt and his friends sometimes went too far with their experimental ideas and innovations and in their sales pitches; but their struggles help to illuminate the day-to-day concerns of those who were trying to change the world.

For a time, Groenevelt's trial for malpractice became remembered in Europe as an example of the conservative nature of the London physicians. While authors writing in English have often been given to contrasting the cutting-edge scientific ideas of English physicians like William Harvey and his discovery of the circulation of the blood to their more "conservative" colleagues in France, people on the Continent often saw things the other way around. One French medical dictionary early in the nineteenth century included a discussion of Groenevelt's use of cantharides (Spanish fly) and camphor, concluding that although his remedy was now in doubt, it was a useful and, better, heroic method (such methods being in fashion when the dictionary was written). Despite the success Groenevelt had with his remedy, the entry went on, the London College of Physicians sentenced him to Newgate in 1693 (the date is mistaken); and although he was acquitted, the trial ruined him. The moral of the story is that "the advancement of science is hindered both by abuse and by enthusiasm alike."[1] Even some Englishmen with Continental educations found Groenevelt's life to have had the same moral: while the conservative College of Physicians ruined Groenevelt with their prosecution for malpractice, he "taught his envious Prosecutors the Safety and Value of his Practice."[2]

What does such a life matter? Why choose to devote a detailed study to a person who, by comparison with the great minds and powerful figures of a heroic age, is only a short and insignificant footnote in what is often portrayed as the exciting annals of the birth of modernity?

More than fifty years ago, in another period as full of anxiety about the future and confusion about the meaning of the past as our own, several eloquent authors of historical literature drew attention to the importance of examining the ideas of those people whom they called "minor writers." One of the most influential historians of the generation, Arthur O. Lovejoy, wrote that historians of literature ought to try to understand "the ideas and feelings which other men in past times have been moved by, and . . . the processes by which what might be called literary and philosophical public opinion is formed." In trying to understand the temperament of an age, a "minor writer may be as important as—he may often, from this point of view, be more important than—the authors of what are now regarded as the masterpieces."[3] To buttress this view, Lovejoy in turn quoted the Edwardian editor of the works of the seventeenth-century English minister George Herbert: "The tendencies of an age appear more distinctly in its writers of inferior rank than in those of commanding genius. These latter tell of past and future as well as of the age in which they live. They are for all time. But on the sensitive responsive souls, of less creative power, current ideals record themselves with clearness."[4] Since at least the beginning of the century, then, many historians have followed this advice to look at the words of people other than "geniuses" in order to discover the framework of ideas and opinion in the past. There is nothing unusual about writing about ordinary people.

By today's standards of historical writing, however, a well-established cleric of noted literary talents like George Herbert scarcely qualifies as a "minor" figure, or someone of "inferior rank." There is an understandable desire among many of the best historians today to investigate the history of groups of people who have not yet had their chroniclers, or to analyze the slow but fundamental changes of society, economy, or culture. Yet if Groenevelt never came close to achieving the reputation of a Herbert, neither does he clearly represent a large group, nor does his single life shed much new light on the causes of massive social changes. The life of a village healer or bonesetter, or a traveling cataract remover or mountebank, would make a better study of the average medical practitioner in the seventeenth century; and probing the attitudes of patients toward the host of medical practitioners available to them would make a better study of the structure of ordinary people's mental habits.[5]

Perhaps the best justification for studying such a person as Groenevelt—if justification is needed—lies in the power of a genre sometimes now called "microhistory." Inspired by modern ethnographers, many historians have written detailed accounts of the lives of people previously hardly known to historians, people who by the very fact that good evidence about their lives survives are neither average nor typical, presenting us with lively stories that illuminate little corners of humanity which could hardly have been imagined before: millers reading borrowed books to develop their own ideas about God and nature before becoming caught up by the Inquisition; peasants put on trial for faking their identities; artisans with their eyes on God living through a period of civil war and religious upheaval; a Chinese scholar in Europe locked up in an insane asylum; even rowdy young apprentices killing cats.[6]

As in these other instances, Groenevelt's story can shed light on the life and attitudes of the period not because he was average or typical but because in the echoes of his life one can hear the sounds of many others, too. Time takes all things, and no modern magic allows us to conjure up the real voices or shapes of people from the seventeenth century. All we have left are words and objects, largely in the form of ink on paper: the tangible signs of vanished spirits. Yet with a bit of sympathy, and a collection of words, we can begin to sense something of the world in which Groenevelt and his acquaintances walked. As we do so, we shall find that one cannot fruitfully separate the world of ideas from the world of circumstance (or, as historians of science sometimes put it, the "internal" from the "external" worlds). Nor can we forsake an understanding of how people practiced medicine and surgery. Instead, following Groenevelt's "science in action" will be our task.[7] We shall also come to see how deeply Anglocentric current accounts of early modern medicine have been. Groenevelt made his way to London, and in doing so he brought with him some of the finest learning the Continent offered. The practices that flowed from his experiences were not well regarded by many of his English contemporaries. And yet the story of his struggles in London is not exactly one of a cultural clash between nations (or of scientific "national styles"), since Groenevelt also had English defenders of his views among people who shared many of the values of the Dutch. We shall therefore have to look at his life not only from a perspective situated west of the Dover cliffs but from one east of the sandy beaches that stretch along the European coast of the North Sea, too: from the lowlands that sat at the crossroads of northern Europe.

Trials of an

ORDINARY
DOCTOR

CHAPTER 1

Medical Malpractice in the Seventeenth Century

JOANNES GROENEVELT found himself at the center of one of the great medical controversies in London during the 1690s. A patient of his, Mrs. Withall, claimed to have ended up bedridden as a result of a secret remedy given by Dr. Groenevelt. She and her husband and neighbors made their complaint against him known to the Censors of the College of Physicians of London, a group of physicians who had the legal authority to regulate medical practice and practitioners in the City of London and within seven miles of its walls. Withall lodged her complaint just at the moment when the censors and other officers of the London college were trying to restore their lapsed authority. As a law-abiding physician, Groenevelt belonged to the London College of Physicians, although he remained only a licentiate rather than sitting among the full voting members, the fellows. Members ordinarily received the benefit of the doubt when confronted with charges of bad practice. In this case, however, the censors of the college investigated Withall's complaint and eventually brought charges of malpractice against the doctor.

For his part, confronted with Withall's charges, Groenevelt first tried to demean the character of the women witnesses against him; when the censors refused to listen to character assassination, he then tried to explain his medical method. But the censors did not want to hear about his ideas or justifications. By continuing to argue for his views when the censors seem already to have made up their minds that his practice had been a bad one, Groenevelt only showed himself to possess a disobedient character. Even so, although they formally found him guilty of malpractice, the censors could not agree to sentence him. One of them, Edward Tyson, even changed his mind, deciding that Groenevelt's practice had not been so evil. Tyson had had his own troubles with the college censors.

Thus, the sad case of one of the patients on whom Groenevelt used a new remedy became caught up in the institutional and intellectual conflicts of the London physicians. Groenevelt bore the brunt of the censors' anger against what they thought to be bad medical practice and bad personal behavior on the part of some of the members of the college. They tried to make an example of Groenevelt. But they had picked on someone who refused to think that he could be in the wrong on this matter, someone who would never agree to accept the judgment of his lawful superiors when he believed them to be accusing him unjustly. Groenevelt's uncompromising nature, together with the censors' own judgment of his wrongdoing, eventually caused the debate about his care for Mrs. Withall to develop into a great struggle over contemporary medical ideas and practices in London. It became a battle pitting the English medical establishment against a Dutch doctor and his London allies. His case came to divide deeply the London physicians at a crucial moment.

But before examining the ramifications of his case, let us turn to an examination of the record of Groenevelt's malpractice.

The complaint against Dr. Groenevelt was very grave indeed. On 27 July 1694, Suzanna Withall and three of her women neighbors came before a formal meeting of the Censors of the College of Physicians of London to lodge a complaint. Established in 1518, the College of Physicians had obtained the right to limit the practice of "physic" to its own members and to oversee the practice of medicine in London. By the end of the sixteenth century, the four "censors" and the president of the college ordinarily sat as a body once or twice a month from the early autumn to the late spring, both to examine candidates for the fellowship and licentiate (the two main categories of membership) and to hear complaints against people practicing badly or without their permission. When the censors investigated cases of malpractice or illicit practice, they could call witnesses and the accused before them to hear testimony, and they could hand down sentences. The number of meetings of the censors' board each year varied considerably depending on how vigorously the college officers wished to pursue complaints. In the later seventeenth century, the committee met often in the college's new buildings in Warwick Lane, sitting in a large upstairs room. The president presided in dignity in an ornate chair with a canopy, the censors to his left and right asking questions of witnesses, the registrar seated nearby scribbling notes of the proceedings which provided the basis for the transcript of meetings he later entered into the official "Annals" of the college. All wore their long red gowns and powdered wigs, covered by the square bonnets of the university graduate.[1]

In the mid-1690s, the president and censors tried actively to impose some order on medical practice and practitioners in London, and they took a special interest in complaints about malpractice. For instance, in early 1694, they heard testimony against a French surgeon called Francis Pursenett du Mongean: he stood accused of extorting from Mr. Herman Grafflyn large sums of money after Grafflyn had agreed to a course of treatment which so weakened him that he could not even get out of the bed at the inn to beg for water. In another case, a German Dr. Marholts was said to have administered a medicine that made Lieutenant Colonel Bridewitch vomit blood until he died.[2] The president and censors also took much care to investigate the case of the London empiric William Rivett. ("Empirics" like Rivett were practitioners who had no formal medical education but depended on previous experience; by the seventeenth century they had become identified in many minds with quackery.)[3] One Stephen Fargie told the censors that Rivett had been responsible for the death of Andrew Cork, who had lived in St. Anne's, Blackfriars. Cork, Fargie thought, had been in a deep consumption and very weak. When Rivett attended Cork, however, Rivett let large quantities of blood by opening a vein several times and also gave Cork strong medicines to take, which purged him upward and downward. Most medical practitioners at the time used venesection, emetics, and purgatives, but they were supposed to use them with care, taking into account the patient's condition. After interviewing Rivett, the president and censors decided that he did not know enough about what he was doing; they also looked into his prescriptions. When Rivett refused to come before them for further investigation, they found him guilty of malpractice, fined him £20, and ordered him to Newgate—the infamous prison of murderers, highwaymen, and rogues of all sorts—to be held at their pleasure. Such a verdict brought Rivett to his knees, and after he begged not to be sent to Newgate, the president and censors released him with only the fine and two promises: not ever to practice again in London, and never to bother the relatives of the unfortunate Cork about the remaining money they owed him for his services.[4]

Groenevelt had already found himself accused of bad behavior, although not malpractice. In August 1693, Mrs. Katherine Hawes complained to the censors about the way Groenevelt arranged his fees. Groenevelt had practiced surgery on Mrs. Hawes's husband to extract a bladder stone. The doctor was to have been paid £20 for his work. The day after the operation Mrs. Hawes had paid him £8 and obtained in return a letter from him saying that if her husband died within a month, Groenevelt would repay the amount. Sadly, Mr. Hawes had died five days after the operation. Yet despite their agreement, Groenevelt presented the new widow with a bill for a further payment of £3 6s. for expenses, "though the Dr. owed her, as appeared by her Book for Cloathes, etc. four pounds." That is, Groenevelt had apparently paid the £3 6s. for another surgeon's help with the operation or postoperative care, while Mrs. Hawes had spent somewhat more for the bandages and other expenses incurred; she also thought that Groenevelt owed her the £8 she had already paid. More seriously for Groenevelt, Mrs. Hawes also claimed that he had refused to allow her to consult with other physicians about her husband's recovery. Groenevelt denied preventing her from consulting others, admitted that he had taken in hand £8 of the £20, and agreed that he had given Mrs. Hawes a written promise to return it if her husband died. The censors' committee decided on a Solomon-like reply: Groenevelt was to pay the assistant surgeon's bill out of the £8 he had received, and of the approximately £4 remaining, he was to repay her about half, 40s. The decision seems to have satisfied both parties.[5]

In 1694, the censors' committee tried so hard to remove medical abuses from London that they continued to meet regularly through that summer, a time when many physicians, like the English gentry, left the city for the countryside. Mrs. Withall was able, therefore, to bring her complaint of being badly treated by Groenevelt before the censors' board in July.

According to the account of her testimony later written into the Annals by the registrar, Dr. Thomas Gill, Mrs. Withall told the censors' committee a story about the quackish behavior of one of their own members, a case not unlike that of Rivett. Although she had not died from Dr. Groenevelt's treatment, he had caused her to become a weak, pained, and bedridden woman. Having called him in to cure her of pain in her "lower parts" following the delivery of a child, Withall took a medicine Groenevelt gave her, which resulted in painful urination, debilitating discomforts, and violent sweats. Groenevelt had made Withall an invalid, unable to care for her seven children or husband. And he had done this out of ignorant and, she thought, illegal practice. The president and censors of the college agreed. Dr. Groenevelt, is seems, was a dangerous and undisciplined man—just how dangerous is best left to the words set down in Mrs. Withall's complaint.

According to the registrar's words, Mrs. Withall humbly informed the censors that matters had begun innocently enough. Having "received a hurt in her Labour," she "was advised to send for one Dr. Groenvelt." She "related her Griefs" to him and asked him to give her something "that might recover her." The doctor said that he would do so. From a later record, it appears that she first called for the doctor about 20 March 1693 and that she had previously consulted a leading male midwife for her complaint, Dr. David Hamilton, apparently without success.[6] So far, Withall was doing what typified the medicine of the period: people did what they could by themselves before sending for help and then called in someone who they determined would give them what they wanted.

Once Mrs. Withall decided she wanted treatment from Dr. Groenevelt and he agreed to treat her, they had to settle on a price. According to her recorded testimony, she had agreed to pay him £4 10s.: a considerable amount of money. Since the daily wage of building craftsmen in southern England at the time amounted to 18–20d., £4 amounted to about two months' wages for a good wage earner (at 20d. per day, six days per week): a large sum indeed.[7] On the other hand, other practitioners also charged about what Groenevelt did or more. An apothecary named William Eels charged Thomas Sharpe £20 for five months' treatment (or £4 per month); another, John Hobbs, charged Mrs. Powell £13 14s. 8d. for treating her husband (who died).[8] In fact, many of the complaints heard by the censors' committee of the College of Physicians show that plenty of practitioners charged higher prices than Groenevelt. One Gaspar Reinhold Baddingbroek went to a Huguenot refugee named James Feuillel la Saufay, who had been recommended as someone who could cure Baddingbroek's rheumatic pains. Saufay gave him some red powder, folded into two pieces of paper, which only caused Baddingbroek to get sick and faint, while making his gums and mouth sore and his breath stink. When Baddingbroek refused to pay Saufay for the powder, however, Saufay sued him for nonpayment, demanding 12 guineas (a guinea was £1 1s.); Saufay later had Baddingbroek arrested for a debt of £15.[9] The censors wanted to know what Groenevelt charged, but since they seldom brought up the matter of price again, they seem to have been content that Groenevelt, unlike Saufay, did not ask an unreasonable amount.

On the other hand, they clearly wanted to know from Mrs. Withall how Dr. Groenevelt had been paid. She testified that she gave him half the fee then and there, with the other half to be paid "when he had performed the Cure."[10] Many practitioners, like Groenevelt, obtained their fees in this manner. One Dr. Briggs did so in late 1700, for instance.[11] Such a manner of payment secured at least part of the costs for practitioners if their patients later refused payment. Patients themselves may have considered that they could better control the medical relationship if they controlled the final payment, although we have no direct testimony about this. Some patients even seem to have thought that payment alone ought to guarantee a cure. In 1688, for example, William Davis complained to the censors that he had paid £3 10s. to one William Harder to cure his throat but that Harder's treatment had done no good despite payment.[12] To the leaders of the medical profession, however, like the president and censors of the College of Physicians, bargaining over payment smacked of the shopkeeper. They preferred to act like gentlemen and take an honorarium after having assisted someone rather than charging fees, much less demanding half the money up front.[13] As we shall see, they made sure to put on record the accounts of the other witnesses about Groenevelt's billing practices, presumably because it indicated that he had some of the trappings of a quack.

Having set down Withall's testimony about how Groenevelt obtained half his money in advance, the registrar went on to record what she said about his treatment. According to Withall, soon after she paid Groenevelt half his fee, he returned with "a Dose of Pills" (small round balls held together by a glutinous liquid containing medicine which Mrs. Withall was to eat). The Annals then moved on immediately to note that Withall suspected that this dose "was not proper for her Distemper" and entreated him "to give her nothing that had poison in it." The registrar's account goes on to say that he "assured her there was none in them, and they were prepared according to Art": that is, prepared according to the best medical knowledge. "If he gave her any thing that was not duly prepared, she might apply herself to the College of Physicians, whereof he himself was a Member, and she should have redress," the record goes on at third hand. Unfortunately, according to the transcript of Withall's account, "she had no sooner taken" the pills than they "instantly put her into such a racking Torture, and miserable Condition, as cannot be expressed." When the doctor returned soon after to check on her and heard her complaints, "he told her that [the pills] were of such vertue, that if the College knew the worth of them, they would value them at a high rate." Nevertheless, the registrar wrote, Groenevelt took the remaining pills (since Mrs. Withall had not been able to eat them all) and threw them into the fire.[14]

But Groenevelt and Withall did not have their conversations alone. As usual in the period, Withall's case had been conducted in front of friends, family, and attendants. Among the others, "the nurse being present carefully preserved" one of the pills thrown into the fire. Mrs. Withall recollected that this pill had afterward been shown to "severall able Physicians, and others, who all agree[d] that they were for the most part Composed of Spanish Flies, and other things altogether improper for her Infirmity."

Spanish flies were also known as blister beetles, since their most common use was externally, in plasters meant to cause blisters (to allow the shedding of excess humors from the body). Later in the century, Nicolas Lémery recommended the external use of cantharides behind the ears and shoulders for diseases of the eyes and nose, apoplexy, and paralysis and applied to the legs for rheumatism and sciatica.[15] The beetle known in English as Spanish fly had the Latin name of cantharides and contained both a yellow and a green oil, the second of which gave its color to the whole powder;[16] moreover, their glittering green wings retained their color after powdering: they were probably the "shining greenish things" noticed by the nurse. (According to Groenevelt, the English knew two kinds of beetle as Spanish fly, a smaller kind being cantharides proper, and a larger kind—called *Buprestis* in Latin and "burn cow" in English—also going by the name.[17] The most thorough contemporary study of the cantharides beetle proper clearly dealt with a species now known as *Lytta vesicatoria*.)[18] But more important, Withall would have shared the popular wisdom about how taking Spanish flies internally would stimulate the sexual organs. The Roman poet Ovid had written: "You ought to drink the juices of cantharides since they will make you a parent."[19] In the early eighteenth century, the president of the College of Physicians, Sir Hans Sloane, received a long report from someone who found an elderly male visitor to his home giving his wife several doses of Spanish flies to get her to lie with him. "I have since inquired of this, and find it's common for the Boys to buy it at the apothecarys and give it [to] the maid. Oh! horrid thing that renders Conversation dangerous."[20]

Withall believed that taking pills made with Spanish flies by Dr. Groenevelt's "illegall (and as she humbly conceive[d]) ignorant undertaking" had "utterly ruined her." She explained to the censors that her present condition was one of "extream weakness" and "so great an Indisposition" that she was "no way able to stand, go, or dress her self" and was growing "every day worse." Groenevelt, she said, had not only "undone" her but her husband and seven children, too.[21]

The local records do not show us anything further about Suzanna Withall. Not even her recent childbirth had been recorded by the parish clerk.[22] Perhaps she was therefore not a member of the Anglican church but a dissenter. She lived with her family in what is now the borough of Southwark, a densely packed neighborhood of ordinary working folk and shopkeepers and the poor.[23] Later references to her living space indicate that she had at least one room with a bed and fireplace—and probably an additional room or two, with a cooking area available nearby if not in her lodgings. She may, like

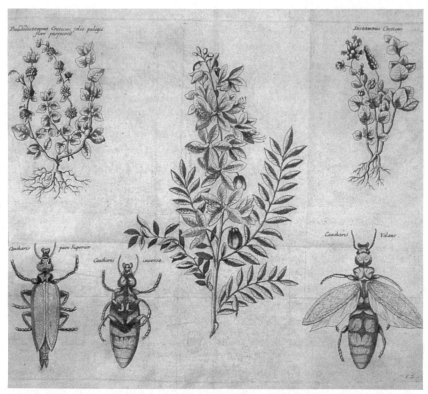

FIG. 1. *The cantharides beetle is depicted from above, from below, and with wings open, together with the plants on which it is commonly found. From Joh. Daniel Geyer,* Tractatus physico-medicus de cantharidibus *(1687), by permission of the British Library.*

other women, have engaged in various kinds of employment, but the college records identify her as the wife of William Withall, a chapman—that is, a petty trader who might keep a small booth or sell little books, forks, knives, cooking utensils, pills, and other inexpensive household goods door to door from a pack he carried on his back.[24] The college officers treated her as a humble but respectable person, one of the ordinary people who had sufficient means for themselves and their families; she had certainly been able to call on more than a little cash or credit to pay for her medical help, from doctors and midwives to nurses.

To support her testimony, Withall brought other witnesses, people who had attended her during Groenevelt's treatment, one of whom had first spotted the Spanish fly in the pills. The three supporting witnesses were women from

Withall's neighborhood, the parish of St. Mary Overy, otherwise known as St. Saviours' Southwark (a parish just on the south side of the Thames over London Bridge). In the original complaint, only their names are mentioned, but further identifications are given in a later document. One was Prunella Beckett, a nurse; a second was Hannah or Joanna Walding (not unusually, her first name is given both ways in the documents) wife of William Walding; and the third was Jane Daylight, a midwife (and according to a later deposition, a Quaker).[25]

Prunella Beckett spoke first after Withall. She gave further information about Withall's original illness, according to the registrar saying that Withall had suffered from a "soreness in her lower parts, which she complained of after her lying in, which the Dr. did say was an ulcer." Here we get a glimpse of the differences in diagnostic categories of ordinary people and physicians: Beckett and Withall only knew that she had a soreness, and they attributed it to the results of having a child, whereas Groenevelt diagnosed a specific medical condition, giving no cause. The patient and her attendants probably thought Withall's own general description of her problem a sufficient guide for deciding on a course to take, such as calling in Dr. Groenevelt. But at a later time, when questioned by the censors about his diagnosis, Groenevelt more precisely said that he had determined that Withall had an ulcer in the "neck of the Bladder."[26]

Nurse Beckett added other details as well about the negotiations over treatment. According to her, Groenevelt said he could "take away" the ulcer in three days, and he agreed to do so for £4, of which he got half (40s.) in hand. The registrar also noted that she testified that Groenevelt said that if he did not cure Withall, they should complain about him to the college. The officers of the college may have been especially sensitive about this because they had recently passed a statute forbidding members to use their membership in the college as anything but a license to practice: that is, Groenevelt should not have implied that his license from the college meant that the censors endorsed his practice.[27]

Finally, Nurse Beckett gave the censors more details about the course of treatment and its outcome: Groenevelt brought Withall eighteen pills to take, of which she took fifteen; Nurse Beckett crushed them ("bruised" them) with a spoon to help Withall swallow them, upon which occasion she noticed in them "some shining greenish things," which she told Mrs. Withall she thought were Spanish flies; and after Withall took the pills, she "had occasion often to make water, which was at first with great pain, and bloody, and afterwards she made perfect blood to the quantity of six quarts, or thereabouts."[28] The details of Beckett's account confirm her own medical abilities, showing someone trained to watch over the condition of patients; Beckett also seems to have been the first one to suspect the main ingredient of the pills and to have warned Mrs. Withall, presumably giving rise to Withall's questions to the doctor about whether the pills contained any "poison."

Another witness, Hannah Walding, "confirmed all that Prunella Beckett had said," according to the registrar. He noted her words on only two matters, which he considered important. On the subject of the ingredients in the pills, the registrar heard Walding confirm that they contained Spanish flies. "Dr. Groenevelt did tell her" this himself, he wrote. He also added her voice to those who believed that these pills had caused Withall's later troubles: "[E]ver since Mrs. Withall did take the pills, she hath been troubled with great pains and burnings in her back, with Convulsions, and violent sweats."[29]

Then the third witness spoke, midwife Jane Daylight. She claimed to have been present to hear the agreement between the doctor and his patient and added that the doctor promised to return the first payment if he did not cure Mrs. Withall. The registrar also noted that Daylight confirmed that Withall had taken fifteen of the eighteen pills brought to her, seconding the testimony about Withall's urine getting red and then turning to "perfect blood" after she took them. Moreover, Daylight told the censors, soon Withall's chamber pot contained "a small lump of flesh." When Daylight saw that, she told them, she "did desire that the Dr. be called for." Groenevelt came, explained how good his medicine was, but at the same time threw the remaining pills on the fire, one of which Daylight herself fished out of the fire and wrapped in paper. This pill was "preserved by the nurse" (presumably Beckett). At some point the pill came into the hands of Mr. Withall, who presented it to Daylight, who broke it open and, like Beckett, thought that it must contain Spanish flies "because there was shining glittering Greeness in it" just like that of Spanish fly, the registrar wrote. He also noted that Daylight said Withall's husband had also told her that he had taken the pill to the nearby hospital of St. Thomas "to show it to the Physicians and Chirurgeons there."[30]

The testimony of the unfortunate Mrs. Withall and her three corroborative witnesses seemed straightforward and convincing to most of the censors. A few confusions arose over time about who did what, and when, but at least the registrar had confidence that they all told the same story. When Withall's own account is taken together with the others, it appeared that Groenevelt had, for a fee—half of which he got in advance—administered to a woman with pains in her "lower parts" eighteen pills containing Spanish fly. Both the nurse and the midwife believed that Spanish fly had been in the pills, and all the women believed that these had been the cause of Mrs. Withall becoming bedridden. Since many people knew of the use of Spanish fly as a blister or as an aphrodisiac, thought of its internal use as risky at best, and could identify it without great difficulty, it seemed sensible to suspect that it was indeed the pills containing Spanish fly, administered in a large dose, which caused Mrs. Withall much pain and bloody urine and apparently caused her such other harm that she still suffered the ill effects, being "undone." Given the gravity of the charges, the president and censors of the College of Physicians immediately ordered that Dr. Groenevelt come before them to answer the complaint.

Groenevelt's testimony would have to wait, however. Like many physicians of the period, he spent at least part of the summer out of London and traveled to visit patients elsewhere in the country. In August 1694, he happened to be in Newcastle. When the censors met on the appointed day of the next week and found him absent, they ordered the college's beadle to summon him when he returned. Groenevelt seems not to have returned by the next meeting of the censors two weeks later, or the censors' meeting two weeks after that, either—or maybe Groenevelt had heard of Withall's testimony against him and had simply been able to avoid being dunned by the college's beadle. Then came an annual period during which the college officers had other business to attend to in organizing the meeting around Michaelmas (usually on 30 September, but in 1694 on 2 October) at which the college elections took place. At that meeting, a number of new men took office as president, treasurer, and censors; and in mid-October, someone who would turn out to be a thorn in Groenevelt's side, Richard Torlesse, gained entry to the inner circle of eight college elders, called the "Elects." It was not until shortly after the end of October, then, that someone (perhaps the one censor to remain from the previous year, Samuel Collins the younger) recollected their past business with the doctor, and the president and censors ordered their beadle once again to summon Groenevelt.[31] At a meeting on 7 November, called especially for the purpose of hearing his reply to the charges against him, the censors finally took up their business from three months earlier.

The three women who had previously testified on Withall's behalf came again, plus another, Barbara Curtis, although Withall herself did not. Since three of the four censors, together with the president, had just been elected to office and so had not been present at the hearing in July, the registrar read out the testimony of the witnesses from the Annals. The previous witnesses said that they stood by their words as set down by the college registrar. The censors then asked them to step outside and called Groenevelt into the room and had the testimony read to him. They then ordered him to "give an account of Mrs. Withall's Case, and of the medicines he had given her."[32]

Groenevelt, however, began his reply by angrily attacking the characters of the women who had testified against him. According to the registrar, he tried "by slighting and vilifying them, to render what they said of little account." The president and censors, however, ordered him to confine his remarks to Withall's case. For a time, Groenevelt only replied to what the censors asked of him.

The censors' committee began by asking him about Withall's condition when he first saw her. She had been "a Beddrid woman," he replied, suffering from an ulcer of the bladder. They asked how he knew that, since her illness had resulted from her recent delivery, at which he took no part. According to the registrar, he replied that "he search't her with an instrument which was stained by the matter" coming from the ulcer. (Being a lithotomist and specialist in urinary complaints more generally, he commonly used a silver catheter for diagnosis.)[33] The censors then asked about the composition of the pills he administered and who had made them. He had made them himself, he replied: of bread crumbs and cantharides, five grains to every three pills, prescribing eighteen pills in all for a total dose of thirty grains, to be taken over the course of twelve hours.[34]

When the censors heard his prescription, their behavior or words probably indicated that they thought this practice at least unwarranted. The registrar put matters this way: since the censors "seemed to dislike" his prescribing such an amount of cantharides, "he went about to justify" his prescription. But the president and censors seem to have had little patience for any novelties of his practice, for they apparently refused to listen to his explanation, at which Groenevelt became increasingly vehement. As the registrar simply put it, from his point of view Groenevelt "behaved himself with great Confidence without any respect at all to the President and Censors, telling them he would vindicate this his practise, and if he could not have justice here, he would have it another place, threatening them to write a book against them about it." In the book he threatened to write, he would inform the world of the great number of cures he had performed by his method, even in cases abandoned by eminent fellows of the college whose names the registrar set down: Drs. Edward Browne, Francis Bernard, and Nehemiah Grew. During this outburst, according to the registrar, Groenevelt worked himself into a "passion," boasting of himself and his practice and carrying himself "very rudely, and disrespectfully to the President and Censors."[35] But the registrar did not record any explanations for his practice he might have offered.

When Groenevelt had ended, the women were called back in for cross-examination. After hearing what the doctor had said, Nurse Beckett and Barbara Curtis contradicted him on various parts of his testimony. Beckett stated that Withall had not been bedridden before Groenevelt administered his pills, complaining beforehand only of having pain when making water.[36] Withall's previous condition, she went on, could be verified by Dr. Hamilton, the male midwife: possibly he had supervised Withall's childbirth. (He never did formally testify before the censors.) She and Curtis also noted that Groenevelt had not used "an instrument or probe" to examine Withall but "only his hand"—although the registrar did not note whether the witnesses had paid close attention to Groenevelt's examination of Withall or had simply been in the same room. In a final question put to the doctor, the president himself, John Lawson, asked why he had thrown the pills into the fire. According to Registrar Gill, Groenevelt replied: "for fear of the Clamour of the people."[37]

After excusing the defendant and witnesses, the president and censors debated the issue for a while, finally declaring Groenevelt guilty of "mala praxis" for prescribing "thirty grains of Cantharides to be taken in Twelve hours, or thereabout."[38] A woman had been severely harmed by an unorthodox prescription of a dangerous drug; clearly Dr. Groenevelt had taken great liberties in an undefensible practice. With their declaration, the majority of censors probably considered the matter closed. Strangely, however, the censors did not have the registrar set down a record of any penalty.

It might be expected that the declaration of malpractice by the president and censors of the London College of Physicians would have brought an end to the case, as it usually did. When the committee of censors declared themselves, the only thing remaining in ordinary cases was whether and how they could impose their will on the condemned party. If all went according to the expected course, the censors would decide on a penalty—usually a fine, although, as in Rivett's case, it might be coupled with imprisonment—and the condemned party would admit his or her guilt, agree to obey the sentence, and go away with a promise never to bring trouble to the censors' doors again. In Groenevelt's case, though, things went differently: one of the new censors, Edward Tyson, had some sympathy for Groenevelt or his practice, or both.

A well-known surgeon-physician and comparative anatomist, fellow of the eminent Royal Society of London as well as of the College of Physicians,

Tyson exhibited a strong interest in natural history and in experimental medicine.[39] Until 1699, he served as the anatomical lecturer to the London Barber-Surgeons' Company; he also published in the *Philosophical Transactions of the Royal Society* a number of accounts of other, public, dissections that he performed on various unusual animals, several accounts of which were subsequently brought out as illustrated booklets.[40] Tyson did not believe that the old medical systems were thoroughly sound, nor did he think that new methods of treatment should be condemned out of hand without an explanation and an experimental trial. Moreover, he had had his own problems with the college censors in the past and would continue to do so in the future.

The troubles between Tyson and the officers of the College of Physicians had broken out shortly after the so-called Glorious Revolution of 1688. In early November 1688, William of Orange, military chief of the Dutch Republic and leader of the Protestant struggle against His Most Catholic Majesty, Louis XIV of France, crossed the North Sea with a fleet and army of a size probably not to be seen again until the Normandy landings of 1944. He used his forces to seize the British Crown for himself and his wife Mary Stuart, preventing a repetition of the French-English alliance of the early 1670s which had brought disaster to the Dutch. Leading disciplined and regularly paid troops, and working in concert with a number of British aristocrats who had become disaffected from the government of his uncle and father-in-law, James II, William managed a virtually bloodless takeover. His coup placed firm Protestants on a throne that had been occupied by a Catholic monarch who had ruled in an increasingly autocratic manner—without Parliament and in contempt of the established church—and this at a time when the absolutism of his fellow Catholic monarch, Louis XIV, was at its height. By late February 1689, the revolutionary settlement had decreed William and Mary joint majesties of England, Scotland, France, and Ireland; they were crowned in April.

Almost immediately after William's coup, Tyson helped to make trouble for the officers of the College of Physicians. The new government began by purging the kingdom of many of the charters recently enacted by James II. The College of Physicians had been among the corporations to receive a new charter from the old king, a charter that had given them increased powers over their own members and other practitioners in London. The officers of the college and most of the members (many of whom owed their membership to the new charter) therefore petitioned Parliament to pass a special act exempting their charter from the general abrogation of James' charters. But Tyson had been among the small number of college fellows who objected to this, and he petitioned the Parliament to reject the new charter and restore the old. Such behavior did not make him a favorite of the new guard in the college.[41]

Five years later, in October 1694, the fellows elected Tyson a censor, perhaps because he represented a group within the college who wanted its policies changed. He used his position to try to undermine the revived disciplinary behavior of the college. For instance, Tyson refused to go along with the order of the college to keep its discussions secret from the apothecaries just as the moment the college officers were attempting to prevent the Society of Apothecaries from obtaining new powers from Parliament.[42] When Tyson's colleague, Censor Richard Torlesse, obtained unusual special permission to take the Annals off the college premises to have a copy made of various passages to further one of the projects of the new officers, Tyson also asked to see the Annals privately. This led to a bitter row between Tyson and the registrar: Tyson apparently did not trust Gill to have entered proceedings accurately, while Gill, calling Tyson a "criminall" because of an earlier unpaid fine, thought that Tyson would alter the records on his own. In the course of the argument, John Downes and other fellows accused Tyson of being "the great solicitor, and Fomenter of the Differences, and Divisions in the College"; Tyson in turn accused Gill of calling him "Sirrah Rascall" and of saying that "he would beat his teeth down his Throat."[43]

When it came to looking into the medical practices of others, too, Tyson caused his fellow censors much trouble. For instance, Charles Goodall, one of the most important proponents of a strong college, tried vigorously to get the president and censors to take action for malpractice against one Mr. Wragg. According to the testimony entered into the Annals, Wragg had been called in to treat Mr. Mason, who suffered from a grave fever that confined him to bed. Wragg prevented Mason from calling in any other practitioners, until Mason had almost died. Then some of Mason's attendants obtained the help of Goodall, who brought about Mason's recovery. Angry at having his patient taken away, Wragg sent Mason an "unreasonable bill" for his services and then two days later took the still weakened Mason to the "spunging house by the Counter," a private debtors' prison. Wragg kept Mason locked up for two days and a night at Mason's own expense and then had him thrown in another prison for nonpayment. Mason's neighbor, Mr. Wright, finally paid Wragg off and got Mason out, but Wragg still threatened to take Mason to court. Three of the censors—Collins, Torlesse, and Martin Lister— wrote out a certificate declaring Wragg's practice to be "altogether, unwarrantable, dangerous, and prejudicial to the health of the said Mr. Mason, and the administration of his medicines, they censured [as] evill, and undue," but Tyson refused to sign the indictment. Again, the other three censors "did adjudge [Wragg] guilty of mala praxis, but Dr. Tyson would not, but did think him guilty of illicit [i.e., unlicensed] practice onely." Tyson finally got his way: the censors ordered Wragg prosecuted only for illicit practice.[44] When it came to Groenevelt, too, Tyson refused to treat his case simply as one of malpractice.

For almost a year, Tyson blocked his fellow censors from taking any action against Groenevelt. At the last censors' meeting before the next annual college election, late in the summer of 1695, the censors took up Groenevelt's case again at some length. The other three censors tried one last time to get Tyson to agree to impose a penalty on Groenevelt. But now, after a year of increasing friction, Tyson not only refused to impose a penalty, he even refused to adhere to their earlier collective decision finding Groenevelt guilty of malpractice. The reason he gave for refusing to abide by their earlier decision was that he "questioned the power of the College" to condemn Groenevelt for malpractice.[45]

The case against Wragg showed that Tyson's arm could be twisted to go along with the other censors in imposing fines for illicit practice. Unlike Wragg, however, Groenevelt had practiced with the license of the college, making charges of illicit practice out of the question. If Tyson would not allow his fellows to judge cases of malpractice, and if Groenevelt could not be condemned for illicit practice because he already had the college's license, then no action could be taken against him. The words of Tyson suggest that he simply stood on principle: the college did not have the power to decide cases of malpractice. But perhaps, too, Tyson's principles were affected by his understanding of Groenevelt's side of the story, which the registrar had not bothered to note down. For Groenevelt had a somewhat different account of events and a rationale for what he did. While many of the more experimentally inclined physicians like Tyson accepted Groenevelt's version of events or his explanation for his practices, the majority of censors could not or would not accept either. Both his character and his knowledge had been called into question by the majority of censors. In the following year, when Tyson did not gain reelection to the censors' board, Groenevelt suffered not only their contemptuous words but their punishment as well. In the course of his further problems, however, something of his medical views were entered into the record.

At the end of September 1695, another new group of officers were elected, including four censors who were to continue in office for the next two full years. Tyson was not among them; but Thomas Burwell—who had been president during the revival of college discipline from the end of 1692—and Tyson's adversaries Gill and Torlesse were. The new president was Samuel Collins, who had served as censor the previous two years. At their first monthly meeting, on 4 October, the president and censors looked into business left unfinished because of the disputes between Tyson and the other censors. One of their first actions was to call for a rehearing of Groenevelt's case.[46]

Indeed, at their next monthly meeting the censors again heard from Prunella Beckett, Hannah Walding, and Jane Daylight. The registrar and censor Thomas Gill read out from the Annals their previous testimony about Groenevelt, and each of them stood by their earlier statements. They also reported that two and a half years after her treatment, Mrs. Withall remained "very weak" and very often had "Convulsions." The censors also heard a new complaint of malpractice against Groenevelt from Susanna Smith. Smith claimed that he had caused harm to one Mary Thornton, but she apparently knew few substantive details. She promised the censors "to inform herself more fully" about the case and then return—but she never did. The censors had enough on Groenevelt in the Withall matter and ordered the beadle to call him before them at their next meeting.[47]

On 6 December, Groenevelt gave testimony to the censors yet again; this time he either revealed more about his methods, or Registrar Gill took the trouble to record them. Groenevelt began, in response to questions put by President Collins, to confirm his earlier account. But on this occasion, when the president expressed great surprise that he would administer so much of a dangerous substance like cantharides internally, Groenevelt's explanation was recorded. He claimed that he could safely administer even fifty-six grains of cantharides or more. He did this, he explained, by making up another eighteen pills of bread crumbs and two scruples (that is, forty grains) of camphor, to be given in conjunction with the cantharides. These pills he later called his "antidote of the Cantharides."[48] The method of taking these medicines in combination was first to swallow five pills of cantharides, followed three hours later by five pills of camphor, "and a quart of Drink between each dose." Every three hours the cycle was repeated. He claimed to have given the first three cycles—fifteen pills of cantharides together with fifteen pills of camphor—to Mrs. Withall with his own hands.[49]

He had precedent for administering cantharides internally as something other than an aphrodisiac. Hippocrates had recommended cantharides internally for hydropsy and amenorrhoea (according to Galen, Hippocrates had used only the head, wings, and legs of the beetle); and Dioscorides had advised taking the hard parts of the beetle as an antidote to the poison contained in its juices.[50] Groenevelt knew these precedents and many more.[51] Moreover, some of his Dutch contemporaries were interested in the use of cantharides internally. The well-informed Constantijn Huygens not only described the use of cantharides as a blister to clear eyesight but went on: "I give much good [from Spanish fly], they bite and they sting, but they truly cure people who use them." Cantharides were no bad treatment: "Sick men eat [them] with titillating cures, in place of violent, painful and fruitless ones."[52] More important, not only educated men of the world like Huygens but physicians like Groenevelt's teacher Sylvius, and his contemporary Cornelis Bontekoe, were developing new theories that suggested new uses for medicaments like cantharides.

A little book that Groenevelt had published just before his treatment of Withall offers insights into his reasoning. His theory of the gout was rooted in the doctrines of his medical professor, François dele Boë Sylvius. Groenevelt wrote that the four humors present in the body had qualities: "bitter, salt, acid," and others. In healthy conditions, all these qualities were properly mixed together, but when one of the qualities was "divided or separated from the rest, and exist[ed] by itself," it caused great pain. In short, when the salt and acrid qualities became separated, the salt fell upon the "sensible parts about the joynts," where it created pain. It happened this way: The salt was "lodged in the serum" of the body, which was acidic. This acidic serum also contained "a certain thicker matter" from which "nodes" and stones were generated. The salty serum was "contained about the extremities of the muscles, tendons, ligaments, *periostea,* and the nervous parts of the joints." When present in large amounts, this thicker salt caused the pain, heat, and endurance of gout. As long as one's diet, exercise, emotional state, and other matters (termed by contemporaries "the non-naturals") were moderate, all would be well. But if excesses led to the generation of less perfectly mixed blood, then the blood would become "corrupted by divers humours," while the unnatural heat rising from poorly mixed blood would grow so high that it would be "forced to undergo a fermentation like new beer," which forced "those sharp and foreign juices" deeper into the body. The guts could get rid of excess salty serum via "a watery looseness," the kidneys "by plenty of urine," and the fleshy parts "by the pores of the skin." But the joints had no way of getting rid of the excess salty serum, so that it worked its way "into the inmost recesses and interstices of the nervous parts" of them, causing the pains of gout.[53]

Groenevelt here followed Sylvius's theory. In the chapter on urine in his medical treatise, Sylvius had written that salt made the urine very thick, because when salt was mixed (*concretio*) with the blood, it dissolved in the serum, making it thick. Thick urine was a sign of the thick, salty serum in the blood. The thickening of the serum happened especially in men—who had an abundance of thick gummy moisture (*abundat pituita viscida*)—as well as at the beginning of fevers, especially intermittent fevers. The thick and salty serum sometimes developed into stone and gravel, which blocked the ureters, a problem that was hard to remedy, since once the passages were blocked, remedies could not penetrate to the site of the blockage to dissolve them.[54] Groenevelt had explored Sylvius's ideas further, deciding that gout was a disease "altogether of the same origin" as the stone and gravel: that is, caused by the salty serum. On at least one occasion Groenevelt recommended treatments straight out of Sylvius's book: we can be sure that Groenevelt had read it carefully.[55]

Of course, the best recommendation for the gout which Groenevelt could give his readers was prevention: people should avoid certain foods (especially "wines which have much Tartar in them"), gluttony and drunkenness, intemperance, studying too hard (especially at night), afflicting cares, and "above all immoderate Venus." But people who already had the gout wanted it cured. One way to treat it was to evacuate the offending humor by the usual methods of vomits, purges, sweats, urination, and bloodletting. But another and better method was to evacuate the salt and tartar by administering "volatile salts," or alkalies, such as salt of hartshorn, greater burdock root, "a decoction of germander, and several things called antipodagricks." In general, "discutients" made from fixed or volatile salts worked best, because they scoured "the impacted humors, and corroborate the weakened parts."[56] In short, Groenevelt elaborated his theory about the causes and cures of gout in terms of the doctrine of acids and alkalies, which had its origin in the early 1660s among Continental iatrochemists influenced by Cartesianism.[57] Dutch savants particularly advocated this theory in conjunction with their ideas about animal physiology as consisting of vessels and liquids.[58] One of the most vigorous advocates of the acids and alkalies theory had been Groenevelt's teacher, Sylvius.

The English, however, had not been nearly as enthusiastic as the Dutch about the theory of acids and alkalies. This was particularly so after the theory had been attacked by Robert Boyle in 1675, who probably aimed his remarks specifically at the teachings of Groenevelt's teacher.[59] Although Boyle exercised his usual caution in carefully saying that, while the doctrine had grave philosophical weaknesses, it might be useful to chemists and

physicians in devising remedies,[60] his opposition to the theory nevertheless
carried great weight in England. Still, the idea that the chemical world could
be divided into acids and alkalies had a power and simplicity that made it
increasingly popular among the public in England. As one practitioner put
it: "It is scarce possible for a Man to converse with Persons that are ill, let
the Distemper be what it will, . . . but they presently tell you, their Blood
is so very acid, that unless the Acidity can be corrected, it is impossible for
'em to be well: And accordingly they fly to Alkalious Medicins, as Pouder
of Pearl, Coral, Crabs eyes, or something of that nature."[61] The popularity
of the acid-alkali theory among the English public caused one of the most
pointed rebuttals to Boyle to be translated into English in 1689.[62] Even some
English physicians began to adopt the theory in the later 1680s and early
1690s. It seems to have been in Thomas Sydenham's circle that the theory
found its most articulate English defenders—a group of people with whom
Groenevelt had associations.[63] So it was that Groenevelt let it be known at
that moment that he, too, advocated the theory of acids and alkalies.

If we turn to a passage in the medical work of another Dutchman who
strongly defended the doctrine of acids and alkalies, Cornelis Bontekoe, we
can better see precisely what Groenevelt was up to.[64] Bontekoe put it bluntly:
some useful remedies can be found among animals, which are useful as
volatile salts. In particular, cantharides were a penetrating salt.[65] He went
on to explain that most chronic diseases were helped by diuretics, since such
diseases were caused by acidified serum (*sappen*). What was needed were
remedies to drive the serum onward by thinning it and causing proper transpi-
ration, circulation, and urination. One of the best diuretics was cantharides,
which were alkaline, although they had to be used carefully so as not to cause
deadly hemorrhaging or satyriasis.[66] The similarity between Groenevelt's
reasoning and Bontekoe's is unmistakable. Both wrote about the importance
of provoking urination in treating chronic diseases and about using volatile
salts like cantharides to thin the thick serum in the blood.

Of course, it is one thing to say that cantharides are a volatile salt and
alkaline, another to go ahead and administer them in large doses. Everyone
knew quite well that they caused satyriasis and had to be handled very
carefully. Prescribing as much as Groenevelt did could certainly mean trouble
for a patient. "By bare application . . . they hurt the Bladder so much as to
ulcerate it," warned one authority.[67] The trick to Groenevelt's new remedy,
then, was the use of cantharides in combination with something that would
"rectify" its bad qualities: camphor.

Camphor had reentered the European pharmacopoeia recently, being refined from the sap of a tree that grew in East Asia. The plant grew in China, Sumatra, and Borneo, but the best camphor came from Japan.[68] That placed the trade in camphor firmly in Dutch hands, and the Dutch sold it to the rest of Europe for a long time.[69] Refined for medical purposes, it took the form of a white, pelucid, very fragrant, and volatile liquid.[70] Because in this form it evaporates quite rapidly, camphor was typically used in salves to soothe hot and inflamed sores or aching limbs.[71] But it could also be taken internally in the form of pills. Later authors noted that camphor behaved somewhat like nitric acid, which the "Lithontriptique de Tulp" used to rectify cantharides— perhaps Groenevelt had some similar ideas. Certainly one of its better-known effects from inhaling or swallowing was the suppression of sexual activity, a property of camphor known to Groenevelt's contemporaries.[72]

Thus, Groenevelt had excellent precedent for thinking along the following lines: The body's vessels needed to be kept open; if they were not, nasty chronic diseases would ensue. Of central importance in keeping the vascular physiology working well was maintaining a correct balance of acids and alkalies. In both the stone and gravel and in the gout, and in other chronic diseases of a similar nature, the breeding of a thick acidic serum caused problems in the vascular circulation, resulting in serious medical problems. The remedies required would have to be diuretic in nature; they would have to scour the vessels in order to reopen them; since the thick serum was acidic, they would have to attack the problem by being alkaline. Cantharides had all the necessary properties and had been recommended by others for careful internal use in attacking complaints like the stone; but it needed to be handled very carefully indeed, especially because of the way it stimulated the sexual organs. However, when it was combined with another diuretic, camphor, its potentially dangerous effects could be canceled out. He had apparently first hit upon the idea of uniting cantharides with camphor in 1679.[73] The result was a powerful, effective remedy for a number of chronic diseases, which by 1691 he believed could be used effectively against gout. This was Groenevelt's special medicine, which he had been reluctant to divulge publicly. He had not prescribed cantharides for Mrs. Withall without reason; and some physicians—Tyson among them—thought that Groenevelt had hit upon an important new medicine.

Groenevelt's explanation of his remedy brought the censors' proceedings against him to a temporary halt. But as we shall see, they slowly gathered their forces and eventually not only repeated their charges of malpractice against him but sent him to Newgate prison, the filthy London jail for murderers, highwaymen, and other desperate criminals. Groenevelt's friends, and the opponents of the college censors, quickly mounted a series of public campaigns that made Groenevelt's case into a cause célèbre. Groenevelt obtained his release from prison, and the resulting series of lawsuits and countersuits eventually created important precedent in English law. The censors had proceeded against him not only because they refused to take seriously the rationale he offered for his medical practice but because they did not consider him to possess the right sort of character. He was certainly not English. Not only did he therefore possess the wrong medical ideas, but he possessed the wrong religion, and his friends were among the London dissenters, experimentalists, and general troublemakers. Equally important, Groenevelt had overstepped his bounds. He had been allowed to practice as a lithotomist: someone who cut for bladder stones. But now this foreign surgeon with a degree had taken it upon himself to practice medicine among the English public, the consequence of which seemed plain.

A superficial reading of the College of Physicians' actions against Groenevelt suggests what other historians have argued: that the state of medical practice was quite dismal at the end of the seventeenth century. Quacks flourished, endangering the health of patients and even throwing unpaying ones in prison or threatening surviving relatives with lawsuits. On such a view, among the numerous quacks could be found an incompetent and careless doctor by the name of Joannes Groenevelt.[74] By administering pills containing large quantities of Spanish fly—a substance commonly known to be dangerous when taken internally—Groenevelt had made a woman suffering from discomforts into a bedridden, languishing invalid. The only general solution to the scandalous state of affairs would be to root out and punish malpractice; in Groenevelt's case, having been found guilty of malpractice, he should have been heavily fined and, if necessary, threatened with prison, as others had been. The censors' deliberate proceedings against him, and his eventual stay in Newgate, had every justification.

But another reading of the case suggests something rather more complicated. In the controversy over the treatment of Suzanna Withall, the medical community of London exhibited deep cultural and intellectual conflicts. The officers of the College of Physicians had singled out an unprotected foreign member to hold up as an example of what would happen to those who behaved in ways of which they did not approve. In part, the resulting conflict pitted Dutch intellectual tradition against English. Yet given the aid Groenevelt found in London among many segments of the public as well as the medical community—including a number of well-educated English physicians—the conflict represented more than a simple clash of national styles. A clash of national styles there was. But Groenevelt's story also illustrates the conflicts of values brought out everywhere by what has come to be known as the "scientific revolution." Ambitious and utilitarian, educated in the latest Cartesian and chemical ideas, and abiding by no old-fashioned boundaries between surgery, medicine, and pharmacy, Groenevelt had come up against the more old-fashioned gentlemen-physicians of the Oxbridge establishment. His allies came not only from the Continent but locally, from among the physicians who most strongly favored the new science as well as from among the more empirical practitioners of the metropolis—surgeons, apothecaries, and unaffiliated people alike. At stake, then, were conflicting values about moral and medical practice, differences that became particularly explosive when set in the context of both the medical rivalries of later seventeenth-century London and the differences in national culture between England and the Netherlands.

The best way to look beyond the issue of malpractice into the deeper implications raised by Groenevelt's case is to do what the censors did not: to give him the benefit of the doubt, to assume that he had done no intentional harm but had good reasons for acting as he did. In short, we need to understand his life and views, the structures and events of his life, how this Dutch physician had come to practice in London and what were his hopes and ideals. We will meet his teachers, friends, and associates in the Netherlands and in London. We will further examine his rationale for practicing as he did. And in the process, we will deepen our awareness of the medical and cultural milieux of the period. We can then later return to the malpractice case and see its ramifications from a variety of points of view. While the controversy over Groenevelt's treatment of Withall provides us with the most dramatic testimony about differences of outlook in the period, it was not the only event in the life of this ordinary physician. The reader may not be convinced that giving a woman with a urinary complaint large quantities of Spanish fly was a good thing; we may, however, come to understand something about the varieties of medical outlook and practice present during the period. A plurality of views resulted in conflict. But they also forced change.

CHAPTER 2

A Place in the World

J OANNES GROENEVELT grew up in a world far from
England, yet one connected to it by history. His place
of birth remained a large and important city in the new
Dutch Republic: Deventer. Although it could no longer compare in wealth
or significance to Amsterdam, Deventer had once been a far more important
place. Until the sixteenth century, it ranked among the considerable cities
of northern Europe, with stronger connections to the German lands than to
the cities of Holland and Flanders. While Joannes grew up in Deventer,
however, the city was rapidly losing much of its last vestiges of regional
importance, becoming transformed into a Dutch provincial town. His outlook,
then, turned not only on Deventer's heritage and resources but on the reformed
religion brought to the city by the Hollanders and on the new sense of Dutch
nationhood being taught to children like him. Joannes could grow up within
the walls of a well-to-do city and take pride in its past; yet if he wanted to
take part in greater events on the world stage, he would have to move away.
When he did, he would always carry with him that sense of unease and
ambition so often found among proud people from the borderlands trying to
make an impression in the metropolis.

The ancient connections between Deventer and England could be seen from
the windows of the house in which Joannes Groenevelt was born and raised.
Across the square stood a very large, brick, late Gothic church dedicated to the
memory of a British martyr, Saint Lebuinus. Constructed in the late fifteenth
and early sixteenth century, this large hall-church was built around the foundations of a Romanesque basilica from the eleventh century, which in turn stood
on a crypt in which the relics of the saint were said to be interred.

The connection between Deventer and Britain marked by the Lebuinus church had existed virtually from the origin of the town. Around 772, the young Liafwin (Latinized as Lebuinus), born in Britain, came to a place on the IJssel River at the invitation of a Christianized widow, Abarhilda. This place became Lebuinus's base of operations as he tried to convert the Saxons, and there he built a rough church. Lebuinus had come over as one among a host of Anglo-Saxons who, a generation or two after invading Britain and taking up the new monotheism, returned across the North Sea to attempt the conversion of their brethren. With the help of the Frankish kings, who made the Christian religion a pillar of their policy, one of the first of them, Willibrord, at the end of the seventh century began to bring the faith to the region around the mouths of the Rhine and Meuse rivers. From the new diocese he founded at an old Roman fortress, now called Utrecht, Willibrord and his successors began to send out energetic missionaries to the north and east. One of them, Lebuinus, settled his church on the banks of the IJssel, around which the little settlement soon known as Deventer began to grow.[1] The missionary earned a safe conduct after suddenly appearing in the midst of an annual council of the Saxons: dressed in long robes and carrying a cross and gospel, he ordered them to accept the word of God, disappearing in an instant before he could be killed. After his death around 777, some Saxons burned his church to the ground, but the missionary Liutgeres followed in Lebuinus's footsteps, erecting a new building around the place of Lebuinus's burial, upon which site the Romanesque stone crypt rose about 937.[2]

Lebuinus's wooden church, and then his crypt, stood near the center of a small settlement on the east side of the IJssel River. As Lebuinus looked farther east, he found a land of gently rolling woods, heaths, and brooks ruled over by the yet mainly unchristianized Saxons, on whom Charlemagne would soon make war; among these people he walked and proselytized. Over the river to the west, the thinly populated, sandy woods and sparse meadows of the Veluwe made a kind of wilderness. Beyond the Veluwe lay Utrecht, and further west yet, the marshes of Holland. Several days' travel to the south, the more civilized Frankish territories that soon became known as Brabant and Flanders yielded good pasture and several large towns. To the north, downriver, the dangerous shallows of the Zuider Zee ("southern sea") stretched away in a broad bay before emptying into the North Sea. The crossing of the IJssel at Deventer linked the Saxon lands of the east and northeast with the Frankish territories to the south and west. It was a fine place to build an outpost, from where one could easily travel throughout northwestern Europe.[3]

Deventer may have drawn Lebuinus because of its importance as a border town, but the large structure later dedicated to his memory—the church on which Joannes Groenevelt looked—signified the dignity and wealth of the city in the centuries after his mission. With expanding population in the surrounding area after Charlemagne's conquests, increased agricultural production, and trade links running from northern to southern Europe, Deventer found itself in the midst of a region that may very well have led the economic expansion of the early Middle Ages in northern Europe. The IJssel served as a highway for boats and thus traffic in goods. It flowed from a major European artery, the Rhine, north into the wide and shallow Zuider Zee. From there, merchants could easily travel by water to the Scandinavian lands and the Baltic, which sprouted important towns and cities of their own. Since from the Rhine boats could put into the Meuse (or Maas) River—which in turn connected to routes extending to the south of France—traffic between the Mediterranean and the North and Baltic seas often went via Deventer and its sister IJssel cities, Zutphen and Kampen, and the nearby city of Zwolle (which lay adjacent to the IJssel on the deeper Zwarte Water, which not only connected to the Zuider Zee but to German Westphalia). Especially after Charlemagne extended the borders of his empire well to the east in the late eighth and early ninth century, and after cities closer to the North Sea coast were raided and wrecked by Vikings in the tenth, Deventer became an important entrepôt in the north-south trade in western Europe. In 896, Zwentibold of Lotharingia awarded the residents of the town special legal freedoms as members of an imperial city (*homines imperatoris*), the city established a mint, and from the mid-ninth to the mid-twelfth century the powerful bishop of Utrecht even resided in Deventer. Together with the decline in Deventer's economic rivals of Dorestad and Tiel, such events made the city a center of commerce.[4]

For reasons of geography and political good fortune, then, this place that the Anglo-Saxon Lebuinus had made his camp grew into an important stop on the trade routes of western Europe. It became even more important in the late Middle Ages. At the turn of the thirteenth century, Deventer joined the league of northern cities known as the Hansa. The Hansa towns regulated trade among themselves and with others and cooperated in political and military enterprises. Deventer and its sister IJssel cities formed the heart of the Hansa presence in the northern low countries, forming one of the western borders of the confederation. As the most important end point in the low countries for Baltic commerce, Deventer hosted five annual fairs in the fourteenth and fifteenth centuries which brought together merchants from the Rhineland, Westphalia, and Holland. In the growing trade wars between the

German and Flemish merchants of the fifteenth century, the Hansa even planned at one point to move its trading headquarters (*kontor*) from Bruges to Deventer.[5]

Fittingly, too, Lebuinus's city lay not only in the midst of an important network of trade but in a region that gave birth to several important religious movements and cultural developments. A citizen of Deventer, Geert Groote, founded a religious movement in the late fourteenth century called the "Modern Devotion." Associated with both the monastery of the Augustinian Canons at Windesheim and with laymen—who called themselves the Brethren of the Common Life, living together in common but not separated from the world as in monasteries—the Devotio Moderna taught humility, industry, and constant emotional and intellectual commitment to God. The movement quickly spread throughout Westphalia to the east, Frisia and Groningen to the north, Utrecht and Holland to the west, and the Flemish lands to the south. The Brethren of the Common Life worked charitably, but rather than preaching (as the revived Franciscan and Dominican orders were doing), the members of this lay group quietly went about setting up schools and writing devotional literature. Some of them established Latin schools in the low countries which became renowned as among the best in northern Europe, including the schools in Deventer and Zwolle. Another follower of the new teachings, Thomas à Kempis, who lived in the monastery of St. Agnietenberg near Zwolle, wrote a work considered one of the greatest pieces of Christian devotional literature, the *Imitatio Christi* ("Imitation of Christ").[6] Although the region was briefly touched by the early religious radicalism of the Anabaptists, who in 1534–35 established a tragic and short-lived independent kingdom in the nearby city of Münster, the ruthless suppression of the movement eliminated any further threat of politico-religious turmoil. Contemplative and learned Christian humanism remained dominant. The lands around Deventer even began to develop their own literary language in the sixteenth century, one somewhat different from the Flanders-Brabant-Holland tongue that gave rise to modern Dutch.[7]

By the mid-sixteenth century, however, the city of Deventer had again become a kind of border town as in Lebuinus's day, rather than the center of a cultural region. Pulled by traditions of trade and politics toward the German-speaking lands to the east and north, Deventer merchants nevertheless found the cities of the west and south becoming more important to their future. By the fifteenth century, the cities of the provinces of Utrecht and especially Holland had begun to rival the IJssel and Friesland cities in the amount of trade they carried. As Bruges and then Antwerp became the dominant trading centers of the low countries, and the Hansa confederation declined in economic and political significance, relations between Deventer and the Dutch cities on the lower Rhine grew stronger. The economy of the Hollanders there had grown specialized: they imported wheat and rye from the Baltic for human consumption and exported meat, cheese, oats, and barley (commonly in the form of beer) to the densely settled cities of the southern netherlands. From this lucrative system of trade, stretching from the Baltic to northern France, a proto-industrial and export-driven economy developed among the Hollanders. Dutch merchants took over more and more of the trade and transportation of the North Sea region. As goods moved increasingly east-west along the Meuse and Rhine to Holland and then north or south along the North Sea coast, rather than directly north along the IJssel, the importance of Deventer slipped. To maintain their wealth, Deventer merchants increasingly had to come to terms with the Hollanders.[8]

It was dynastic and political events of the sixteenth century, however, which gave Deventer's people no choice but to band together with the powerful cities to the west and south. Deventer, Kampen, and Zwolle had been incorporated into the province of Overijssel, which had a weak overlord in the bishop of Utrecht. Then, as a result of a thirty-five-year-long war between the Habsburg provinces of the low countries (including Holland) and the duchy of Gelderland, Overijssel came into the possession of the Habsburg family in the Treaty of Schoonhoven (1527); a year later, the Treaty of Gorinchem forced the heirless duke of Gelderland to make the head of the Habsburg clan, Charles, the heir to all his territories. With the accession of the province of Groningen and the creation of Drente in 1536, and the death of the duke of Gelderland in 1543, the Habsburg chieftain, Holy Roman Emperor, and king of Spain, Charles V, controlled the whole of the low countries.

Charles and his viceroys soon set up councils in each of the provinces to exercise his authority and began ordering their affairs to his own desires. In 1548, he moved the administration of the city of Zutphen and the provinces of Gelderland, Utrecht, and Overijssel (including Deventer) from the West-phalian Circle to the Burgundian Circle, thus uniting them with the provinces to their south and west. In the "Pragmatic Sanction" one year later, Charles forced all the territories of the Burgundian Circle to swear fealty to his son, Philip. Despite continued differences among these possessions, then, by the mid-sixteenth century the seventeen provinces of the low countries had been divided from the German lands and brought into one administrative whole governed by councils in Brussels. Politically as well as economically, Deventer had come firmly into the orbit of the Hollanders and Flemish.[9]

The forced union of Overijssel with Holland, Brabant, and Flanders caused much friction among leading people and towns of the region. When Philip took over the Burgundian Circle on his father's abdication in 1555, he worked vigorously to make a single territory of all his low country provinces. While Philip's uncle inherited the Holy Roman Empire, Philip got Spain and the low countries; but he had also married Mary, queen of England, in 1554, which promised to bring together the lands on each side of the North Sea. England and the low countries would continue to be embroiled in each other's affairs for a long time.

Unfortunately for Philip, Mary died at the end of 1558, and in the meantime he had to attend to affairs in Spain, leaving his low country possessions in the hands of various governors. His attempts to create a more systematic rule in the Burgundian Circle therefore gave rise to further bad feelings among the locals without being tempered by the presence of Philip himself. Among the first things Philip did (in conjunction with the pope) was to reform church government. Protestant heresies had been spreading rapidly in central Europe and France and had even touched Spain and England; Philip wanted to strengthen and reform church government in the low countries to prevent the spread of like heresies there. Without his own presence, however, his reforms failed and brought on the so-called Dutch Revolt, which ended with the independence of the northern provinces.

Events in Deventer not only reflected the problems of the late 1500s, they helped to spur them on. As part of his plans for reform, Philip introduced the Inquisition and decided to bring increased authority to the northeast provinces of his domain by establishing a new bishopric at Deventer. This and other declarations caused great outcries. By 1563, Philip's chief minister in the low countries, Antoine Perrenot, lord of Granville, first archbishop of Mechlin, cardinal and primate of the netherlands' church, had become so unpopular with the nobility of the region that he had to be recalled. The policies of Philip's regent, Margaret of Parma, alienated many nobles further. A league began to be formed among Protestant nobles; in 1565 many withdrew from Margaret's council, and in 1566 the revolt began, accompanied by Protestant uprisings against the church in the form of the smashing of images. Philip sent the count of Alva and Spanish troops to quell the rebellion in 1567, and he almost succeeded. But from protected areas along the coast, William I, prince of Orange, and his successors managed to keep the armed rebellion going until the truce of 1609 gave de facto recognition to the northernmost provinces as the independent Dutch Republic.[10]

In Deventer, the magistrates allowed Protestants to hold religious services

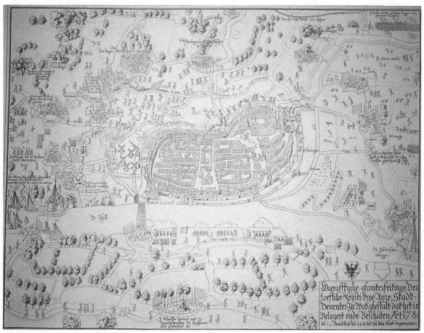

FIG. 2. *A contemporary depiction of the siege of Deventer in 1578. East is toward the top, the IJssel River flowing north-south on the west side of the city.*

in a church during 1566–67, but by the end of the 1560s, the "Iron Duke," Alva, had put an end to this, forcing the magistrates to crack down severely on heterodox views and garrisoning the city with German troops, preventing the city from going over to William's side. Philip finally did install a bishop in the city in 1570.[11] He also forbade students to go beyond the borders of the Burgundian Circle to study, so as not to be infected with heresy, and he planned to establish a university in Deventer. According to his scheme, each of the archbishoprics he established in his Burgundian territories would have a university; the one for the Archbishopric of Utrecht would be in Deventer. He did reinvigorate the University at Louvain and built a new one at Dowai, and discussions about Deventer grew increasingly serious after the rebels set up their own university in Leiden in 1575.[12] In November 1578, however, troops loyal to the cause of the rebels captured the city after a siege of more than three months, just before Philip's new governor, Alexander Farnèse, could relieve it.

The leading rebel noblemen had led the revolt partly in the name of religious peace, but the uprising allowed militant Calvinism to spread throughout the liberated lands, including Deventer. The conqueror of Deventer, the count of Rennenburg, established a formal religious peace in Deventer within six weeks of its capture. At first, most of the citizens remained Catholic, and most of the Protestants began, like the neighboring Germans, as Lutherans. But almost immediately after the declaration of religious peace, small groups of toughs began to attack Catholic churches and clergy. Increasing numbers of people began to attend "reformed" services. Except for the greatest merchants and the working poor, much of Deventer's population began to become Calvinist. When Rennenburg defected to the king's side early in March 1580, the civic guard quickly demanded the right to elect their own officers to prevent the return of the city to Philip's forces; almost immediately thereafter churches, monasteries, and hospitals were plundered, and the Catholic clergy fled. By the end of March, the mainly Calvinist civic guard had taken firm control and forbade not only Catholic but Lutheran services.[13]

As the revolt continued, war came to Deventer several more times. Rennenburg's defection to the side of Philip created an opportunity for Philip's general, Parma, and the northeastern provinces were regained for Philip during 1580, making Deventer a front-line city for the forces of the United Provinces, controlling the important IJssel River crossing. The English governor of the United Provinces, the earl of Leicester (who arrived in the country in 1585 at the head of English troops) purged Deventer's government of the soft middle *politique* magistrates, installing firm Calvinists. But his policies also allowed the local English governors, Sir William Stanley and Rowland Yorke, to betray Deventer and Zutphen in January 1587, and the citizens raised hardly a hand to prevent a return to the Catholic side. Prince Maurice's troops recovered Deventer for the United Provinces in May 1591, and from there he launched his reconquest of the northeast. From 1591 forward, Deventer remained firmly within the entity increasingly called the Dutch Republic.[14] The religious and political reformation had been secured in Deventer by an army from Holland.[15] For another sixty years, with a short intermission, the war would go on, but it would be fought to the south of Deventer. On 15 May 1648, the day after the baptism of Joannes Groenevelt, the leaders of the States of the United Provinces, including representatives from Overijssel, ratified the Treaty of Münster, bringing an end to the eighty-year war fought against Spain, acknowledging the existence of the Dutch Republic and defining its borders.

The Calvinist reformation had come to the region in intimate association with the political rebellion, driving out "papist superstitions" along with Alva's and Parma's soldiers and reordering daily life along more severe lines.

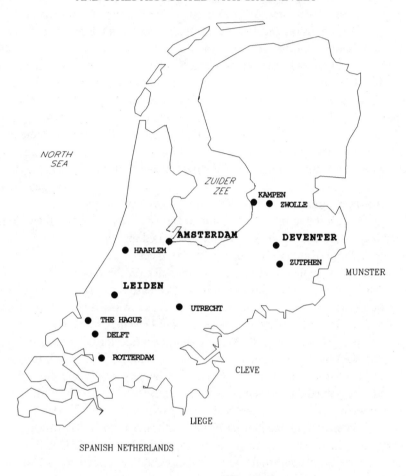

THE UNITED PROVINCES IN 1648

AND CITIES ASSOCIATED WITH GROENEVELT

FIG. 3. *The United Provinces in 1648 and cities associated with Groenevelt.*

No more processions would snake through the streets on saints' days: most religious holidays were eliminated in favor of daily work, while those few that were left (such as Christmas, Easter, and Ascension Day) would be made into more sober days of prayer and thanksgiving. Officially, no one would publicly light candles to help a soul out of purgatory, no stained-glass windows would teach about the Virgin Mary, no miracles would take place, and no more saints—like Lebuinus—would be called upon for help. The old faith would have to be confined to private ceremonies or night thoughts.

Now located in a mainly Calvinist Dutch town of secondary importance, the St. Lebuinus church across from Joannes's house had lost its stained-glass windows and ornaments—and even the name of the British saint buried in its crypt—during the religious purge: the now Reformed people called it simply the Grote Kerk ("big church"). When the citizens of Deventer added to the church in the early seventeenth century, they topped its tall Gothic tower not with a steeple pointing to heaven but with a huge wooden lantern containing a clock: it marked not the timeless world of eternity but the daily round of time.[16] Moreover, the new structure had been designed and built by a famous architect, Hendrick de Keyzer, who hailed not from Deventer but from Amsterdam.

Joannes Groenevelt therefore grew up Dutch and Calvinist. His speech might have the German-tinged accent of an easterner, and he might remember that his native city had once been a free and powerful Hansa town associated with Catholic piety and Erasmian humanism. In later years, he recalled his hometown with obvious pride and love. But Deventer had been swallowed by the United Provinces. A border now existed between Deventer and the Westphalian lands nearby, and between it and the Habsburg Netherlands farther to the south. Much of the trade over the Zuider Zee and along the Rhine now moved in the boats of Hollanders to western cities, especially to Amsterdam, from which cities the Dutch began to build a world empire. Deventer remained a dignified place. But it had become a regional outpost and military garrison rather than a city of international importance. In the shadow of Lebuinus's church, remade in the image of the Calvinist Holland-ers, absorbing the rich but anxious culture of a formerly great city, Joannes Groenevelt spent his childhood.

Joannes Groenevelt was born on the eve of the end of the eighty-year war that created the Dutch nation. The rains fell very heavily that spring, which many poets took as a fateful sign.[17] On Sunday, 14 May 1648, the day before the States General solemnly ratified the Treaty of Münster, the infant's parents took him to the Grote Kerk for baptism into the Reformed faith.[18] His mother, Guedeken ter Klocken, was just past her fortieth year; his father, Frans Groenevelt, was a year younger. Three brothers had preceded him to the baptismal font. The eldest had been twins. They apparently died before adulthood, for they are never mentioned in any other record (although the dates of their deaths cannot be known because the registers of burials from Deventer survive only from 1674 onward). A third son quite clearly died in infancy, for our Joannes received the name of his deceased brother at the baptismal font—a common custom at the time, assuring that deceased family members lived on.[19]

Like most people in the seventeenth century, Joannes's parents had grieved for loved ones many times before, his mother especially. Before she buried three children, she had seen two husbands die. A native of Deventer, Guedeken ter Klocken was baptized as Judith on 9 February 1608, one of five children born to Jos and Jenneken ter Klocken.[20] She first married at the age of twenty-one, to Gelmer Henrick, on 25 October 1629. He must have died a few years after, for ordinary people could not divorce, and Guedeken remarried on 7 June 1636, at age twenty-eight. This second husband, Werner Kremer (a burgher of Deventer), also died, and relatively soon after marriage. The widowed Guedeken announced her third engagement on 3 February 1638, just before her thirtieth birthday. As in the previous marriages, church custom was followed in having the banns announced on at least three Sundays before the wedding; for her third marriage, Guedeken had them announced in her hometown of Deventer, while her fiancé had them read out in his hometown of Zutphen on 11 February. Guedeken and her third husband, Frans Groenevelt, then married in his church in Zutphen (just to the south of Deventer) on 22 April.[21] For some reason, it would be yet another five years before she had her first children. Perhaps she decided to put them off.[22]

Guedeken's third husband, Frans Groenevelt, had grown up in the IJssel city of Zutphen—where the English poet Sir Philip Sidney had died in defense of the town in 1586.[23] Like many young men, Frans Groenevelt put off marriage until he could support a family: in his case, in his late twenties. He had been baptized on 15 December 1609, the only child of Christoffel Fransz. Gronefelt and Johanna (or Janneken) Sprenchels, being named after his paternal grandfather. Like his father before him, he married a woman newly widowed.[24] As a glass engraver, Frans had almost certainly had a long period as apprentice and journeyman, but by the time he married, he undoubtedly worked as a skilled craftsman in the luxury trade. The couple settled in Deventer, in a house "op de Graven": a street just off the large square outside the Grote Kerk.[25]

Guedeken may have engaged in business herself, as Dutch women very often did; but given the Groenevelts' income, she might have remained in charge of the household alone.[26] She also brought some money into the marriage, since at least one property of fields and woods the couple later owned is mentioned as her mother's land.[27] Presumably she had also inherited something from her deceased husbands. Since Frans also came from the family of a citizen, he may have had some assets too, as well as his craft skills. Within two years of their marriage, if not before, the couple had enough money to engage in some modest financial speculation, advancing loans to neighbors and family.[28] By the time of Frans's death, at least, their house had become quite well furnished with cabinets, clothing, linens, and bedding; earthenware, pewterware, copperware, silverware, and glassware; paintings (fifty-two, both large and small); and books (one large Bible, a smaller Bible, two psalmbooks, two Testaments, ten other Dutch books, and a shelf full of Latin works—probably Joannes's schoolbooks); the widow also still had eight tracts of land (mainly pastures and oak woods), a place on the main market square rented out to Jacobus Temmincks, a house on the other side of the IJssel River, their house "op den graeven," and a house where the widow used to live. Of course, she also had large debts (amounting to 6,450 gilders); but the ability to borrow so much also spoke to the family's creditworthiness.[29] Joannes grew up the only son of a substantial, though not rich, family.

The neighborhood in which Joannes played lay roughly in the center of the city. As he stood in the cobbled street passing his front door, looking toward the Grote Kerk, immediately to his right lay an open square bordering the church, and just a bit farther along, the street ended at the steep banks of the IJssel River and the busy docks. On his left, the street ran east toward a wooded square, shops, inns, coffeehouses, and another church. The Assenstraat cut across his street very nearby, traveling through a neighborhood of fine houses to end just west of the grand city weigh house (where the official scales were kept), which looked out over the main market square. Behind him lay a maze of alleys and streets running toward the fortifications on the north side of town. Ahead, he could see houses and shops built on the side wall of the Grote Kerk, which rose up high above them. Just on the other side of the church, a wooded yard provided another open area for play, next to which sat the ornate Stadhuis, the seat of the municipal government. Farther south from the main market square, up a hill covered with more fine houses, yet another large church, with two tall spires, rose on the edge of the city walls. He and his friends could play games in the nearby squares and alleys, run about among the market stalls and shoppers, or scoot up and down on the banks of the river among the skippers and fish vendors. The Dutch generally loved children and indulged them: it was not they but the English who said "spare the rod and spoil the child." Depictions of children's

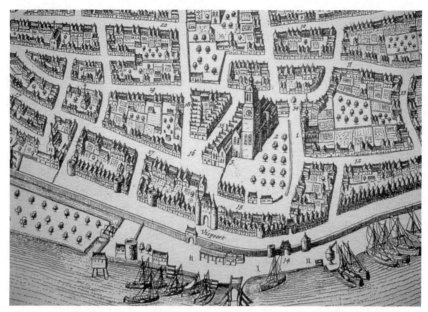

FIG. 4. *Detail from seventeenth-century map of Deventer (with north to the left), show-ing the Grote Kerk just east of the IJssel and the gate at the Vispoort ("Fishgate"). The street on which Joannes lived, "op de graven," is number 18, just to the left of the church.*

games were among the favorite subjects painted on the Dutch tiles that covered hearth and kitchen. Among their many pastimes, Joannes and his friends would have learned how to leapfrog, play ball games and shuttlecock, spin tops, fly kites, jump rope, and roll hoops with a stick.[30]

Joannes's family undoubtedly took seriously the moral and religious in-struction of their son. Bringing up Joannes with edifying stories and moral lessons would have been almost second nature to Frans and Guedeken Groene-velt. The tone of most of these lessons made every event meaningful. A contemporary epigram by Jan Vos drew a moral lesson from his daughter's play:

> My daughter hits the hoop, and struck thus, 't will rotate:
> She finds no end, but runs, till panting ends her cheering.
> Through hoops, eternity children thus indicate.
> The eternal may be gained by sweat and persevering.[31]

Mainstream Dutch culture was, in fact, full of moralizing. As the poem suggests, much of it pointed to eternal verities that could be discovered beneath the surface of everyday life. In a Calvinist society the Bible became the main source for finding deeper meanings in ordinary experience, and so a biblical gloss could be found for almost every event. Emblem books, too, became a popular form of literature, drawing lessons from particular circumstances and illustrating them pictorially. The most notable author of such books was the grand pensionary of Holland in the second quarter of the seventeenth century, Jacob Cats, who not only wrote long didactic poems on subjects like marriage but published a famous emblem book, the *Mirror of the Old and New Time* (1632), which sold huge numbers of copies and is still sometimes read today. Deventer also had its own famous poet: the strict Reformed minister Jacobus Revius, whose *Overijsselsche sangen en dichten* ("Overijssel Songs and Poems") also circulated widely.[32] Mainly composed of religious poems and poems commemorating important people's lives and great events, Revius's book moralized with determination. In one of his shorter everyday poems he wrote:

> Here rests the lazy Melis Brand.
> Here rests? That's hard to understand:
> Here rests, is not the thing to say
> Of one who never worked a day.[33]

Such lessons and moral preaching affected the lives of Dutch people like the Groenevelts by reinforcing the importance of four concepts that have no exact English translation: *keurig, deftig, deugd,* and *gezellig. Keurig* has a dictionary definition of "charming, dainty, trim," but it also means something like the older English meanings of "correct" and "upright." The word speaks to the famous Dutch tidiness and cleanliness, but with reference to persons as well as objects: not only a clean and tidy kitchen can be *keurig,* but one's manner, dress, and speech can be as well. The word thus implies orderliness and an attention to detail in one's character as well as circumstances. *Deftig* is related: it applies to distinguished people or faces, stately houses, or dignified style. It means restraint and reserved elegance: no loud speech, loud laughter, loud dress, or gaudiness—hence the reserved postures and dark clothing of so many contemporary Dutch portraits. *Deugd* can easily be translated as "virtue," but again the term can be applied to parts of life which speakers of English do not always associate with virtue. A person or deed can indeed be *deugdzaam* ("virtuous"), and the cultivation of *deugd* encouraged the many public works of charity for which the Dutch cities were famous—even in a society in which good works did not help earn one's way to heaven. But the Dutch also apply the term to hard work, an organized and well-regulated life, and even (again) cleanliness. If these three words seem to suggest that Dutch life epitomized bourgeois stiffness and order (as has sometimes been argued), they are tempered by another frequently used concept: *gezellig*. The Dutch themselves often attempt to use the English word *cozy* as an equivalent, but that word is not quite adequate. *Gezellig* is the feeling one has when one is engaged in social intimacies, being among friends, enjoying their conversation in good humor, and eating and drinking— without excess. It means something more like "letting one's hair down" than "partying," "cheery" rather than "excited."[34] *Gezelligheid* could be considerably helped by the Dutch love of beer, *jenever* (Dutch gin), tobacco, tea, and coffee, products they marketed to the world. While many of the Dutch behaved in the disordered manner portrayed in the paintings of Jan Steen, public moralizing went along with sentiments that shaped the daily Dutch language, urging people to strive for a quiet, restrained, productive, friendly, correct, cleanly, and joyful life.

Like most Dutch, too, the Groenevelt family attended the Reformed church, just across the square from their home—thrice on Sunday if they were sincere. Services consisted mainly of public readings of lessons from the Bible, with a sermon following. The parents entered public confessions (Frans in June 1641, Guedeken in April 1642),[35] although they left no large sums of money to the church.[36] The Frans Groenevelts, however, lived quietly, and publicly conformed to the Reformed religion.

Joannes therefore grew up a member of the dominant religious group in the northern Netherlands: the Calvinists. Unlike virtually every other country at the time, the Dutch Republic did not have an official religion to which all people had to belong, but the Calvinist faith had the favor of the government and charge of all the public churches. The revolt had been fought in the name of religious peace, and even more important, each city established its own religious policy. Many people remained secretly Catholic, and some even did so openly; various religious sectarians could live, trade, and worship; and, unusual for the time, even Jews were tolerated in some cities, coming to take a very important part in the life of the United Provinces.[37] Nevertheless, to hold almost all public offices, a person had to be a member of the Reformed religion, and many other pressures of daily life existed to push people toward becoming members of that faith.

In Deventer, the Reformed church dominated the city and did not welcome diversity of religious outlook: the city refused to admit Jews in 1654, for instance.[38] When it came to points of doctrine, too, the Deventer church remained rather strict. Although the bitter division within Dutch Calvinism between the Remonstrants and the Contra-Remonstrants had quieted down by Joannes's youth, it remained a source of tension. The religious dispute had centered on the problem of predestination, but in arguing that question, the issue of who would control the future of the Dutch church and even the Dutch nation brought political questions to the fore.[39] Between 1609 and the early 1630s, the religious split led to deep divisions and even fighting in the streets, as well as to the execution of the grand pensionary of Holland and civilian leader of the struggle against the Habsburgs, Johan van Oldenbarnevelt. The altercation began between two professors of theology at the new Dutch university of Leiden, Arminius and Gomarus. Arminius argued that human free will and God's omnipotence and foresight were compatible, especially stressing that Christ's atonement had been for all rather than only the elect, and that although God's grace was necessary for salvation, even Christian believers could fall from grace. To Gomarus, his colleague's views smacked of a Catholic-like emphasis on good works and the associated notion of free will.

The controversy quickly spilled outside the halls of the Leiden academy. Soon after Arminius's death in 1609, a group of his followers drew up a document (a remonstrance) setting out their views. In turn, the Contra-Remonstrants (or Gomarists) organized themselves throughout the country to resist the Arminians and asked that a synod of the church meet to declare the Remonstrants' position false. They even resorted to coercion in ridding parishes of Remonstrant ministers. The leaders of the States of Holland officially preferred quiet on the religious front, but many of them privately favored the Remonstrant position: having an Erastian outlook, Arminianism would have created links between the state and religion amounting to a national church controlled by the magistrates.[40] The leaders of Holland, especially, refused the call for a national synod, and the grand pensionary, Oldenbarnevelt, raised a militia to protect the Remonstrants and their local allies from angry Contra-Remonstrant demonstrations. But the military leader of the United Provinces, the stadholder, Maurice of Nassau, intervened on the side of the Contra-Remonstrants: in 1618–19 a national synod met at Dordrecht (referred to as the synod of Dort) which found against the Arminian position, and after a phony trial, Maurice also had the leader of the States Party, Oldenbarnevelt, executed in 1619. Fourteen years of persecution followed for the Arminians.

In Overijssel, neither side had clear dominance in the early years of the quarrel.[41] Many of the magistrates (*regenten*) of the three major cities of the province—Deventer, Zwolle, and Kampen—favored the Arminians: in some of the cities the Arminians even dominated among the *regenten*. In this preference, they followed the example of places like Amsterdam. On the other hand, while each of the cities sent four or more representatives to the meeting of the local provincial assembly (*landdag*), the other members of the assembly came from the provincial gentry (*ridderschap*) who possessed estates that brought with them the right to sit there. These provincials tended to favor the Contra-Remonstrant position. But when controversial matters divided the provincial representatives, no one felt quite sure how to take a decision: could the towns outvote the gentry, or the other way around, or did a majority composed of people from both groups have to decide, and if so, by how many from each?[42]

In lieu of a clear consensus on religious matters, each place in the province treated the controversy differently. Whereas in Kampen most of the magistrates and ministers favored the Arminian side, by the mid-teens, the Contra-Remonstrants had come to the surface in Deventer. Some of the *regenten* of Deventer favored the Arminians, and one of the local ministers encouraged them to follow Kampen's example. But the other chief ministers in Deventer blocked this attempt—after all, the *regenten* not only sat in the city government but worked with the ministers in the *classis* (or presbytery) which ran the city churches, giving the ministers a great deal of influence. When the leading Remonstrant minister of Deventer moved to Kampen, the Contra-Remonstrants consolidated their position. In 1618, the *classis* of the Deventer church even aided their Contra-Remonstrant brethren in Kampen by sending one of their own ministers to aid their allies there who had broken with the dominant Arminians. The Deventer ministers were among those who ultimately brought the provincial synod over to the Contra-Remonstrant side, and they sent representatives to the Synod of Dort to enter complaints against the Remonstrants.[43] As late as 1631, the Deventer theologian Nicolaus Vedelius published a scathing attack on Remonstrant beliefs.[44]

This great crisis in the Dutch church had passed by the time Joannes Groenevelt came into the world, but its legacy remained in the 1640s and 1650s. By the time of Joannes's upbringing, the "further Reformation" (*nadere Reformatie*) was bringing a variety of sects and freethinkers to the surface, while many of the most serious among the Reformed had become attracted to Pietist notions under the influence of English Puritanism.[45] But echoes of the Remonstrant clash remained. They remained partly in the memories of older people. For example, the grandfather of one of Joannes Groenevelt's friends was Casparus Sibelius, one of the ministers who helped to organize the Contra-Remonstrant movement in Deventer, a person of learning who also helped in the work of writing an official Dutch translation of the Bible mandated by the Synod of Dort (the "States Bible").[46] But the legacy of the dispute also lived on in the strict religious teaching of the local church, transmitted to Joannes in his first schooling.

The child Joannes imbibed the teachings of the Dutch Reformed church from the clergymen who also functioned as schoolmasters. We do not know the details of schooling for young children in Deventer or Overijssel in the seventeenth century, but Joannes's education can be reconstructed in its general shape. To "bring up the children in the true faith of the elect" (including an adherence to the doctrine of predestination) constituted an essential goal of elementary-school teachers, who also taught reading and writing.[47]

Seventeenth-century Dutch children like Joannes began school at the local parish, around the age of five.[48] Unless the school was especially large, all the young children would have been taught in the same room together, rather than in separate classes. The main goals of this education, spelled out in 1612, were to bring children up in the fear of God, to inculcate respect and obedience for public authorities and their parents, to bring them to knowledge, and to teach them good morals and manners. The Synod of Dort added that even poor children should go to school, supported by the local diocese, and it set regular standards for the form and content of education. The organization of the school day reflected the goals of 1612 as ratified by Dort. The day began and ended with prayer, and during the lessons the psalms to be read in church on the following Sunday were studied.

For the first three years, from ages five to eight, the children learned how to read in Dutch—since reading the Bible was one of the foundations of the Reformed faith—and they learned their catechism: religious questions and answers, which had to be memorized by heart. Joannes's teachers used two catechisms that he still possessed in his adult years, valuing them enough to have them shipped over to him in England.[49] One was the so-called Heidelberg catechism, the basic text for the Dutch Reformed faith.[50] Commissioned by the Elector of the Palatinate, and unanimously approved by the Synod of Heidelberg in 1563, this catechism had been quickly adopted among Reformed churches throughout the Continent and accepted at the Synod of Dort as the official catechism of the Dutch church. It divides religious instruction into three parts (sin, redemption, and new life), teaching the Protestant faith in a way that generally avoided controversy and polemics (despite an attack on the Catholic Mass as idolatry in Section 80). After being drilled in the

Heidelberg catechism—129 questions and answers—the children could be sure of knowing the tenets of the Reformed religion. Joannes may have begun to read the Bible directly in school and home at this age, and his family possessed a large Bible, undoubtedly an edition of the Dutch translation authorized by the States General following the Synod of Dort.[51]

Surely Joannes thought deeply about his faith when an epidemic of plague struck Deventer in 1656, when he was eight. During that summer, the pestilence swept away many people: one contemporary estimated that perhaps over half the city's population of slightly less than eight thousand died in the outbreak.[52] If the magistrates enforced the rules they used during another epidemic, in 1665–66, they quarantined in their houses everyone in a residence in which someone had come down with the disease, placing a large "P" on the house to warn others away.[53] When plague epidemics struck, virtually all trade came to a standstill, and many people fled as quickly as possible. The Groenevelts probably moved out of town and into their house across the river, but they remained close enough to town to worry about getting the disease: Frans followed the custom of many of his fellow citizens and drew up a will.[54] He and his family, however, survived to see a day of thanksgiving for the end of the epidemic proclaimed by the city fathers on 9 November.[55]

Probably sometime soon after life returned to normal, Frans and Guedeken Groenevelt decided to send Joannes to school for a few more years. Knowing how to read and having a basic indoctrination in his religion, Joannes now learned how to write in Dutch. Children from families who did not have to set everyone to work as soon as possible commonly went on in Dutch school from ages eight to nine; like many others in a city with a long educational tradition, Joannes probably continued until the age of eleven or twelve. In a city such as Deventer, too, the children might also learn some arithmetic at this age.[56]

Joannes not only acquired additional skills in this further schooling, he drank in more deeply the dominant elements of his national culture. Probably one of the texts he used at this time was the history he later mentioned as among his books. The title is referred to too cryptically for us to be sure of its full title ("2de deel der spaense Tyde," or "second volume on the Spanish time").[57] But in all likelihood, this was the *Spiegel der Jeught* ("Mirror for Youth"), which first appeared in 1615, the major text used to teach Dutch children their history, or one very much like it. The second part of the "Mirror" was subtitled "A Short Account of the Chief Tyranny and Barbarous Cruelties Which the Spaniards Here in the Netherlands Had Imposed on

Many Thousands of People."[58] Such books taught Dutch schoolchildren about Spanish atrocities and the glorious struggle for freedom and nationhood waged by their grandparents. Whatever the exact text he used, we can be sure that the young Joannes learned from his books the lesson he also imbibed from the world around him: as the new Israel, the Dutch nation had been chosen by God as the city on the hill, serving as a beacon to the godly and a model for the rest of humanity.[59] He could be proud to have been born into a nation chosen by God for greatness.

Reinforcing the teachings of history was the deepening understanding of the articles of his Reformed faith. The Calvinism defined by the Synod of Dort made five points clear: original sin has spiritually incapacitated all people; God has, however, unconditionally chosen a few on whom he has bestowed his grace and who will therefore be saved (the elect); consequently, Christ's saving work has power for the elect alone; the elect cannot turn aside the saving grace given to them by God; the elect have been chosen by God from the beginning and will be saved, forever. On the questions of free will and predestination, then, the Synod of Dort had been clear: God alone had at the beginning of time determined who would be saved, so that neither a willingness to be saved nor good works could earn election. So, too, the synod had been clear on God's free gift of salvation for the few alone. The elect had been chosen by God from all time, for all time, and could not even cast off his saving grace if they wanted to. All others had been condemned to the eternal hellfires because of Adam's original sin. The doctrine of predestination might have caused the young Groenevelt to examine his conscience thoroughly in order to find whether he was of the elect or not.[60] On the other hand, the doctrine might well have increased not Joannes's self-doubt but his self-confidence.

The second catechistic book possessed by Groenevelt, a kind of supplement to the Heidelberg catechism, explained these refinements of the Dutch Reformed faith. Written by Petrus de Witte and first published when Joannes was four, this "Catechism on the Heidelberg Catechism" explained how only the elect members of the Reformed religion possessed the one true faith, calling Catholics, Anabaptists (or Mennonites), and others no better than Mohammedans—the worst abusers of faith De Witte could imagine.[61] Joannes would begin life knowing that he had been brought up in the only true faith and that members of other faiths could not be trusted.

Joannes Groenevelt therefore grew up a child of the Dutch "Golden Age." Born at the end of the war that created his country, having escaped a grave

epidemic, able to read, obedient and well mannered, and well grounded in
the proud faith of the elect, Joannes epitomized many Dutch children. His
generally comfortable but militant world produced in him a religious member
of a powerful young nation. Growing up in the shadow of the new clock
tower of the Grote Kerk where the remains of the Anglo-Saxon Lebuinus
lay, hearing the hours regularly struck, and seeing the clear white light of
northern days shinning through church windows uncolored by stained glass,
Joannes undoubtedly found stability in the faith of the elect. As long as he
abided in his faith, all would turn out as God willed. In the meantime,
he would study his books. But even an ordinary childhood could have its
uncertainties: plague, or the violent world beyond his city's walls, threatened.
At the same time that he absorbed the religious, moral, and patriotic values
of the Dutch nation, then, his sense of place remained strong. The city that he
would remember so fondly retained a sense of pride and some independence. It
had grown around the church of a British saint, in which place Joannes had
been baptized. English soldiers had come to protect Deventer before their
officers betrayed it in 1587. The religion into which Joannes had been born
had been brought to the place by a Briton; and though his religion had been
shaped by the militant severity of the Synod of Dort, some people were
already yielding to the more introspective strains of Pietism, formed in part
under English influences. Whether he knew it or not, his world and that of
the English had already crossed many times, as they would again.

CHAPTER 3

The Education of a Dutch Physician

To succeed in his world, Joannes Groenevelt would not only have to keep his faith, he would have to work hard. Although born into the Dutch Golden Age, he lived near its end: the future would be hard. Left without a father in his late teens, he could soon see, just beyond the walls of his hometown, enemy armies that ravaged the land and people and shriveled the local economy. Looking out on a world in which Death came when he pleased, the young man prepared himself as best he could for the struggles ahead. His work would not be that of a craftsman like his father. For some time, it would be the work of mastering difficult texts and learned traditions. He grew up in perhaps the most highly educated society of the time and had excellent opportunities for study. As a youth, he attended the local gymnasium and then the Illustrious School, one of the best higher schools in northern Europe. He then went on to attend the medical faculty of the University of Leiden, renowned for its professors and graduates. As he progressed through his education, he became acquainted with some of the more serious intellectual debates of the time, including those surrounding the philosophy of Descartes. His abiding faith would not be allowed to rest on simple certainties. Because of an epidemic in Leiden, he had to take his medical doctorate elsewhere—in Utrecht—but there, too, he found a fine medical teacher. For his medical degree, received just two months before his twenty-second birthday, he produced a thesis on a chronic disease that troubled many people, especially men: bladder stones. It was one of the most thorough discussions of the disease produced in a Dutch university. He would turn out to be one of the learned elite of Europe: a university-trained physician.

The kind of education he obtained made him an excellent scholar, but not just for the sake of scholarship. His early Latin-school education continued to shape him morally as well as intellectually, and his medical studies at Leiden united the study of medical texts with the experience of clinic, anatomy theater, and chemical laboratory. His education had not been for the sake of learning alone but for use. The kind of education he received, shaped as it was by Dutch Christian humanism, by the Reformed church, and by clinically oriented medical professors, would make him somewhat different from the university-educated physicians he later encountered in England. Despite the high quality of his education, excellence had no absolute standard: the young Groenevelt grew up not only learned but Dutch.

After his years of schooling in the Dutch language and Reformed religion, around the age of eleven or twelve, Joannes stood at an important crossroads. His parents had to make important choices about his future. For a boy of his age, they might have found a master to whom he could be apprenticed to make him into a craftsman like his father or into a tradesman or merchant. Or they could prepare him for a different calling. From the late Middle Ages, the local leaders of the low countries had developed a fondness for Christian humanism, rooted in impressive scholarship. The Reformation itself had depended upon the development of a deep appreciation for the revelations of philology, a way of knowing which came from an understanding of the original languages in which Scripture had been written. While the pursuit of letters provided hardly a crust of dry bread by itself, many people of even modest wealth and influence thought it important to be able to discuss learned matters with intelligence, and so they had their sons well educated. For some who needed to earn a living, formal education also provided the foundation for a good future. While the sons of the wealthy and powerful often chose to study law, medicine and the ministry could provide a more modest livelihood for the sons of middling sorts.[1] The study of all of the three higher faculties demanded a foundation in the liberal arts, the teaching of which was in Latin. Given the moral, social, and economic value of learning in the Netherlands, then, Guedeken and Frans chose to send their only child to the local Latin school.

Deventer had a long tradition of excellent Latin education. In the fifteenth century, the Deventer Latin school had a fine and widespread reputation. The famous papal legate and philosopher Nicholas of Cusa even set up a scholarship in Deventer for poor boys who wanted to attend its school.[2] Part of the chapter of St. Lebuinus, the Latin school had teachers from among both the clergy and the Brethren of the Common Life. It was in Deventer that the great Desiderius Erasmus began his Latin education; toward the end of his stay, the rector of the school, Alexander Hegius—a friend of the renowned northern humanist Rudolph Agricola—introduced the study of Greek for the first time north of the Alps. The city also boasted several printers before 1500, and Deventer presses worked closely with the school, being responsible for nearly half of all Dutch fifteenth-century school grammars.[3] The tradition of learning continued into the sixteenth century. An anonymous manuscript of 1551/2 noted that Deventer was said to have had thirteen hundred students studying Latin, having already trained three thousand. It was here that Philip II had planned in the 1570s to establish a new university, and here that at about the same time a pious Catholic noblewoman, Anna van Twickelo, provided an endowment for a university in the memory of her son.[4]

To this high tradition of humanist schooling, the Reformation brought only a few changes when linking the local schools to the Reformed rather than the Catholic church.[5] The schools did drop lessons in music (which had been a staple of the medieval and humanist schools but was seen as sinful by the strict Reformed). By the seventeenth century, the earlier emphasis on reading and writing Latin was further extended, and Greek and logic were now offered in the higher classes. (Unlike the lower, Dutch-speaking schools, the Latin schools also continued not to admit girls). By Joannes's time, a school board governed the Dutch school and two Latin schools: the "Triviale" School (or gymnasium) and the "Illustre" School (or athenaeum). The school board was made up of two magistrates, two ministers of the Reformed church, and two members of the city assembly. They decided on general policy and appointed the teachers (ordinarily clergymen in the lower schools and professors in the athenaeum) and a rector for each school (who was usually one of the best-educated local ministers). The board took special care to insure that all the teachers showed up on time, maintained sobriety, and at all moments exhibited other signs of good character and seriousness.[6] In stressing moral rectitude on the part of teachers and students, the Deventer schools were like the schools in other Dutch cities.[7] Moreover, under the influence of the strong-minded Contra-Remonstrant minister, moralizing poet, and school board member, Jacobus Revius, the Deventer teachers all had to subscribe to a document stating the articles of faith as defined by the Synod of Dort.[8]

While the States General of the United Provinces did not issue general regulations for all the Latin schools in the country (as the Calvinist ministers had urged after the Synod of Dort), several provinces issued their own regulations, and the Deventer Latin schools conformed to the general pattern.[9]

Like other Latin schools, Joannes's Triviale School was divided into five classes, each lasting a year, with the "first" being the most advanced. The students were to speak only Latin in school. As in their elementary-school days, students continued to be trained in good manners, with severe punishments for failures; and religious training remained important. Lessons would take place six days a week, in four roughly two-hour blocks with a two-hour break for lunch, the day beginning about seven o'clock in the morning and going until around five in the afternoon (or from eight to six during the winter, when the sun rose late). The school year broke for a month's summer vacation from the main Deventer fair to about 25 August, a month's winter vacation from a week before Christmas to after 25 January, half-week vacations for Easter and Pentecost, and local feast days.[10] On Wednesdays and Saturdays, instead of new lessons the boys had religious services, review and practice sessions, and disputations—the exercise of formal debate on specific questions before a public of teachers and students, undertaken by the older boys. The students also underwent periodic examinations, with promotions and prizes being awarded with much ceremony. The fees for such an education would not have been negligible but within the reach of a well-to-do craftsman like Frans Groenevelt.[11]

In the first classes, reading and reciting of Latin made up the day, with new words and the elements of grammar being slowly introduced. Dutch children learned their Latin grammar from Gerhardus Joannes Vossius.[12] From the list of books that Joannes Groenevelt later possessed, we can guess that he began his Latin with readings from Cato and Cicero; he certainly used the plays of Terence.[13] As they progressed, the students were also gradually introduced to writing Latin prose and poetry. Joannes possessed two textbooks that anthologized the major poets.[14] In more advanced classes, he turned to Caesar.[15] After a year or two, students could also begin Greek, and in the final two years they would study logic as well. He learned his Greek from Homer and a Greek grammar.[16]

But tragedy struck the Groenevelt household while he attended Latin school. In early 1664, just short of Joannes's sixteenth birthday, his father died at the age of fifty-five.[17] Joannes undoubtedly suffered not only a personal sense of loss at the death of his father but also many anxieties about his future. According to the will Frans had made out during the plague of 1656, all his estate was to go to his widow and his surviving children after an inventory of the estate to determine its worth. Since passages in the will were underlined, someone apparently went through it to check its provisions.[18] An inventory was made of what Guedeken possessed, showing a well-furnished house and various properties as well as debts.[19] Since Dutch women usually kept possession of the properties they brought into a marriage and half of what had been accumulated during the marriage, Joannes probably inherited the remains of his father's original estate plus half of what had been formed during his marriage.[20] On the last page of the inventory, Joannes's mother stated that for the "fatherly good" of her son, she placed him under the care of two guardians (*mombers*): Joan de Wilde and Henricus Ter Borch (later a burgomaster).[21] These steps seem to have been taken to set aside Joannes's portion of the inheritance and to put it under the care of his guardians, who would administer his estate and pay him an allowance from it. Given later events, the income seems not to have been large enough for him to live from his inheritance alone but certainly sufficient for him to continue his studies.

But Joannes not only lost a father early in his teens; the world beyond soon threatened, too. Not only his country but his native city were put at risk when the English took up arms against the Dutch Republic. Since the death of the stadholder William II in 1650, the country had been run by the *regenten* of the major cities and some of the nobles, without a stadholder. (Technically, the stadholder ruled a province in the name of the king, but during and after the Dutch Revolt, when there was no king, the stadholders were the military leaders of the country, sometimes with ambitions to become princes in their own right.)[22] The magistrates of Deventer solidly supported this "States Party," led by the grand pensionary of Holland, Johan de Witt.[23] But the king of England, Charles II, took offense at the way Their Noble Great Mightinesses (as the States General styled themselves) dealt with him and with the education of his nephew, William of Orange, the posthumous son of William II. Moreover, trade conflicts had also created a great deal of friction between the two nations, so that the English Parliament urged Charles to attack the Dutch. In 1664, unannounced, English ships attacked the fort and island of Cape Verde operated by the Dutch West India Company off the Guinea coast of Africa, while English colonists seized islands in the West Indies and New Amsterdam (renaming it New York, after Charles' brother James, the Lord High Admiral and duke of York). In reply, Their Noble Great Mightinesses secretly ordered the Dutch Mediterranean fleet under Admiral De Ruyter to counter the English move off Guinea. When Charles received definite news in early December that De Ruyter had taken over all of the Guinea coast from the English, he flew into a rage, and formal war soon commenced.[24] It lasted from 1665 to July 1667, ending with the Dutch gaining the upper hand in the spice islands of the East Indies and the English retaining New York.

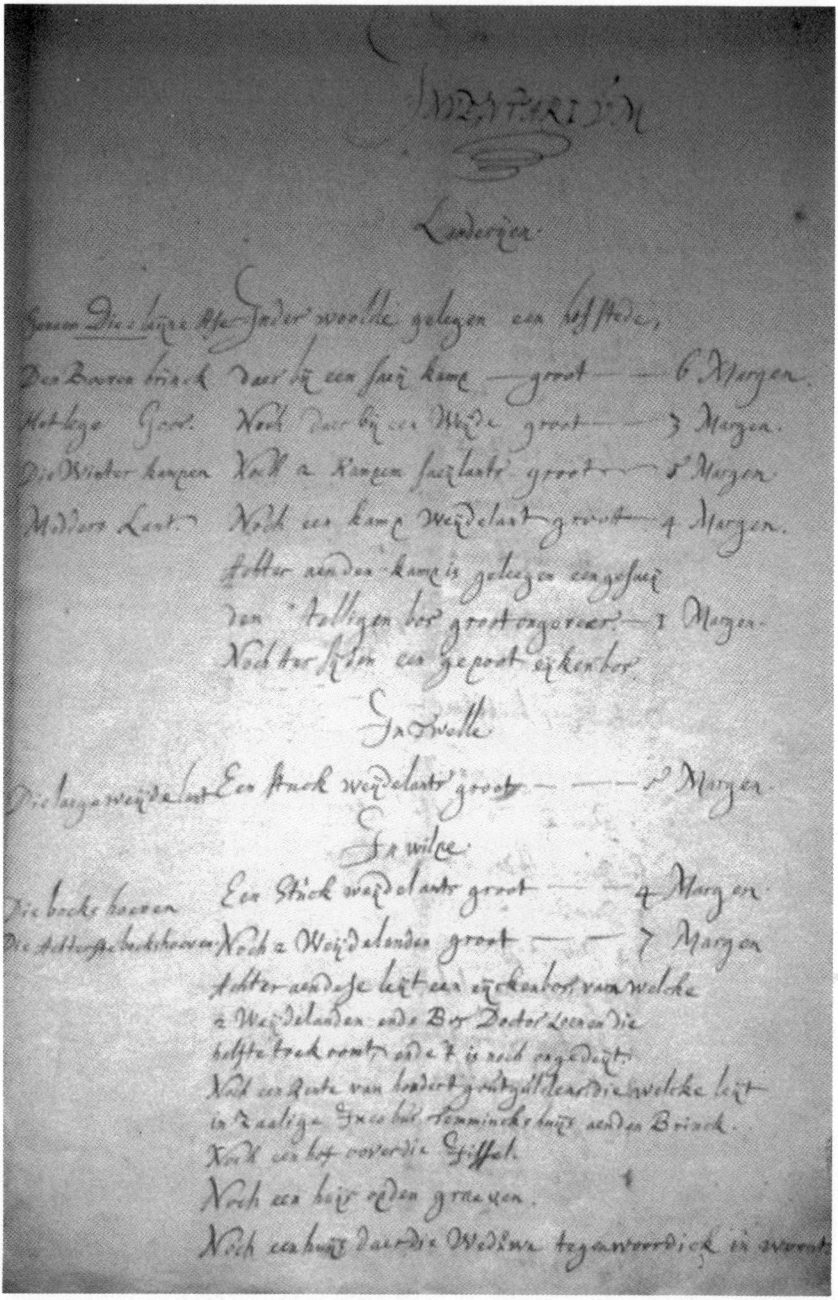

FIG. 5. *First page of the inventory of the widow Groenevelt's possessions.*

All these battles off Africa, America, and Asia, and even those off the coasts of Holland itself, would have seemed far away from Joannes and his kin in Deventer except for one thing: the English successfully bought an ally in the bishop of Münster, whose territories bordered Overijssel and Gelderland on the east. Having let its defenses decay since the peace of 1648, and having sent most of its troops to the navy for use against England, the Republic found itself virtually helpless to prevent the bishop from seizing most of those two provinces late in the summer of 1665. What remained of the Dutch army retreated behind the IJssel, leaving Deventer one of the few redoubts of the Republic on the eastern side of the river, as it had been during the 1580s. The arrival of a French army on the side of the Dutch late in 1665, and the alliance between the Republic and the Elector of Brandenburg in February 1666, forced Münster to withdraw and make peace that spring. But for the moment, during 1665 and the first part of 1666, Deventer became the easternmost bastion of the Republic in yet another war. On top of everything, plague again struck the city in 1665–66. When siege and plague ended, the province of Overijssel lay in financial ruin.[25]

It would be nice to know just what Joannes Groenevelt thought about the war and plague surrounding him in the mid-1660s and how he and his mother lived during the time. It cannot have been easy. We only know that he did his best to go on with his studies. He was old enough for military service, but the Dutch armies mainly employed the poor or soldiers from other countries; the seventeenth century was not yet a period of citizen armies. In the midst of the conflict, then, in the middle of January 1666, he matriculated to the higher Latin school, the Illustrious School, or athenaeum.[26]

In the early seventeenth century, a number of Dutch cities established athenaeums. The first had been at Harderwijk (1600), and the second was in Deventer (1630). Other cities soon followed their example: Amsterdam (1632), Utrecht (1634), Dordrecht (1636), 's Hertogenbosch (also known as Den Bosch, or Bois-le-Duc; 1636), Breda (1646), Middelburg (1650), Nijmegen (1655), Rotterdam (1681), Maastricht (1683), and Zutphen (1686).[27] More than Latin schools, staffed by professors and offering advanced studies not only in the liberal arts but in the higher faculties of theology, law, and medicine, athenaeums amounted to small universities with the important exception that they did not grant degrees; when the schools at Utrecht and Harderwijk did get the right of promotion (in 1636 and 1648, respectively), they became universities in fact.

The Deventer magistrates and ministers may have hoped to turn their

Illustrious School into a university, too. For its first professors, they tried
to attract famous scholars from German lands, including Joannes Henricus
Alsted, whose expectation of the imminent thousand-year reign of God on
earth had great influence throughout Europe and among English Puritans.[28]
Although in the end Alsted turned the magistrates down, for a while the
renowned philosopher and personal friend of René Descartes, Henricus Renerius, taught philosophy at the Deventer school (from the autumn of 1631 to
January 1634) and attracted Descartes himself to Deventer—where Descartes's illegitimate daughter, Fransientgen Regnier Joachims, was born in
July 1635. Following Renerius, one of Descartes's main opponents, Martinus
Schoock, was brought in as a professor of philosophy later in the 1630s,
perhaps to root out Cartesian influences. The Deventer school was not only the
second athenaeum founded in the Netherlands, then, but earned a reputation as
being one of the best, if conservative, schools in the country during the mid-
seventeenth century, with its professors participating in some of the great
philosophical debates of the time. It attracted many students from around
the Republic and abroad, and although by the time Joannes enrolled the
number of students had slipped from its peak of 1650–54 (of about 150), it
remained a large and important institution of higher education.[29]

Joannes spent almost two years refining his education in the Deventer
athenaeum before he left for further studies in university. His matriculation
depended on his having finished the Triviale School and of being a firm
adherent of the Reformed religion. The schedule of teaching in the athenaeum
much resembled that of the gymnasium, with the professors lecturing publicly
during set hours every Monday, Tuesday, Thursday, and Friday, keeping
Wednesdays and Saturdays for repetitions and disputations. In their public
lectures, the professors treated the most important authors of the subject
under discussion. In addition, the professors gave private lessons (*collegia
privata*) to students with a special interest in their subject, for which they
used compendia of various writers and in which they might introduce authors
and ideas far beyond the set curriculum.[30] For example, the professor of
philosophy was supposed to systematize Aristotle's logic, physics, and metaphysics for the students; but under the first professor of the subject, a philosophy student defended a thesis on the superiority of Ramist over Aristotelian
logic, which undoubtedly originated from the private lessons.[31] The students
would work with a professor in a special faculty and also follow the required
public lessons in philosophy, theology, and Hebrew.[32]

Joannes Groenevelt became acquainted with all the faculties at the athenaeum. In law, the professor was Willem Tichler, an undistinguished jurist

but a good friend of some of the local magistrates.[33] From some of the books in Joannes's possession, it is possible to infer that Tichler taught not only standard Roman law but the law of the city of Deventer, too.[34] Although the athenaeum had a professor of medicine from 1638 to 1647, it had dropped the subject by Joannes's time, perhaps because the magistrates could not afford to invest in the anatomy theater, cabinet of specimens, and instruments that would have been necessary to teach the subject by modern standards.[35]

It is therefore not surprising that the evidence from Joannes's books suggests that he followed the courses in philosophy and especially in theology most seriously. The professors of these subjects taught them in an orthodox fashion but also introduced the students to some of the contemporary debates that challenged established opinion. Formally, philosophy remained the servant of theology at the school: all the professors in Groenevelt's time subscribed to a document detailing the articles of faith determined by the Synod of Dort and, aside from one person, had not tried to make philosophy an independent subject, as did the followers of René Descartes.[36] The senior professor of philosophy, Rutger Loenius (or Van Loenen), who was also the city physician of Deventer, taught logic, metaphysics, and physics. While nothing is known from his hand, he seems faithfully to have given the public lectures on Aristotle, as required.[37] Joannes possessed a standard summary of Aristotelian natural philosophy, perhaps used by Loenius.[38] Perhaps, too, Loenius was Joannes's mentor at school: a patch of oak woods which his mother owned had come into the possession of Loenius, perhaps for tuition.[39]

The second professor of philosophy while Groenevelt attended the athenaeum seems to have been more interesting: Theophilus (or Gozewijn) Hogers. Hogers taught rhetoric and history. On the one hand, the evidence from Joannes's books suggests that Hogers taught the usual fare: ethics from authors who based their views on Aristotle's *Nichomacean Ethics,*[40] and ancient history from the long-standard accounts of Valerius Maximus and Justinus's epitome of Pompeius Trogus's *Historiae Philippicae,* and a chronology developed by the first professor of philosophy in the athenaeum, Henricus Gutberleth.[41] On the other hand, Hogers was a close friend of Rabo Herman Schele's, one of the formulators of the States Party ideology that predominated in the 1660s.[42] Several of the leading members of the States Party, including the grand pensionary De Witt (with whom Hogers was also acquainted), had Cartesian sympathies, and it is unlikely that Hogers could have taught without mentioning some of Descartes's principles, at least in his private lessons. Groenevelt later possessed the works of Descartes, and he might very well have been introduced to some of his ideas in Deventer.

Certainly there is good evidence for a liberalizing of the Deventer school's curriculum in theology during Joannes's time. His professor of theology was Antonius Perizonius, a moderate Cartesian and a friend and advocate of Joannes Coccejus, professor of theology at the University of Leiden.[43] Coccejus emphasized not a theology growing out of philosophy but one rooted in the notion of God's covenant with humanity. Because the Coccejeans tried to separate theology from philosophy (just as the Cartesians tried to separate philosophy from theology), and because they therefore rejected Aristotelian terminology in the interpretation of Scripture, they could freely support new philosophical views, such as Cartesianism.[44] But the emphasis on biblical rather than philosophical interpretation also led Coccejus to stress the Greek rather than Hebrew version of the Bible, the Septuagint. The difference in language implied a difference in critical methods of study. During the Jewish Diaspora following the time of Alexander the Great, a large group of Jews had settled in Alexandria and adopted the Greek language. Sometime during the period from the third to first century B.C.E., they translated the Bible into Greek: because of the tradition that the translation was made by seventy-two elders in Alexandria during the reign of Ptolemy Philadelphus (284–247 B.C.E), this edition of the Bible was called the Septuagint (LXX). While the Christian Latin Bible had been translated by Jerome from contemporary Hebrew texts (around 400 C.E.), earlier Christian authors like Origen had worked from the Greek. Moreover, the oldest extant Hebrew manuscripts of the Bible available to Groenevelt's contemporaries dated from about the seventh century C.E. Since the Greek Septuagint had been used by the founders of the Christian church, and since extant versions of it existed from a date almost one thousand years before the oldest Hebrew Bible, some scholars began to work with the Greek rather than Hebrew Bible in the sixteenth century; Coccejus made it the foundation for his critical study of the Bible. Which version one used made an important difference for determining various issues: not only for biblical chronology but for determining the holiness of the Sabbath and other issues that gave rise to public controversy.[45]

Joannes Groenevelt therefore studied theology with a Coccejean, a member of the most important group of academic revisionists within the Reformed church. He possessed a Dutch edition of the Septuagint, suggesting that he studied the new textual criticism with Perizonius seriously.[46] Moreover, Perizonius emphasized teaching the New Testament from the Greek, too, which, while not as radical as using the Septuagint, nevertheless had important critical implications.[47] Joannes had a New Testament in both Greek and Latin.[48] Given their epistemological orientation, Coccejeans like Perizonius tended toward a philo-Judaic biblicalism rather than the rigid confessionalism of people like Witte, who had written the commentary on the Heidelberg catechism that Joannes had studied earlier. In short, the critical philological studies of the humanists which had helped to spur the Reformation in the low countries now challenged some orthodoxies of the Calvinist church itself. Joannes was moving away from the stricter views of his earlier catechism.[49]

Whether Joannes made theology or philosophy his main subject of study is unknown. But he spent an ordinary amount of time in the athenaeum for a student who graduated, and for that he would have had to have performed before the school a disputation based upon a set question in one subject. In Deventer, as at the Dutch universities, Joannes would—with the help of a professor—write a short Latin treatise on a subject, with a series of corollaries or questions at the end, and have the work printed. The students had to have at least twenty copies of their theses printed and had to circulate them to the members of the school board, the magistrates, the local ministers, and the professors of the school, additionally depositing one in the school library.[50] Then the student would defend his thesis and answer any questions about it or its corollaries in a public disputation. Unfortunately, almost none of the Deventer theses survive from the seventeenth century, including that of Joannes, so we cannot know what question he chose to debate, nor whether he was innovative or traditional in his handling of the subject. We can be sure, however, that if he completed his studies in this way, as he must have, then he was well acquainted with the elements of his nation's academic knowledge and forms.

As important to Groenevelt's life as the education he got at the Illustrious School was his becoming acquainted with, or further acquainted with, four schoolmates who would continue to play an important role in his life in later years. All had entered school just ahead of Groenevelt, and three came from families of slightly higher social rank than his. The oldest were Casparus Sibelius à Goor and Herbert Dapper. Born in 1646, Casparus Sibelius was the son and grandson of ministers. His grandfather, after whom he was named, had been an important clergyman in Deventer, a friend of the powerful Revius and an early supporter of the Illustrious School.[51] Just over a year older than Groenevelt, Sibelius had also begun his studies at the athenaeum a year before Joannes.[52] Herbert Dapper, who was also a year older than Joannes, came from a very substantial family in Deventer, which not only possessed wealth but consistently held places on the city council.[53] The next two were one year younger than Joannes but had entered the athenaeum half a year before him: Willem ten Rhijne and Henricus van Duren. Probably born in 1649, Ten Rhijne's father was a glassmaker (and so in a trade similar to that of Groenevelt's father);[54] Van Duren, like Dapper, came from a very wealthy family that had long served in the city government.[55] These four youthful friends of Joannes were the ones we know he kept in touch with in later years.

After a year and a half spent in the Deventer athenaeum, in 1667, aged nineteen, Joannes Groenevelt left for the University of Leiden, renowned throughout Europe. After the August vacation he went to his church, told them that he was leaving for Leiden, and obtained a certificate (dated 9 September) stating that he was a member in good standing of the Reformed church of Deventer.[56] Probably not having a lot of money, he traveled to Leiden directly rather than taking in various sights on the way. We can guess at the route he traveled: by boat down the IJssel to Kampen, from there over the Zuider Zee to Amsterdam, and from Amsterdam to Leiden via Haarlem by canal boat. The trip would have been relatively inexpensive: a few stuivers to get to Kampen, about 15 stuivers to cross the Zuider Zee, and about 20 to get from Amsterdam to Leiden.[57] He entered his name in the book of matriculants at the university on 13 September.[58] His expenses probably came to somewhere in the range of 150 to 200 gilders per year, paid for from his inheritance.[59]

   The city of Leiden lay in the heart of the heavily populated province of Holland, the most powerful member of the United Provinces. The largest city in the province after Amsterdam, with a population of about sixty-five thousand, many of whom composed a poor urban proletariat, its wealth depended mainly on the manufacture of cloth. Located in the Middle Ages on the lower Rhine, Leiden maintained a water outlet to the sea despite projects that altered the course of the main river. Immigrants from the religious troubles in the southern netherlands and England—including those known to Americans as the Pilgrims—settled in crowded little houses and narrow back streets in Leiden and worked the looms from morning till night. Windmills ringed the city walls, fulling cloth and grinding grain, while printing presses stamped out both great books and ephemera. Students who came to the university also brought money to the city, although far less than the weavers.[60] Like other students from out of town, Joannes paid for lodgings and probably meals in a rooming house. In his case, the widow Geltons provided his accommodations. In addition to the young Groenevelt, nine other students jammed into her house, all about the same age as he. Like most students, too, they lived with others whom they knew from some other network: all but Joannes studied letters or the law, and most in the house were from the eastern part of the Netherlands—in fact, six of the nine came from Overijssel, and three had been to the Deventer Illustrious School.[61]

The great majority of students from Overijssel who sought a university education migrated to Leiden, not only the oldest and largest but the most famous of the five Dutch universities.[62] The university had been founded in 1575, after a long siege by the Spaniards which, had it ended with the taking of the city, might have broken the Dutch Revolt.[63] After the siege, William the Silent had proposed that the States of Holland and Zeeland establish a university in Leiden in order to educate the sons of what was becoming a new country. The story that William had offered the city magistrates either a period of no taxes or a university as a reward for their endurance, with the city fathers choosing the latter, is probably apocryphal. But it does speak to the deep-seated learning that many Leiden *regenten* and local noblemen possessed, especially the Lord of Nordwijk and military governor of Leiden, Jan van der Does (or Janus Dousa), one of the first curators of the school. Dousa, a fine scholar and poet himself, recruited famous scholars the likes of Lipsius and Scaliger to the new university.[64] The States of Holland and Zeeland established a group of governors of the university chosen not from among the Calvinist clergy but from among themselves: three curators chosen by the States of Holland and Zeeland for life, and the four annually elected burgomasters of the city of Leiden. Planned from the beginning to train students in theology, law, medicine, and the arts, the university gradually grew in size until, by the time Joannes matriculated, it contained several hundred students, many of them from abroad, and fifteen faculty supplemented with a number of irregular teachers.[65]

Empowered during a period in which the revolt still proclaimed religious peace and in which its leaders sought a broad-minded Christian humanism, the curators, backed by the States of Holland, largely successfully exercised their authority in such a way as to keep the university up to date and undoctrinaire. Although events following upon the Synod of Dort purged the university of some of the less orthodox curators and professors, the university remained fairly liberal in spirit even then. The professors had to be members of the Reformed church, but the doors of the university were open to students of any faith, including Jews. And although, especially after the Synod of Dort, the curators did not wish to endure too much public controversy over religion or philosophy and so prohibited publishing for or against Cartesianism in the mid-1640s, new opinions, including Cartesian ones, continued to be discussed. In fact, the new rules of the university allowed Cartesianism to

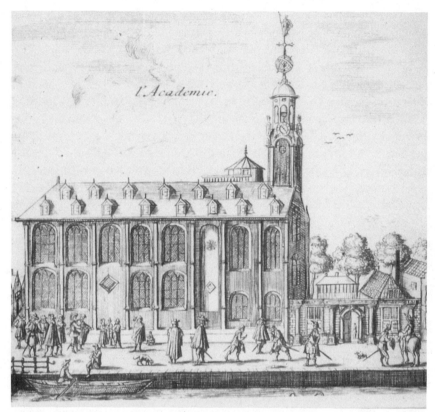

FIG. 6. *The main university building in Leiden. From "Les Délices de Leyde" (1712).*

flourish, despite the strong objections of those like the conservative Deventer minister and Leiden teacher Revius.[66] The students led the way, making matters difficult for philosophically conservative professors: in 1659, the States of Holland had to issue an edict forbidding their stamping and banging in lectures, orations, or disputations.[67] From the mid-1660s to 1672, during the time that Groenevelt attended the university, the ferment of new ideas at Leiden reached a peak, with the curators not attempting to limit any kind of teaching, public or private.

Having obtained a firm foundation in Latin literature, history, philosophy, and theology, it was time for the young Groenevelt to concentrate his studies in an area that would earn him his bread. Given his studies at Deventer, which concentrated in philosophy and theology, one might have expected him to enroll in the faculty of theology. But he did not. Instead, he matriculated in the medical faculty. This is especially surprising because the Illustrious School had not taught any medicine during his years there, although the senior professor of philosophy, Loenius, had also served as city physician. Very few students from the Illustrious School went on in medicine. Indeed, among the university graduates from the city of Deventer, the percentage who had graduated in medicine was the lowest of any of thirty-eight Dutch cities.[68] But among Groenevelt and his four friends, all but one went on to take graduate degrees in medicine, two switching into medicine after beginning in theology.[69] Switching from theology to medicine was relatively common, being a course taken by the likes of Isaac Beeckman or Groenevelt's own medical professor Florentius Schuyl. One might serve God in another way by serving his people as a physician to their bodies as well as their souls; and since medicine in part still meant telling people how to live their lives according to an appropriate regimen, it had a pastoral function.[70] Theology still remained a contentious field, and the ministry did not often offer good prospects of material success. Perhaps one of Groenevelt's guardians even suggested that being a physician would be a good career for him. Then, too, his family was personally acquainted with some of the local physicians: not only had a piece of his mother's lands come into the possession of Loenius, but the family owed debts to both Dr. Jordens and Dr. Meilingius.[71] Moreover, Groenevelt's friend Ten Rhijne provided an even more immediate example, having left Deventer during the plague to study medicine at Franeker—he would soon join Groenevelt in Leiden.[72] The little group from the Illustrious School already had a sufficient background in philosophy for studying medicine. So for the young Groenevelt, medicine it would be.

As at the Deventer Illustrous School and other Dutch universities, the Leiden professors lectured on Monday, Tuesday, Thursday, and Friday, with Wednesdays and Saturdays being reserved for academic exercises such as disputations, meetings, graduations, and public ceremonies. They also gave private lessons. In addition to the professors, a number of other people taught Leiden students as private lecturers, occasionally with the license of the faculty. Customarily, the students performed two public disputations during their regular course of study (called *exercitii causa,* these theses were sometimes the work of the sponsoring professor and so published under his name at a later date); for his graduation exercise, the student underwent a private examination and a public defense of a printed thesis of his own (*pro gradu*).[73] The graduation theses also commonly had corollaries appended on a variety of subjects in the general field which represented the views of student and professor. Aside from the printing of theses—an innovation of the Germanic-speaking lands—and the precise form of academic ritual, this system of lectures, private tutoring, and disputation typified university education throughout Europe in the period, and it would have been entirely familiar to the athenaeum-trained Groenevelt.

What made medical teaching at Leiden unusual was the addition of clinical and chemical teaching to the lecturing and debating. Clinical and chemical knowledge could be acquired in other university towns, too, but in Leiden the professors themselves taught these subjects, not just private teachers. The Leiden professor could therefore expect his students to bring their clinical and laboratory experience into the classroom, and their philosophical learning into the clinic and laboratory. This integration of practical experience with university lecturing attracted large numbers of medical students not only from the Republic but from all over Europe.

For several decades, the medical faculty at Leiden had been one of the most innovative of the period; during Groenevelt's time there, it reached a high point. The anatomy theater, along with the library and the fencing school, stood in a part of the nearby church of the Béguines (the Falibagijnen-kerk) which the university had taken over. Public anatomical demonstrations took place there in years when the bodies of criminals could be obtained, during the cold winter months when bodies deteriorated less rapidly. During the rest of the year, paintings, maps, and engravings hung below the stands, and human and animal skeletons stood on the railings representing various themes, even Adam and Eve. Many of the skeletons also held flags with Latin mottoes reminding visitors of the shortness of life and other moral lessons.[74] "I was much pleasd with a sight of their Anatomy Schole, Theater & Repository," wrote the English visitor John Evelyn. "[It] is very well furnish'd with Naturall curiosities; especially with all sorts of Skeletons, from the Whale & Eliphant, to the Fly, and the Spider." The way in which the small spider had been prepared impressed Evelyn very much. But more: "Here is the Sceletus of a Man on Horse-back, of a Tigar, and sundry other creatures: The Skinns of Men & Women tentur'd on frames and tann'd: Two faire and entire Mummies, Fishes, Serpents, Shells, divers Urnes; The figure of Isis cut in wood of a greate Proportion and Antiquity; a large Crocodile; The head of the Rynoceros; The Leomarinus, Torpedo, many Indian Weapons, Curiosities out of China, and of the Eastern Countries; so as it were altogether [impossible] to remember all, or take particular notice of them." Evelyn even noted that a knife had been kept for display which had been successfully removed from a man's stomach after he had swallowed it—an impressive operation for the time.[75]

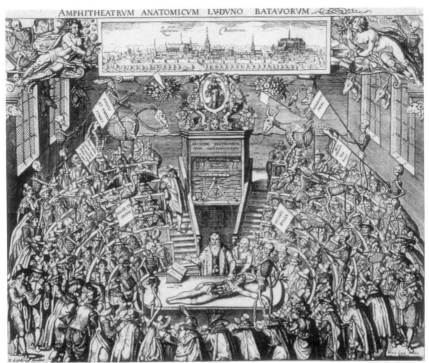

AMPHITHEATRVM ANATOMICVM LVGDVNO BATAVORVM.

FIG. 7. *Leiden anatomical theater, B. Dolendo after J. C. Woudanus. The illustration shows both the skeletons and a public anatomy lesson; in practice, the skeletons would have been removed during demonstrations.*

Inspired to imitate the best medical teaching of the famous medical school of Padua, the first Leiden curators had also quickly set about establishing a botanical garden. The garden, located behind the main university building, grew rapidly and introduced students not only to medicinal plants but to plants from all places in the world. The garden "was indeed well stor'd with exotic Plants," noted Evelyn.[76] Botanical lessons taught the medical students about the plants used in medicines and introduced them to moral lessons about nature as well: often, the garden was spoken of as an imitation of paradise.[77] To the back of the garden stood a building that housed the less hardy plants in the winter and provided space for further natural curiosities.

Additionally, and even more unusual for the period, the curators of the Leiden school had worked closely with the magistrates of the city to integrate some of the medical teaching into one of the city hospitals, the St. Caecilia

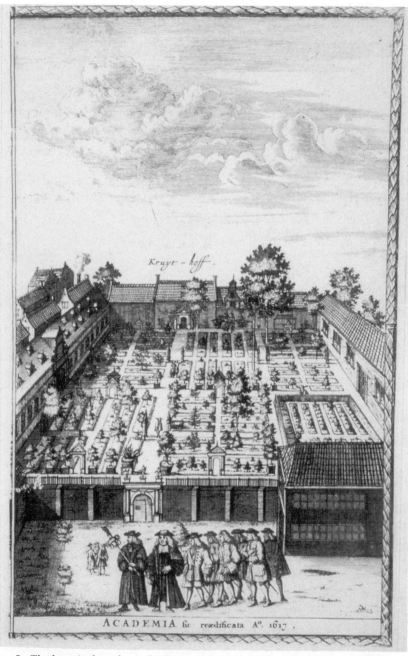

Fig. 8. *The botanical garden in Leiden, engraved in 1617; to the left is the building in which delicate plants could be housed over the winter and additional natural curiosities were displayed.*

Hospital, a former plague house and madhouse. In St. Caecilia's, the medical professors had carried on clinical teaching since the late 1630s (the *collegium medico-practicum*), introducing their students to various diseases and remedies. Here, suffering and its relief could be observed closely, and the professors and students could afterward dissect the bodies of those who died. Even more surprising, inspired by Paracelsianism, plans for the university from the beginning also included teaching in chemistry—although, like clinical practice, it would have to wait until a couple of decades before Groenevelt's arrival.[78] In short, the medical teaching of the Leiden school emphasized both an acquaintance with the details of nature and edification.

Because of the several teaching forums, medical students at Leiden tended to devote more of their attention to anatomical, botanical, clinical, and chemical studies than to the niceties of medical philosophy still so important at ancient universities like Paris, Oxford, and Cambridge. The example of Sir Robert Sibbald, an important Scots physician who began his medical studies in Leiden in 1660 and 1661 (just a few years before Groenevelt's arrival), is representative. He studied anatomy and surgery under "the learned Professor Van Horne" and attended some of his anatomical demonstrations; botany he learned under Adolph Vorstius. Sibbald also "studied the institutions and practice, under Sylvius, who was famous then." He went on: "I saw twenty-three human bodies dissected by him in the Hospitall which I frequented with him." He learned from his fellow students, too, including the later famous Nicolaus Steno, who, Sibbald wrote, "dissected in my chamber sometymes, and showed me there, the ductus salivalis superior, he had discovered." Additionally, Sibbald "frequented ane apothecaryes shop, and saw the materia medica and the ordinary compositions made," and he studied chemistry with private teachers: "a German called Witichius, and after he went away, under [Christiaan] Margravius [or Marggraff]." Busy with all these practical studies, Sibbald occasionally also made time for studying medical texts: "Sometymes I heard the lessons of [J. A.] Vander Linden, who was famous for critical learning."[79]

The emphasis that Sibbald and his fellow students placed on learning by doing and observing tended to take time away from the study of classical medical texts and the frequent practice of disputation. Consequently, when the Oxford-educated physician John Locke attended the disputation of a graduating doctor in Leiden in 1684, he seems to have been a bit disappointed. Those who took up the arguments against the intending graduate were "usually friends of the respondent," and those Locke saw "dispute, that they might not mistake, had their arguments writt down." Locke concluded, "I suppose their studys tend most to practise, for in disputing noe one that I heard urged any argument beyond one or 2 syllogisms."[80] That is, pushing arguments to their logical conclusions in competitive oral argument was not what the Leiden medical school stressed, making it seem rather intellectually lightweight to more traditionally educated men. In the English context Locke stood for philosophical and medical innovation; but even for people like him, the shift in emphasis in the curriculum at Leiden from speculative to experimental philosophy, tending "most to practise," made for a number of intellectual differences. The difference between England and the Netherlands in expectations for university studies in medicine would help to create difficulties for Groenevelt in the future.

Four renowned professors taught medicine in Leiden during Groenevelt's time there: François dele Boë Sylvius; Joannes van Horne (or Hornius); Florentius Schuyl; and Charles Drélincourt (or Carolus Drelincurtius). The most important teacher at Leiden, and the one who left the greatest influence on the young Groenevelt, was Sylvius, an excellent clinician, chemist, and anatomist.[81] From a Flemish family—one that he liked to think had a noble descent—Sylvius was born in 1614 in Hanau, near Frankfurt, where his grandfather's family had fled to escape the war in the southern netherlands. He studied in the northern netherlands, Germany, and Switzerland, finally graduating from Basel in 1637, a place where a tradition of teaching medical chemistry remained alive. He settled briefly in Leiden shortly after, and in 1639 and 1640 he gave private lectures in anatomy and physiology in the gallery of the botanical garden. There he demonstrated the circulation of the blood recently proclaimed by William Harvey of England, being among the first to do so on the Continent.[82] Sylvius also became acquainted with René Descartes, who spent some years in Leiden during this time. The chemically inspired Sylvius added Cartesian-like mechanisms to his accounts of the physiological workings of the body.[83] When no prospect of a regular teaching post at Leiden offered, Sylvius left for Amsterdam in 1641, where he developed a very successful practice amidst some of the most notable experimental physicians and surgeons of the period. In Amsterdam he also befriended the influential German iatrochemists Johann Glauber and Otto Sperling.

Sylvius acquired an excellent reputation as a practitioner, and in 1658 he returned to Leiden as the professor of practical medicine—at the high salary of 1,800 gilders—and taught there until his death in 1672. In addition to lecturing, Sylvius developed clinical medicine at St. Caecilia's, where he promoted a Socratic method of teaching, asking the students questions about what they saw and knew, and having their corrected responses direct the

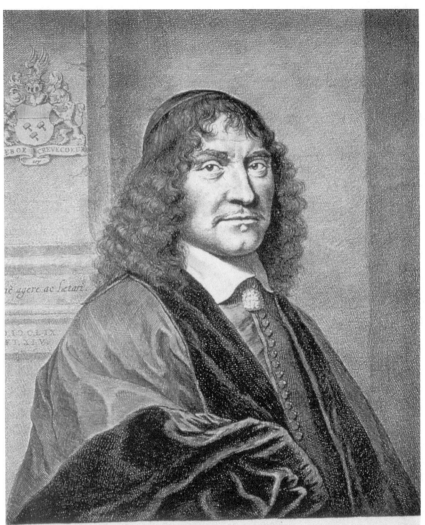

FRANCISCUS DELEBOE SYLVIUS, MEDICINÆ
PRACTICÆ IN ACADEMIA LUGDUNO-BATAVA PROFESSOR.

C. van Dalen Junior delineavit et sculpsit

FIG. 9. *Groenevelt's teacher, the famous François dele Boë Sylvius.*

care of the patient. He visited the hospital with the students early every morning and got the curators of the university to agree to pay for the expensive chemical drugs he administered to the patients. As Sibbald correctly recollected, Sylvius and his students anatomized patients who died in the hospital in order to determine the cause of death and to establish correlations between symptoms and changes in the organs. He also taught chemistry privately in his house, where he built a laboratory;[84] in 1666 he further acquired the position of professor of chemistry (the first ever in the university). He advocated strongly the idea that effervescence typified the chemical physiology of the body and that everything could be divided into acids and alkalies, the alkalies especially causing disease, which were to be countered with acidic remedies. A generation of experimental physicians followed him in uniting chemistry, anatomy, and practice, including Groenevelt. By far the greatest number of Groenevelt's medical books dealt with medical practice;[85] some were explicitly chemical.[86]

Groenevelt also had much to do with the professor of anatomy and surgery: Joannes van Horne (or Hornius). A graduate of the famous school of Padua in 1643, Van Horne became a professor at Leiden ten years later, after many academic travels. He was both a first-rate anatomist and an excellent teacher, inspiring several famous students with whom he worked closely (such as Frederick Ruysch, Nicolaus Steno, Renier de Graaf, and Jan Swammerdam); for the young Swammerdam, for example, Van Horne not only encouraged his anatomical investigations but paid for his student's materials, let him use his house for the work, and dissected alongside his pupil. In this case, the work resulted in a magnificent new study of the human female organs of generation.[87] Groenevelt later remarked on having seen several stones that had been removed by Van Horne "of blessed memory" from the skull of the deceased Leiden professor of philosophy, Adam Stuart.[88] Groenevelt's list of books shows few signs of pursuing anatomical studies with vigor, but he did possess a few standard works on the structure of the body and two on the growth of the human fetus.[89]

Sylvius's protégé and outspoken Cartesian, Schuyl, taught theoretical medicine, replacing Sibbald's teacher, J. A. van der Linden, who had died in 1664. From 1667, Schuyl also took over the teaching of botany. Groenevelt knew his botany and recent summaries of medical theory, from Fernel to Harvey.[90] The young Groenevelt had little to do with Drélincourt, who came only at the end of Groenevelt's stay: Drélincourt had been a royal physician to Louis XIV until he moved to Leiden to take up a professorship in February 1669.[91]

The authors that Groenevelt's teachers tended to emphasize confirmed the suspicions of the European old guard: they were mainly not the established medical philosophers but the new investigators, authors who pursued chemical, natural historical, and mechanical researches, whether ancient or modern. The principles of two philosophers stand out from the rest as lying behind many of the new authors and student theses of Groenevelt's day: those of Hippocrates and Descartes.

For many learned people of the late sixteenth and seventeenth century, Hippocrates represented not only a source of knowledge but a model of method. Thought to have been a Greek physician who lived just before Plato—that is, in the late fifth and early fourth century B.C.E.—Hippocrates produced a great number of writings (which are now considered to have been set down by a number of different authors, often in later years). While known in the Middle Ages, Hippocrates' works underwent a great revival in the sixteenth century, superseding Galen in the number of editions of his writings by the 1570s.[92] For many learned physicians of Groenevelt's time, these treatises seemed to portray a physician with keen observational skills, who reported in an undogmatic manner the details of the symptoms of disease and the natural environment surrounding the patient. From these details, Groenevelt's contemporaries argued, Hippocrates had extracted principles of diagnosis, prognosis, and treatment which had eternal value, principles set down as aphorisms rather than logical arguments: he had not reduced medicine to a single method nor tried to force the facts to fit a theory as later physicians, especially Galen, had done. (To biblical Protestants, an obvious parallel presented itself: as Jesus often spoke in parables, so Hippocrates sometimes spoke in aphorisms; and just as the medieval theologians had diverted the original Christian religion into a dogmatic theology, so Galen had corrupted Hippocrates' teachings with his systematizing.) In short, the Hippocratic method stood for unbiased, direct, detailed observation and the gradual development of aphoristic truths of practice from this elementary experience rather than for reasoning or imagining from first principles.[93] The Hippocratic method fit well with many of the ideas of the new science of the period, and it also supported the intellectual foundation for both the chemical and natural historical work from which so many new discoveries came.

Hippocratic observations and principles pervaded Leiden teaching. Groenevelt himself had among his books a Latin and Greek edition of Hippocrates prepared by former Leiden professor Van der Linden.[94] As part of the requirements for a Leiden M.D., before a student could defend his printed thesis, he would be assigned two aphorisms of Hippocrates in the morning which he would have to explain in an hour-long disputation in the afternoon.[95] Sibbald came back from Leiden a convinced Hippocratic and natural historian.[96] From the time of Paracelsus, the chemists had also held up Hippocrates as a hero; Groenevelt's friend Ten Rhijne would soon work with Sylvius on a thesis *sub praeside* for public disputation which interpreted the Hippocratic text "On Ancient Medicine" as anticipating chemical theories.[97] That Professor Schuyl stole Ten Rhijne's thunder in a posthumous publication of his own[98] shows how deeply many people wished to connect modern approaches like chemistry to the inspiration of Hippocrates, the original source of all medical knowledge.

Ten Rhijne's rival, Schuyl, is not only a good example of the importance of practical ancient authors to Sylvius and his pupils but also an indication of how influential were modern authors like Descartes. Although French by birth and language, the philosopher René Descartes spent his most active intellectual years in the Netherlands. As a young man, he had come north in 1617 to learn the art of modern warfare in the armies of the stadholder, Maurice of Nassau; here he met the Dutch teacher-philosopher-engineer Isaac Beeckman, who convinced him both that one could indeed hold that the world was made up of material bits (Beeckman being an atomist) and that a mathematical approach to natural philosophy would best lead to philosophical certainty.[99] After various travels in arms and a return to France, Descartes came back to the Netherlands again briefly in 1628 and then moved there permanently in 1629 until he left to become tutor to Queen Christina of Sweden in 1649. Descartes gained many supporters for his philosophical projects among his friends and acquaintances in the Netherlands, who turned his views into a system acceptable for university teaching.[100]

Among Descartes's most influential supporters were the physicians. The support of his friend Henricus Regius, the Utrecht medical professor, unfortunately brought him trouble when Regius and his students got into tangles with the theology faculty at Utrecht, leading to a general sentiment against Cartesianism on the part of orthodox Dutch Calvinists, although Descartes's philosophy continued to be valued by many in the university.[101] In Leiden, after an initial condemnation in the 1640s, Cartesian teachings were generally tolerated. Some members of the philosophical faculty sympathized with Descartes's positions, and the medical faculty, centered around Descartes's acquaintance Sylvius, apparently actively encouraged their students to dig into Descartes. One of the most important medical Cartesians was Sylvius's student Cornelis Bontekoe. And it was probably Schuyl's publication of a posthumous Latin edition of one of Descartes's controversial works, *De homine* ("On Man"), in 1662, some time before the original French was published, which caused Sylvius to encourage Schuyl to study medicine. Schuyl had been a philosophy graduate of Utrecht, although he had studied some medicine at Leiden, and he taught for several years as a professor of philosophy in the athenaeum in 's Hertogenbosch before Sylvius brought him back to Leiden about a month after Van der Linden's death, arranging for his quick graduation in medicine and appointment as Van der Linden's successor.[102]

Descartes was known for many philosophical innovations, but for two in particular which undermined orthodox philosophy: his method of reasoning, and his promotion of the idea that the universe was entirely filled by inert corpuscles, so that change in all things except the human soul could be ascribed to matter in motion. His method of reasoning sought to provide certainty—clear and distinct ideas—through a process of inductive reasoning rooted in undoubtable axioms. Descartes's epistemology was not of special interest to the medical faculty, since they were convinced Hippocratics and chemists. They even reinterpreted Descartes's method to provide a crucial place for experimentation in discovering truth. Descartes's suggestion that the universe could be described as inert matter in motion, and that there could be no empty space (since he united matter and space), was of more importance, since it gave support to those who were already trying to describe the world in materialistic terms. Since Descartes himself developed a deep concern for physiology, the ways in which he described the body as a mechanical system also held great interest.[103] For Sylvius and his students, Descartes's matter theory and theories of physiology held great interest, since they gave a final blow to Aristotelian matter-form theories and physiologies rooted in innate "faculties," and seemed to explain what lay behind many chemical processes. Naturally, Groenevelt owned an edition of Descartes's works.[104]

The studies of Joannes Groenevelt therefore focused on gaining medical experience in the clinic, in the anatomy theater, in the botanical garden, and in the chemical laboratory; this experience was coupled with Hippocratic method and Cartesian natural philosophy. It was an avant-garde medical education indeed.

In the midst of his medical studies, two friends from Deventer joined the young Groenevelt in Leiden: Willem ten Rhijne and Herbert Dapper. In later years, Groenevelt wrote of Dapper as his "loving intimate" and Ten Rhijne as an "intimate friend," and Ten Rhijne in turn later wrote of his "friendship" with Groenevelt.[105] Ten Rhijne had left the Deventer Illustrious School before

Groenevelt but had first gone to the University of Franeker (in August 1666).[106] Franeker had been the second university founded in the Netherlands, and while not as large or distinguished as Leiden, it possessed a very good faculty, including a number of chemically oriented medical professors.[107] Ten Rhijne did not take a degree in Franeker but moved on in his studies. He received from the Reformed church in his hometown a certificate of good standing on 10 February 1668 to take with him on his trip to Leiden. On the same day, Dapper received a similar certificate.[108] Together, Ten Rhijne and Dapper traveled to Leiden, where, three weeks after their departure, they inscribed as students.[109] Ten Rhijne enrolled in the faculty of medicine, Dapper in theology, but Dapper would soon switch over to medicine as well. While they did not room in the same house as their friend Groenevelt, Joannes must have taken comfort in having old friends studying in Leiden with him, even more because they studied the same subject.[110] As we have seen, Ten Rhijne worked very closely with Sylvius in preparing a printed thesis on Hippocrates, and he produced a second thesis under Sylvius preparatory to his final disputation as well, although he took his degree at Angers, where the fees were cheaper.[111]

It must have caused Joannes Groenevelt some anxiety again when his medical studies in Leiden were interrupted just before his graduation. He spent almost two years studying medicine in Leiden, and from the evidence of his thesis, he had been making rapid progress with the help of Sylvius and Van Horne toward completing a study of the special subject of stones in the body. But in 1669 he left Leiden and enrolled in the University of Utrecht.

In all likelihood, Groenevelt left for Utrecht because of an epidemic in Leiden which closed the university.[112] People spoke of the plague, although the disease seems to have been something else, perhaps epidemic malaria.[113] Whatever its cause, from August 1669 to January 1670, about forty thousand people fell ill, and at its height the dead reached two hundred to three hundred per week. The disease especially struck members of the higher social classes: magistrates, ministers, and merchants. Seven of the fifteen professors in Leiden died during the epidemic, at least five definitely of the disease, including Schuyl and Van Horne. Sylvius lost his only child (just a few months after the death of his young wife) and lay gravely ill himself, although he pulled through with the help of mineral water from Spa. During the fall, when the epidemic was at its height, the university closed its doors.[114] In all probability, then, Groenevelt was almost ready to take his graduate exams and defend his thesis in the fall of 1669, and as a person without a large income he could not wait precious months for the university to reopen. Nor did he want to risk disease in Leiden. Instead, he traveled to Utrecht to complete his M.D.

Groenevelt signed the Utrecht register in 1669;[115] if he did arrive there when Leiden shut down in the fall, he would have spent about six months there in all. Utrecht was a smaller university, with just two medical professors: Henricus Regius (Hendrik de Roy) and Ysbrand van Diemerbroek. Almost thirty years before Groenevelt's time, Regius had made trouble by espousing strong Cartesian views, which the senior professor of theology, Gisbertus Voetius (Gijsbert Voet), took to be an attack on the Aristotelian positions defined as the foundation of Calvinist orthodoxy at the Synod of Dort. The resulting dispute brought Descartes's philosophy into general distaste among the orthodox.[116] Eventually, Regius himself moved away from thoroughgoing Cartesianism. Groenevelt owned one of Regius's works, although it was his book on medical practice, not his early Cartesian physiological text.[117] The other professor, Van Diemerbroek, taught practical medicine and is best remembered for an excellent account of the plague of 1635.[118] He followed his predecessor, Willem van der Straaten, in giving clinical instruction in a hospital—it was Van der Straaten's clinical teaching that had caused rival Leiden to introduce its own hospital study. Twice a week, Van Diemerbroek taught students in the Catharijne hospital, but his clinical teaching was often hampered by a lack of patients there, forcing him to rely on imagining cases for the students to discuss.[119] Thus, while the Utrecht medical faculty was not as distinguished and as practical in its orientation as that of Leiden, Groenevelt found there sympathetic professors to help with his thesis and to examine and promote him.

During his stay, Groenevelt was not friendless in Utrecht. A former schoolmate from Deventer, Casparus Sibelius, had only recently left his theology studies in Utrecht, but he apparently introduced Groenevelt to some of his connections there: Joannes joined Sibelius's student society even though he, unlike Sibelius, did not have a family coat of arms to enter in their book.[120] Another friend from Deventer, Henricus van Duren, arrived in Utrecht to study law about the same time as Groenevelt.[121] Van Duren also served as Groenevelt's "paranymph":[122] that is, Van Duren organized all the celebrations surrounding Groenevelt's graduation and sat with him during his disputation to support him morally, intellectually, and, if need be, physically.

After a total of two and one-half years of medical study in all, then, Groenevelt finally received his M.D. on 18 March 1670. He performed at least adequately in the orals and wrote an excellent treatise on bladder stones.[123]

Compared with the one other thesis on stones completed at Utrecht before his own, and the nine other ones on the subject completed at Leiden before his, Joannes Groenevelt's was far and away the most learned.[124] The other theses ranged in length from seven to eighteen pages; on this count alone, Groenevelt's twenty-page text made his unusual. Few of them gave as many or as specific references to other authors as Groenevelt's.[125] All mention the chemical causes of stones. All also discuss remedies, mainly the use of diuretics—several in conjunction with lithontriptics (remedies meant to break up the stone in the body so that it can be evacuated by urination)—to try to cause the stone to be evacuated by profuse urination.[126] The thesis of Ioachimus van der Heyden came the closest to Groenevelt's. Completed in Leiden in 1667, the year Groenevelt arrived, it was thorough and detailed, and in discussing the quarrels between the Galenists and chemists ("Dogmaticos et Hermeticos"), it comes down solidly on the side of the chemists. Even more striking, Van der Heyden, like Groenevelt, mentions seeing Smalzius extract twenty-six stones:[127] the young Groenevelt and he had witnessed the same demonstration as students at Leiden. Notably, however, even though Van der Heyden's major adviser had been the professor of anatomy Van Horne, he avoids any but the most general discussion of surgical procedures.[128] In this respect, Van der Heyden's thesis stood with all the others. The only medical student to deal adequately with the various surgical techniques for removing bladder stones was Groenevelt, and he wrote about them at length.

Dated 17 March 1670, published by the printer to the university, the thesis had a traditional format, although its length made it one of the thicker contemporary theses. Printed in closely spaced Latin, quarto in size (that is, made of folio sheets folded in half and printed on all four sides), it consisted of twenty pages of text divided into twenty-three propositions and seven final corollaries that he publicly defended, plus three additional pages at the end containing three laudatory poems by friends: a short one in Latin by one "M.M.," a long one in Latin by Groenevelt's paranymph Van Duren, and a short one in Dutch by a law student, Everhardus Berdenis. He dedicated it not to a patron, as was common, but to God, country, parents, and teachers.[129] It was his own work, although he mentions the help of his Leiden professors; Van Diemerbroek seems to have had little to do with the thesis other than to chair the promotion committee.[130] In developing his arguments, he drew on major ancient and medieval authors such as Galen, Aëtius of Amida, Avicenna, Arnold of Villanova, Nicolaus Florentinus, and of course Hippocrates; Renaissance medical writers like Antonio Benivieni, Geronimo Cardano, Felix Plater, Jean Fernel, and Heironymus Fabricius ab Aquapendente; botanists like Pietro Andrea Mattioli and Rembert Dodoens; surgeons like Gulielmus Fabritius Hildanus and Ambroise Paré; chemists such as Joseph du Chesne (Quercetanus), Lazarus Riverius, and Daniel Sennert; and modern Dutch authors like Pieter Forestus, Joannes van Heurne, and Johann van Beverwijck.

The framework of Groenevelt's thesis was quite standard. He began with a general problem: stones can be found throughout the human body. Why? He then narrowed the problem to an investigation of stones that occur in the kidneys and bladder (thesis 1). After a discussion of various opinions on whether stones were a disease or the cause of disease (2), he decided for stones being a number of diseases (3). After defining terms (4) and noting that the stone forms from the material that is in us (5), he moved on to examining the efficient cause of stones: the force that brings them into being. Groenevelt dismissed traditional academic answers, such as Fernel's (6, 7). He preferred the answers of the chemists, such as that a stone is caused by a collection of tartar from wine, especially from the crude wine from Spain, Crete, and other places, or by concretion of semen exposed to cold air (8). ("Tartar," which collects in wine barrels during fermentation, had been one of the favorite explanatory terms of the chemical physician Paracelsus and his followers.) Groenevelt developed this line of inquiry further by discussing the views of three important and more modern chemical authors: Quercetanus, Hildanus, and Sennert (9).

The proximate efficient cause of stones, he argued, was concretion: the stony material in the blood serum was segregated at the kidneys and sent to the bladder via the ureters; some of it was not ejected and accumulated, forming the nucleus of a stone around which further concretions occurred; the stones were not formed by the urine becoming cold (10). Children could inherit from their parents a kind of urine which coagulated easily (11). Stones grew around the nucleus as more matter accumulated (12). Whether they grew or not depended upon diet, exercise, and other of the six "non-naturals" (13). Stones differed according to their location in the body: he himself had seen Sylvius in 1667 remove from the right kidney of a body of a woman a hard, angular stone partly stuck into the kidney's flesh; he had also seen ureters solid with stones, and in another corpse, stones in the gall bladder. Stones also differed according to their number: he had seen the Haarlem surgeon Smalzius remove twenty-six stones from a patient's bladder.[131] Stones differed further according to their size, color, shape, and substance and consistency (14). Groenevelt then explained how to diagnose stones properly, warning that the inexperienced could cause harm through manual diagnosis and especially through probing the bladder with a catheter (15). Then he took up the prognostic signs (17). While prevention was the main task of the physician, patients wanted remedies, and he discussed several of the best known (18). Then he examined the physical treatments of venesection (bleeding from a vein) and clysters (medicinal enemas) (20, 21). The efficacy of lithontriptics was hotly debated, and Groenevelt thought that few of them worked, but he discussed some of the remarkable effects cited by various authors, and the hopes of the chemists for discovering such remedies (22).[132] Finally, and unusual for a medical thesis of the time, he discussed the various methods of surgery for removing bladder stones (23).[133] The corollaries that follow were mainly chemical and physiological: on wine, fermentation, that all the humors of the body originate in the arterial blood, and so on.

Doctor Groenevelt, then, had become one of the most learned experts on a common and intellectually challenging disease. He had proved that he could investigate a problem thoroughly, using not only lectures and texts but personal experience as well. He had learned the latest medical theories, but he had also imbibed the best of Dutch clinical and surgical medicine.

Just short of his twenty-second birthday, Joannes Groenevelt took his place among the learned. His education had edified him morally, taught him how to comprehend texts, and skilled him in methods of modern medical research. He now commanded Latin perfectly and had an acquaintance with Greek and a bit of Hebrew; he understood not only the doctrines of his faith but the words and reasons on which they were based; he could construct an argument and find the weaknesses in that of an opponent; he followed philosophical debates about how the world was made and what method would best reveal nature's secrets; he had a sound acquaintance with the most highly regarded medical authors and knew how to find information in them and synthesize the results; he was formally acquainted with the chemical laboratory and hospital clinic; he diagnosed diseases, predicted their courses, and selected the best methods of treatment; and he could combine all these skills to gain useful human knowledge.

In some particulars, though, he had quite naturally come out not a universal medical scholar but a learned Dutchman. In his religion he remained a Calvinist, who took the Bible as the word of God and looked to the primitive church for guidance in his faith; but he also knew enough about the ways in which his ministers had constructed their knowledge to be aware of the difficulties of finding certainty from ancient statements written in difficult languages. In his patriotism, he could be proud to be Dutch, a member of a free republic that had, with the help of God, fought off Spanish despotism and English rivalry; and yet he remained a son of Deventer at least as much as a citizen of the United Provinces. His educational journeys had not yet taken him far afield, but they had brought him to major cities in other parts of the country, making him quite aware of the differences between his hometown and the rapidly expanding commercial cities of Holland and the ancient cathedral city of Utrecht. In his academic knowledge, he knew how to read the medical texts and how to debate an opponent; but he also had been taught to concentrate a large part of his time and attention on developing skills that would make his practice better. Now free to pursue his life as he chose, the young Joannes Groenevelt had become a man of letters who had joined an international elite; but in his heart he remained a neighbor to his family, friends, and fellow citizens of Deventer, which always retained a special place in this thoughts.

CHAPTER 4

Learning to Cut for the Stone

EDUCATED IN THE latest Dutch medical ideas and practices, the young Dr. Groenevelt now sought to find his place in the world as an independent practitioner. Compared with the large and flourishing cities of Holland which he had seen, Deventer was a small town with few opportunities for setting up practice as a physician. The economic powerhouse of Holland, Amsterdam, would therefore be the place he chose to practice. A city of many doctors, surgeons, and apothecaries, it was also a city of good relations between the medical groups, and plenty of people who wanted and could afford the services of educated practitioners lived there. The practical medicine he had studied at Leiden flourished in the hard-headed mercantile capital of northern Europe. Personal connections between the medical professors of Leiden and the leading lights of the Amsterdam physicians also remained close.

But it was not easy for a newly minted M.D. to establish himself in a good general practice, even in expanding Amsterdam. Probably to carve out a niche for himself, Groenevelt specialized—at least in part—in the medical practices examined in his Utrecht disputation. He joined with a surgeon, Henricus Velthuis, who operated to remove bladder stones, while he, the doctor, supervised the diagnosis as required by the laws of Amsterdam. In the process of working with Velthuis, however, Groenevelt learned how to practice the operation himself. This was unusual: although a few surgeons went on to study medicine and take M.D.'s, even fewer physicians took up surgical practice. Moreover, Groenevelt learned how to perform according to the latest technique, introduced to the Netherlands by the Paris surgeon Philippe Colot. The practical orientation of his medical studies had made Groenevelt the sort of practitioner who was willing to adopt any new method that seemed sound and promised to be of value to patients, even if he had to take up the knife himself.

Unfortunately for him, however, his years in Amsterdam coincided with the most disastrous years of the young country's history: the war begun by the English and French in 1672, in alliance with the bishop of Münster. Amsterdam escaped occupation—barely—but the economy was shattered, while political power in the country shifted dramatically with the brutal butchery of Johann de Witt and his brother and the revived leadership of the house of Orange. On top of all the general disasters, Groenevelt's partner Velthuis died in May 1674. Within a few months, then, Groenevelt would leave his country and try to establish himself elsewhere: in London. But for a time he successfully negotiated the medical marketplace of Amsterdam while at the same time extending his medical abilities.

In less than two weeks after his graduation, the new medical doctor had returned to his home of Deventer and appeared before a magistrate. He thanked his guardians, promised never to sue them for anything pertaining to his minority, and obtained their discharge.[1] Presumably, whatever remained of his portion of his father's estate now came to his hands.

Once he earned his independence from his guardians, Joannes Groenevelt had to find a way to live from his newly acquired medical knowledge. His father's estate would give him some support for a while but would not keep him comfortable for life. He did not elect to stay in Deventer and set up a practice there. The war of the mid-1660s had left the local economy in ruins. The political divisions in the region over whether to support the twenty-year-old William III of Orange's claim to the stadholdership or to continue supporting the States Party (who wanted no overlord) were deepening in 1670 and within a year would even lead to skirmishes between rival militias in Kampen and Zwolle, although Deventer remained firmly within the States Party camp and relatively calm.[2] In the further distance, the acquisitive Louis XIV of France made it clear that he looked forward to absorbing large parts of the low countries into his kingdom. The general economic and political situation must have seemed ominous in a border town. A more immediate concern was that without good connections the young Groenevelt would have found it difficult to set up a practice in the local medical field.

The people of Deventer, like others from the eastern parts of the Netherlands, seem to have been somewhat less enthusiastic about receiving their medical care from learned physicians than were their western counterparts. Physicians practiced almost entirely among urban residents, while Deventer remained a relatively small city with rural hinterlands. The city also had far fewer immigrants from the south than the large cities of Holland, with many families having lived in Deventer for generations. People therefore had long-established networks of assistance to call upon when they needed help, including medical help. Even when they turned for medical help beyond their own family, friends, and neighbors, they continued to rely mainly on surgeons, apothecaries, and unaffiliated practitioners for most of their care rather than the fewer and more recently established physicians. But even the members of the surgeons' guild (which included the apothecaries) did not become wealthy, if the evidence of their guild is any indication: the guild's possessions were not nearly as extensive or as expensive as in the west of the Netherlands.[3] Deventer therefore never seems to have had a large popula-tion of physicians.[4] Certainly, it never saw the growth of an association of physicians (a *collegium*), as did several other cities in the Netherlands. As one of Groenevelt's friends wrote when later leaving Deventer to try his medical fortunes elsewhere, "Medicine is little esteemed in our city and the province of Overijssel," thus those who exercised it lived poorly.[5]

The town did have a couple of city physicians. Such a post had been common in Dutch cities for some time: it made the doctor an adviser to the magistrates on any matters pertaining to the health of the populace and granted him a salary in return for those services and his diagnosing and prescribing to the poor for free.[6] Holding such a position gave the physician an effective endorsement from the magistrates and so could help increase the city physi-cian's personal reputation and private practice, too. But even town physicians, like Groenevelt's philosophy professor Loenius, sought to supplement their salaries and fees with other tasks as well—in Loenius's case, he took up a position in the local Illustrious School. A few other physicians practiced on their own in Deventer but seem to have used their family connections to get enough patients to keep a practice. Groenevelt's friend Herbert Dapper practiced medicine in Deventer beginning in 1671, but he came from an influential family and quickly gained election to the city council as well.[7]

Given the old-fashioned ways and weak economy of Deventer in 1670, and his family's lack of political connection or social influence, the young doctor would have to look elsewhere to set up a practice of his own. Despite his fondness for his hometown, then, he decided to seek yet further opportunities before he could return and make a living practicing medicine in Deventer. His other medical friends did the same: Ten Rhijne practiced for a while in Amsterdam before leaving as a physician for the Dutch East Indies; Sibelius, too, practiced for some years in Amsterdam before moving back to Deventer.

No documents clearly show Groenevelt's movements for the two years after his return to Deventer in March 1670. It is just possible that he traveled to Louvain, in the Spanish Netherlands (now Belgium). The suggestion for this comes from a 1753 English translation of a book of Groenevelt's. Groenevelt's 1714 Latin text on which the translation is based very closely followed a book by the Louvain medical professor François van den Zype (Zypaeus), published two and a half decades before; the second anonymous English translator of Groenevelt's book said that it had first been drawn up by "that great Physician Zypaeus, one of the most celebrated of the Royal Academy at Paris . . . for the Use and Instruction of his private Pupils, of whom Dr. Groenevelt was one."[8] There are problems with this assertion, however. Zypaeus is not known to have had any connection with any of the Paris academies. In 1670, moreover, he had just matriculated in Louvain as a poor student and so would have been Groenevelt's junior; the Louvain records do not mention Groenevelt's matriculation there at all.[9] Louvain did then have a famous medical professor in the person of Vopiscus Fortunatus Plemp (Plempius), who had taught practical medicine there since 1634.[10] Groenevelt also later owned a French-Flemish dictionary, while his friend Ten Rhijne spent some time at the Hôtel Dieu in Paris sometime around 1670.[11] It is therefore possible that Groenevelt, too, wanted to explore some of the latest ideas and practices outside the Netherlands and to improve his French, the language of the Dutch social elite, and that he therefore spent some time in Louvain or Paris. But all this must remain speculation.

The next place after Deventer where we can trace Groenevelt with certainty is Amsterdam. He was there on 4 March 1672, when he married a twenty-two-year-old woman of that city, Cristina de Ruiters.[12] The marriage took place in one of the Reformed churches in Amsterdam, with his mother and her father, Jan Jantsz. der Ruyter, present. Cristina is an unusual name for a Dutchwoman of the period, and she had been baptized in the Lutheran church.[13] Perhaps, then, she came from one of the many immigrant families to crowd into Amsterdam in the seventeenth century.[14] Whatever her background, she had converted to the Reformed faith by the day of her marriage. What kind of dowry she brought to the marriage is unknown, but since her first child would not be born for three years, there is no sign that the marriage was forced by necessity or based on anything but mutually consensual love. The fact that Joannes Groenevelt took a convert as his wife also strongly suggests that he was no longer overly chauvinistic about his nation or religion.

Marrying in March 1672 undoubtedly means that Groenevelt had been in Amsterdam for some time: he at least had to have had time to meet and to court Cristina. And his willingness to take a wife probably also means that he had by then established a solid enough medical practice to earn a household income, which also supports the notion that he had been in Amsterdam for some time. He (and his friend Ten Rhijne) soon joined the Collegium Medicum there, perhaps as early as 1670. The record book of the *collegium* does not give the date of entry of the members—only the date and place of their medical degrees—and neither Groenevelt nor Ten Rhijne is otherwise mentioned in its records, so we cannot know the date they joined the society. Groenevelt is, however, listed as the first of the members to have obtained a degree in 1670, strongly suggesting that he had come to Amsterdam shortly after having earned his M.D.—perhaps after a short trip to Paris.[15]

Amsterdam, the chief city of Holland, had in the late sixteenth century surpassed Antwerp as the main entrepôt for trade in northern Europe. Having at first welcomed the duke of Alva, who was trying to restore the authority of King Philip, when Alva's military fortunes declined and Amsterdam found itself surrounded by rebels, the magistrates arranged a treaty with William the Silent in 1578 which brought Calvinism and municipal elections to the city. Since the rebel Dutch had blockaded the Scheldt River, Antwerp's outlet to the sea, trade that had gone to Antwerp now came to Amsterdam. Soon the city's merchants tightly controlled the Baltic trade, parts of the Mediterranean trade, long stretches of the African coast, some of the West Indies and parts of the coast of South America, and many of the riches of the East. By Groenevelt's time, its population had exploded, reaching 200,000. Its people and riches became the main bulwark of the rebellion, with its leaders taking the most important part in deliberations of the assembly of the States of Holland, and the States of Holland taking the leading part in the meetings of the States General. The Amsterdam magistrates opposed the ambitions of the House of Orange to become princes over the Netherlands, so that the city was besieged by William II in 1650; fortunately for the rulers of Amsterdam, he died of smallpox not long after. From then onward, the majority of the magistrates firmly supported the States Party against the Orangists until the disaster of 1672.

While the culture of this bourgeois society stressed edifying and utilitarian projects, it also encouraged learning and toleration. The city possessed a theater, the renowned stock exchange, hundreds of coffee- and alehouses, and various learned societies, as well as hospitals, old-folks' homes, and workhouses. The Amsterdam *regenten* also tolerated open Lutheran and Jewish worship, as well as Catholic and heterodox Protestant services as long as they were private: the city became well known as a place where virtually all peoples and beliefs could be found, no matter the degree of their heresy. Rooted in the idea of religious peace, this open-mindedness also had its utilitarian side. One of the major intellectual figures of Amsterdam early in the seventeenth century, Caspar Barlaeus, set out to prove in his inaugural lecture at the Amsterdam athenaeum that there existed "a sound relationship between commerce and the study of literature and philosophy," so that trade and philosophy encouraged each other.[16] The magistrates themselves not only supported various scholarly projects, including a botanical garden, but encouraged all sorts of new intellectual developments. Some were themselves true men of learning, like Johannes Hudde: an excellent mathematician, he also developed methods for making single-lens microscopes, which he taught to the soon famous Jan Swammerdam and Antoni van Leeuwenhoek.[17]

The opportunities for medicine in this city of immigrants were great, and it attracted a large number of practitioners. Indeed, one could find about one university-trained physician for every thousand residents of the city, the highest ratio of its kind for any place in the country—probably one of the highest in Europe.[18] When one adds to the number of physicians the three hundred to five hundred surgeons and apothecaries, the hundreds of midwives, and the plentiful unaffiliated chemists, traditional healers, and empirics, the "doctor"-patient ratio becomes at least two or three times higher. The Amsterdam medical marketplace was so richly endowed partly because large numbers of residents and visitors had money enough to pay for care from a full-time practitioner, and partly because the mercantile economy of the city accustomed them to doing business with "professional" people they did not know or knew only slightly, as long as such professionals had a good reputation and behaved correctly.

Given such a competitive and relatively anonymous environment, Groene-velt joined forces with others like himself by becoming a member of the Collegium Medicum, the local learned society of physicians which supervised medical practice in the city.[19] Sixteenth and early seventeenth-century physicians had, together with the apothecaries, been members of the grocers' guild (*kramersgilde*). After many petitions to create a society of physicians, to establish a medicinal garden, and to issue an official pharmacopoeia that all apothecaries would be required to follow, the plague epidemic of 1635 finally provoked the magistrates to action.[20] Established at last in 1638, the Collegium Medicum brought together the university-trained physicians in Amsterdam and forbade all others to practice in the city. Under the leadership of Dr. Nicolaas Tulp, who later became a burgomaster himself, the *collegium* issued a pharmacopoeia, organized regular anatomical lessons for the surgeons' guild, inspected the shops of the apothecaries and supervised the training of their apprentices, and founded a botanical garden.[21] It also required all who would practice medicine in Amsterdam to do so only with its permission. Those with university degrees, like Groenevelt, could become members: in the sixty years to 1700, 330 physicians joined the Collegium Medicum. Perhaps, too, Groenevelt's former teacher Sylvius's connections with the Amsterdam social and medical elite helped his students to gain useful introductions in the city—many of the members of the *collegium* had Leiden degrees. Again Groenevelt was not alone, since one of his Deventer friends, Willem ten Rhijne, also joined the society at about the same time. Through the Collegium Medicum itself, physicians could develop good medical and business contacts and find out about the latest developments.

Moreover, despite having separate institutions, cooperation between Amsterdam physicians, surgeons, and apothecaries was generally very good. For instance, the physician Paulus Barbette, a friend of Sylvius's, worked closely with Amsterdam surgeons like Job van Meek'ren and published several books; his posthumous *Praxis Barbettiana* (1669) was edited by one of Sylvius's pupils and became a standard text on surgery.[22] Another of Sylvius's pupils, Frederik Ruysch, became the lecturer on anatomy to the Amsterdam surgeons' guild, in 1669 became an anatomical examiner of the midwives, and in 1672 began formal teaching to them. Ruysch took over the instruction of midwives from the deceased Hendrick Roonhuyze, another noted surgeon who worked closely with physicians and published several books. Roonhuyze's son bought the secret of the obstetrical forceps from the English physician Hugh Chamberlen, Sr., in the mid-1690s, selling it in turn to Ruysch.[23] The opportunities to practice medicine in such a freewheeling and open-minded place as Amsterdam may have been daunting at first. But it was in such an environment that Groenevelt began his practice, and in which he soon began a professional association with the surgeon Henricus Velthuis.

The young doctor entered into a joint medical practice, an arrangement he would later pursue in London as well. The older and more experienced practitioner with whom he first exercised medicine was not, however, another physician but Henricus Velthuis, a surgeon. What brought them together was the subject of Groenevelt's thesis—bladder stones—coupled with a change in how the Amsterdam burgomasters regulated surgery for them.

Groenevelt's thesis had not been a mere intellectual exercise. Large numbers of people in early modern Europe suffered the excruciating torments of stones in the body. Although it is impossible to develop figures on the incidence of bladder stones (or vesical calculi, to give them their Latin name), the condition was clearly a common complaint, as it still is in parts of the developing world today. The learned Erasmus experienced stones; he in turn reported that his acquaintance, the famous English physician Thomas Linacre, died of the complaint.[24] Michel de Montaigne was another literary lion who suffered from bladder stones, first feeling the symptoms when about forty-five years old. His *Journal de voyage en Italie* is an account of travels in which he sought relief from his suffering in mineral water baths.[25] The English Royalist poet John Dryden endured "the gravel" that often accompanied bladder stones;[26] so did Oliver Cromwell. Isaac Newton died from bladder stones, and eighteenth-century statesmen like Benjamin Franklin and Robert Walpole felt its sharp and hot pains.

General opinion agreed that if a closely watched regimen was not followed, a stone might develop. Both males and females developed stones in the bladder, although the larger and shorter urethra in women allowed them to expel the stones safely during urination more often than in men and boys. A report in the *Philosophical Transactions* described a very large stone evacuated from a woman's bladder, and the English diarist Samuel Pepys recorded with frustration that his mother had voided a stone, "which she hath let drop into the Chimny; and could not find it to show it me"; his aunt at Brampton "voided a great Stone" about two weeks after.[27] The "oldest, largest and most famous bladder stone from East Anglia" was removed from a woman, Ann Raisin, after her death in 1662, which King Charles II himself asked to be shown even in the midst of a visit to the Newmarket horseraces: over 10 by almost 8 centimeters (about 4 × 3 inches), it weighs 964 grams (just over 2 pounds).[28]

The condition was often preceded or accompanied by "the gravel," in which the urine contained abundant sandlike particles and a thick white slime that could be voided only with difficulty. "I felt how a great quantity of small stones, gravel and dregs passed away with the urine," is how Erasmus described it to his physician shortly after a fit of stones. "That urine I did not keep, to my regret, though I kept that of the following day, which resembled milk with small pieces of stone. The deposit was plastery. Meanwhile I had a very disagreeable feeling [*sensus molestissimus*] in the bladder."[29] Such a condition would often be accompanied by "strangury," in which "the Urine comes away by Drops only, accompanied with a constant Inclination of making Water."[30]

A retained stone would usually grow in size, irritating the bladder and

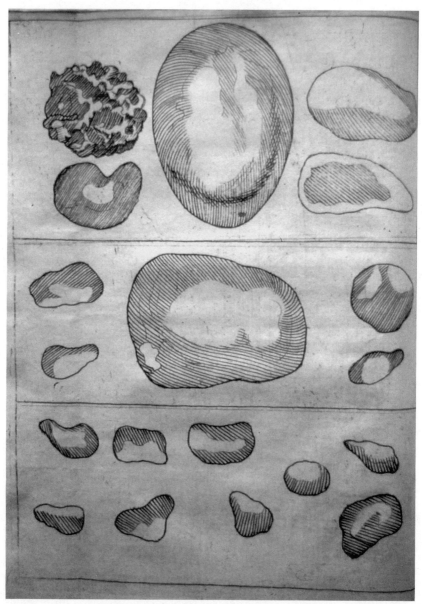

FIG. 10. *Stones, from Groenvelt's* Dissertatio Lithologica, variis observationibus et figuris illustrata (*1684*).

sometimes causing ulcers there. During attacks, the victim would often have to remain in bed, sometimes for many days at a time, and the pain could cause vomiting and the loss of appetite. As Hildanus wrote: "What paine the sick man suffers thereby, it is scarce credible."[31] The physician Sir Thomas Browne wrote of Anthony, bishop of Norwich, "Upon every attempt to go abroad in his coach [he] makes bloody urine and is much payned after, so that it may hazard his life to undertake a London journey."[32] Stones also occasionally dropped into a position that blocked the passage of urine from the body, causing further pain and discomfort. As Montaigne described the symptoms: "You sweat in agony, turn pale, turn red, tremble, vomit your very blood, suffer strange contractions and convulsions, sometimes shed great tears from your eyes, discharge thick, black, and frightful urine, or have it stopped up by some sharp rough stone that cruelly pricks and flays the neck of your penis."[33] If the stone was not passed and continued to grow, it could eventually cause death. Robert Hooke noted the last sufferings of John Wilkins, bishop of Chester and fellow of the Royal Society: "Lord Chester desperately ill of the stone, stoppage of urine 6 dayes. . . . [He] dyed about 9 in the morning of a suppression of urine."[34] Isaac Newton died after two weeks of suppressed urine due to stones, during which time the pain "rose to such a height that the bed under him and the very room, shook with his agonies, to the wonder of those that were present."[35]

Fear of "the stone" could certainly cause shudders of dread to run through anyone. When Pepys began to feel a "rage" in his back, he had to go home and lie in bed for a considerable time before the pain abated, and so he feared a return of stones: "Anon I went to make water, not dreaming of anything but my testicle, that by some accident I might have bruised as I used to do—but in pissing, there came from me two stones; I could feel them, and caused my water to be looked into, but without any pain to me in going out—which makes me think it is not a fit of the stone at all . . . and therefore I hope my disease of the stone may not return to me, but void itself in pissing; which God grant—but I will consult my physitian."[36]

Because of the frequency of the complaint among well-to-do people, contemporary medical interest in bladder stones was high, especially in regions of Europe which had been influenced by the medical chemists. Chemical medicine has often been associated with strong Protestantism; whether or not there is a causal relationship, it was in the region near the Rhine, including the Netherlands, where from an early date people could find chemistry taught as a medical subject.[37] The medical chemists took a deep interest in worms and other things that seemed to breed in the body, including stones, since traditional medical theories seemed little able to account for their presence. One list of works on bladder stones contains roughly two hundred titles with both a place of publication and a date of 1680 or earlier which contain some discussion of urinary calculus or its treatment; of these, over 80 percent appeared in regions with Germanic languages.[38] The newer universities in northern Europe required their students to publish the theses presented for their degrees, including their M.D.'s, which certainly inflates the figures for the Germanic regions. Nevertheless, the universities in those regions had also incorporated chemical medical teachings into their regular curricula, and the faculty there consequently had the greatest interest in urinary calculi. The very influential Flemish iatrochemist Joanne Baptista van Helmont wrote a treatise on stones in 1644, which was widely read.[39] An excellent account of bladder stones had been published by the Dutch physician Johan van Beverwijck.[40] An English chemical physician, Thomas Sherley, wrote *A Philosophical Essay: Declaring The Probable Causes, whence Stones are produced,* which took up the views of Van Helmont "and other great wits": "That stones, and all other sublunary bodies, are made of water, condensed by that power of seeds, which with the assistance of their fermentive Odours, perform these Transmutations upon Matter."[41] Sherley combined this basic Helmontian theory with Cartesian corpuscularianism, and he frequently quoted the English chemist and natural philosopher Robert Boyle. Boyle's own interest in experiments into how stones were formed in the body provided Sherley with a respectable source for pursuing the subject.[42]

In addition to the large number of medical treatises published on kidney and bladder stones, the *Philosophical Transactions of the Royal Society* of London also contained many discussions, such as Frederick Slare's articles on experiments done on stones found in the body,[43] various members' essays on unusual calculi they had found during dissections,[44] and surgeons' reports of unusual stones removed by operations.[45] A Dutch imitation of the *Philosophical Transactions,* published by Steven Blankaart, similarly contains many reports of calculi. Among the more sensational entries are a stone as big as a pigeon's egg found in the gall bladder, a stone in the nerves of the eye found by two doctors, an abscess and stone found under the tongue, and an anatomy of a six- or seven-year-old boy who died of stones.[46]

According to modern ideas, there is no single cause for the complaint: it might be due to infection or to diet; the fact that early modern Europeans drank very little plain water unless by necessity, preferring to take liquid mainly in the form of beer, ale, or watered wine (until in the mid-seventeenth century the fashion for drinking coffee, tea, and mineral water spread), probably contributed to their problems by causing chronic dehydration.[47] Hippocrates and Galen thought that stones were coagulated under cold conditions from raw and thick phlegm,[48] caused in turn by what were called the "non-naturals," the six things apart from the natural structure of the body which affected a person's temperament: air, meat and drink, exercise and rest, sleep and waking, expelling and retaining of superfluities, and affections of the mind.[49] Groenevelt's contemporaries continued to stress irregular or dangerous use of the non-naturals as the root cause of bladder stones, although they rejected coldness as the immediate cause.

For instance, the noted early seventeenth-century authority on bladder stones, Wilhelm Fabricius von Hilden (Hildanus),[50] argued that a "grosse and slimy phlegme" coagulated into vesical calculi owing not to cold but to a "preternaturall heat of the inward bowells." Thus, he recommended avoiding foods either that could cause the "grosse, thick, and slimy humor" or that produced heat in the liver, kidneys, and intestines. That meant keeping away from milk and "all white meats, except Butter; Cheese also and Fish, especially such as live in pooles, mud, and stinking waters, and want scales; the extremes, heads, and bowels of all beasts, and all slimy things, for which very cause Veale and the flesh of Kids, Lambs, and all other beasts newly weaned, if often used, is dangerous to Calculous persons." Moreover, whatever was "hard, grosse, and hardly digested" was to be avoided; "All salt and smoked flesh and fish, the flesh of fallow Deare, red Deare, wilde Boare, Goats, and Beares, all unleavened bread, and whatsoever if fried in Butter or Oyle," as well as pasties, peas, beans, lentils, rice, millet, coleworts, raw fruit, and other such foods. Hot things, like pepper, ginger, cloves, cardamon, bayberry, leeks, garlic, and onions, and strong and hot wines might also cause stones. Finally, people had to avoid idleness, much sleep, "tipling by night," immoderate and violent exercise, hot baths, "long keeping the bed after a sickness, and the like" if they were to prevent stones.[51] The famous French surgeon Ambroise Paré recommended a similar regimen.[52]

Groenevelt, on the other hand, rejected both the ancient idea that cold caused the stone and the more modern idea that heat caused it.[53] No one has heat in his body like that of a furnace, which would be necessary to turn matter into stone like bricks, he argued; if slimy phlegm was made into stone by only a moderate heat, then the stones would be dissoluble in water, like clay; and if stones were caused by a "continuing heat," then continual fevers would follow. No, heats in the body did not cause the stones but were rather caused by the presence of calculi.[54] He also argued against the idea that stones could be caused by occult qualities of some kind, or by "a certain salt and lapidific sort of Spirit, and a certain natural hardning Volatile Earth, as they call it, of the Urine, which produces a new substance, which they call *Duelech* in the Reins [kidneys] and in the Bladder, after the same manner as Sticks, Trees, Animals cast into the waters of some Springs are said to be turned into Stones." If this theory, advanced by Hildanus and others,[55] were true, the petrifying spirit would turn the "Kidneys and the rest of the Body into a Stone."[56] Instead, he thought that several parts of the urine concreted around a kernel of "a certain salt and earthy part," causing the growth of stones in rings, like onions. The kernels settled out like butter separates from whey, because in the churning of the vessels the matter that made up the kernels was unapt for motion: "A not unlike separation is also made in new wine, as the most Ingenious *Des Cartes* does most learnedly demonstrate."[57]

But despite differences from other investigators as to the immediate cause of stones—or the material and efficient causes, to use the philosophical language of the time—when it came to the "remote and mediate causes whereby the matter of the Stone is communicated to the mass of blood," Groenevelt agreed that "the inordinate use of victuals, and intemperance" were to blame. Eating bread that is not well fermented or not baked with moderate heat, or bread that is "very fine, and having too much of a clammy and sweetish quality"; cheese; "too constant use of Beef, Pork, and Goats flesh, and meats very salt and smoked"; fish without scales; too much water-fowl; or drinking new beer that has too much hops; thick and standing water; cold water after a sweaty exercise; tartarous wines; and sweet wines: all can lead to stone (although "small Wines do rather preserve from the Stone"). Other non-naturals could lead to stone, too: thick, rainy, cold air; immoderate sleep, sloth, or too much exercise soon after eating; salaciousness; traveling in snow; retained urine and excrement; violent and exorbitant passions of the mind or sadness, anger, and fear; and heredity. "Unto these Causes the Astrologers add a Conjunction of Saturn with Mercury in the eighth House, under which they say the child which is born will be troubled with the Stone. But whether the influence of the Stars can have such effects upon mans body, I leave it to the Learned to determine."[58]

Diagnosis also presented challenges. Many urinary complaints might have similar symptoms to vesical calculi. The great astronomer Tycho Brahe, for instance, may have died of prostate problems, which caused him to be unable to urinate after a prolonged eating and drinking party (etiquette called for not rising to pass water until after the head of table)[59]—but the symptoms could be the same for calculi. For Pepys, pain in his genitals and the evacuation

of stones brought fear. The symptoms of calculi were several: a white slimy
humor seen in the urine close to the bottom of the urinal after it stood a day
or night unstirred; a vehement pain in making water; urine coming out only
a bit at a time; somewhat bloody urine; an inflammed bladder; the patient
commonly milking the penis in order to make water, something especially
useful for diagnosing children; gravel or little stones occasionally in the urine;
the patient crossing his or her legs and pulling up on the belly when urinating;
the patient feeling a weight in the belly; too frequent urges to make water;
stiffness of the penis without a venereal appetite; and a frequent desire to
drink. But while these symptoms would indicate the possibility of stones,
only physical diagnosis could confirm their presence. For this, the physician
or surgeon had to feel whether there was a hardness when he stuck his oiled
finger in the patient's anus and pointed up toward the pubic bone, or when
he explored the bladder with a sound or catheter.[60] Groenevelt agreed that
the pathological signs of stones, even those described by Hippocrates, were
equivocal, so that the only certain diagnosis came from having the physician
or surgeon feel the stone itself with the finger or a catheter.[61] Despite the
recent impression that only surgeons touched patients to diagnose illnesses
in the sixteenth and seventeenth centuries, vesical calculi were one of the
conditions in which some physicians, at least, were beginning to use physical
diagnosis.

Once the vesical calculi had been diagnosed, various remedies might be
tried to expel them from the body. When Wilkins was lying on what would
be his deathbed, his friends recommended several recipes to him. Joseph
Glanvill suggested drinking a decoction of four oyster shells quenched in a
quart of cider after they were roasted to red hot.[62] Sympathetic remedies like
Glanvill's, containing calcined or crushed shells, had a very long history,
being recommended as "lithontriptics." Joanna Stephens' secret lithontriptic,
which she sold to the English Parliament in 1739 for £5,000, disappointed
the members of Parliament when they found it to consist only of the usual
ingredients: soap and calcined shells.[63] Many medical books contained various
other recipes for lithontriptics. An anonymous English practitioner from the
late seventeenth century who copied medical recipes into a notebook included
two lithontriptics. One recommended dissolving "a large proportion of Crabs-
eyes powder'd, in a good White-wine vinegar." Another "often try'd medicine
for ye stones" of the kidney or bladder was to take one pint of pure white
or Rhenish (Rhine) wine and one pint of water in which the herb fennel had
been infused, and to add an ounce of "well cleans'd" wood lice and a lemon;
after letting this mixture sit in a sealed ("well stopped") vessel for four or

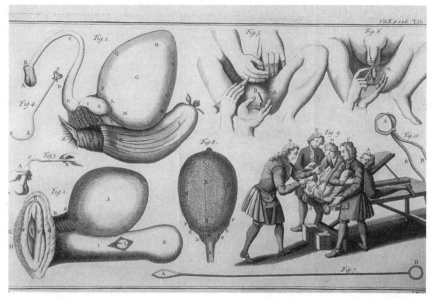

FIG. 11. *Method of Celsian lithotomy, from Lorenz Heister,* A general system of surgery *(1739). In the lower right one can see the patient being held in place in the lithotomy position while the surgeon prepares to insert the knife; the upper center shows
where the cut would be made "on the finger"; in the upper right is shown how the
stone is scooped out after the incision has been made.*

five days, the patient was to take four ounces of it at a time twice a day.[64]
The idea was to ingest something that would cause the stone to break up—
by herbs, chemicals, or the power of sympathy—so that it could be evacuated.

The medical faculty of Leiden became involved in a discussion of one
rare lithontriptic in 1653, about fifteen years before Groenevelt's study there.
The young Henrik Wolraet, count of Waldeck and Culemborg, had suffered
from terrible pains from the age of six, which were finally diagnosed as
bladder stones when he was ten. His doctor took the young count all over
the Netherlands to get advice from the most respected people of the day,
including a learned opinion from the Leiden faculty on the "method of
Laurenbergius." This remedy consisted of *"lapis e Gusarata"* (stone of Gujerat, in India), *"lapis Judaicus," "lapis Manati sive Tiburonum,"* and dried
shark's brain. The Leiden faculty did not know what exactly the stone of
Gujerat was (it may have been a variety of Oriental bezoar, a stone found
in the stomach of the wild goat of Persia); according to the ancient doctor
Dioscorides, the Jewish stone came from the East Indies; and the stone of

Manatus they decided came from the head of an Indian "fish" (apparently a sea cow).[65] Such a remedy seemed fit for a count: rare and expensive. It is notable that the concoction consisted mainly of various stones from animals that lived quite happily with them in their bodies.

By the late seventeenth century, however, many physicians had become skeptical of stone-breaking remedies. Wilkins' friend Dr. Jonathan Goddard therefore recommended another kind of remedy for his suffering, something other than a lithontriptic: "Blisters of Cantharides applyd to the neck and feet or to the vains."[66] Goddard's method was apparently not intended to break the stone but to cause the fluids in the body to rush outward, making the patient void the stone. Other remedies to flush stones by inducing strong urination also had a long history. Already by Montaigne's time, at the end of the sixteenth century, "taking the waters" at a spa, both by bathing in them and by drinking them, was a frequently recommended remedy of this sort, clarifying the urine, kidneys, and bladder by chemically dissolving the stones and gravel or by mechanically flushing them.[67]

In Groenevelt's view, pharmaceutical remedies could best be used preventively, to cleanse the body of the thick humors that accumulated in stones. These remedies especially included mild cathartics (purging medicines that cleansed the stomach, guts, and blood) and vomits. If matter that might turn into stones had already accumulated in the kidneys, then diuretics and mineral waters could be used to flush them clean. If stones had already formed, small ones could sometimes be gotten rid of by the use of freshwater baths and emollient herbs, and by relaxing the passages with lithontriptics, followed by the use of diuretics. Lithontriptics might work to break up the stones if they were brittle, Groenevelt thought. For this purpose he liked Virga Aurea, Arnold of Villa Nova's Probatum, and powdered millipedes. The patient's imagination might also positively affect the breaking up of brittle stones. Remedies could also be prescribed to lessen pain. But clearly, prevention through the regulation of the non-naturals was better by far than all remedies.[68]

When remedies failed, as they so often did, women might have their urethras dilated to help pass a small stone, but women with larger stones and all men had no other choice but to suffer further tortures or have the stone cut out. Such an operation was dangerous and without anesthesia was very painful, making it a remedy of last resort. But once the stone had formed, as Matthew Bacon wrote to Sir Henry Walgrave in 1653, there was no solution but to take courage and get cut for it—after finding an excellent surgeon, of course.[69] Lithotomy, as such surgery was called, could clearly make a deep impression on the patient. In 1717, the French court composer

Marin Marais wrote a *piéce de caractère* for clavichord and viola da gamba titled "A Picture of a Lithotomy" (*Le tableau de l'opération de la taille*), perhaps after he had undergone the operation himself. He musically described seeing the apparatus, trembling in expectation, resolving to mount the apparatus, arriving at the top, having the apparatus lowered, thinking solemn thoughts; then having his legs and arms bound by silken cloths, the incision made, the forceps inserted, the stone drawn out, fainting, and bleeding; being unbound and taken away to bed; and recovering.[70] The piece takes about five minutes altogether, the second half being devoted to the more pleasant sounds of the convalescence, and the lugubrious beginning takes about a minute, so that the quick, screeching notes associated with the surgical part of the operation occupy only a few bars. In its timing, the piece is about right: in the early eighteenth century, the English surgeon William Cheselden was said by a regular observer to seldom exceed "half a Minute" in the cutting and removal of the stone.[71]

As the physical signs of such trauma, souvenirs of operations in the form of the stones themselves were often kept by the patients or surgeons or by the hospitals in which the operations took place. (Many older institutions still have collections of stones squirreled away in back rooms.) Ruysch used bladder stones to form the foundation of his dioramas made from hardened body parts and the skeletons of fetuses.[72] Pepys had the operation at the end of March 1658. He found a fine operator in the surgeon Thomas Hollyer, lithotomist at St. Thomas's Hospital from 1644 to 1683;[73] and he received good pre- and postoperative nursing care from his relative Jane Turner, who had herself been successfully operated on by Hollyer. For years afterward, Pepys celebrated the anniversary of his successful operation with feasting and thanksgiving—even when the anniversary brought news that his mother and father were gravely ill and would soon be dead. Two years afterward, he paid 25s. for a case in which to keep his stone; when in April 1667 the Lord Treasurer lay in bed suffering from the condition, Pepys paid him a visit with stone in hand, to show that his own could be extracted safely.[74] After trying various lithontriptics to no avail, the aforementioned count of Culemborg's physician finally decided that he had to undergo lithotomy; after a successful recovery, the count paid the goldsmith Hendrick Step 6 gilders and 10 stuivers for a silver box in which to keep his stone.[75]

But perhaps the most remarkable story of an extracted vesical calculus is that of the Amsterdam smith Jan de Dood, who removed it from himself.[76] Poor De Dood (his name translates as "the dead") had suffered greatly from bladder stones and twice previously had been cut for them successfully.

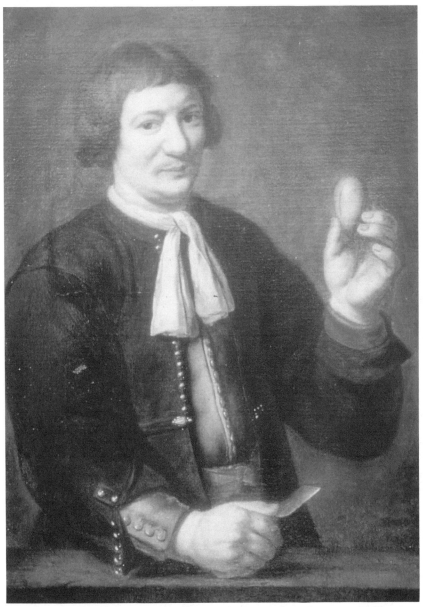

FIG. 12. *Portrait of Jan de Dood holding his knife and stone. Courtesy of Rijksuniversiteit Leiden, Laboratory of Pathology.*

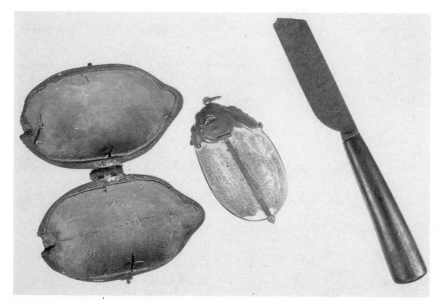

FIG. 13. *The surviving knife, stone (reinforced by metal), and case (for the stone) of De Dood. Courtesy of Rijksuniversiteit Leiden, Laboratory of Pathology.*

When another bladder stone developed a few years later, De Dood submitted to the knife yet again, but this time the surgeon did not have success in pulling out the stone. De Dood would have to be cut yet again; but rather than call the surgeon back, De Dood sent his wife to the market and got his brother to assist him in making the incision himself, fishing the stone out of his bladder with his own fingers. News of this event quickly spread throughout Amsterdam, and when skeptics raised their heads, De Dood gave an account to a notary under oath, saying he had done the deed on 5 April 1651. A version of the notary's document circulated as a broadside, on which a life-size representation of the extracted stone and De Dood's knife were also printed. The famous Amsterdam physician and burgomaster Nicolaas Tulp believed De Dood and placed a Latin account of the self-extraction in the 1652 edition of his *Observationes Medicae,* the frontispiece of which depicts the event.[77] Even later poems celebrated De Dood's feat. His portrait, knife, and stone, encased in leather, remain in the museum of pathology of the University of Leiden.

As these accounts of Pepys, the count, and even De Dood emphasize, people could be operated on successfully for bladder stones. But clearly, the operation was dangerous—so much so that a controversy developed over various surgi-

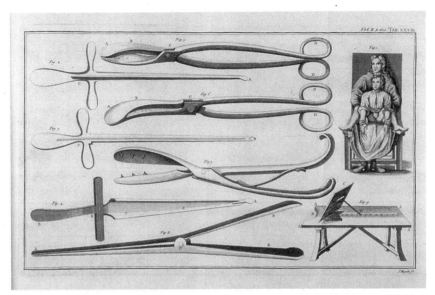

FIG. 14. *Instruments, operating table (lower right), and method of holding a child in the lithotomy position (upper right). From Heister,* A general system of surgery.

cal techniques in Amsterdam in 1667 and 1668, leading to a new city ordinance, which is what brought together Groenevelt and Velthuis. The medical controversy occurred just as Groenevelt arrived in Leiden, and it may even have been this that led his teacher Sylvius to suggest that he look into the subject of bladder stones for his medical thesis.

Two versions of lithotomy were then in use in Amsterdam, the "minor" and "major."[78] Both took a perineal approach: that is, the stone was removed through the perineum, the region between the genitals and the anus. Rochus van Dijk practiced the "apparatus minor," like some other Dutch surgeons such as the lithotomist Jacobus Sasbout Souburg of Dordrecht.[79] Also known as the "Celsian" operation after the Roman author who first discussed it, or as cutting "on the stone" or "on the grip" from the method by which it was done, the minor operation could be done with no instruments save a knife and sometimes a scoop.[80] Hildanus describes this operation plainly. The patient would be put on a fitting diet for several days before the operation. Then, when he or she had reached the right frame of mind, "the Patient being bound" in the lithotomy position (sitting, with the knees pulled up to the shoulders and legs spread), "the Chirurgian putteth the first, or middle-finger of his left hand," oiled or greased, into the patient's anus, "and with

his right hand thrusteth downe the lower belly towards the Bladder." These
two movements forced the stone toward the surgeon's finger. "The Chirurgian
having found the Stone by his finger in the fundament, thrusts it downe" to
the "neck" of the bladder (where the urethra exits), at the same time pressing
the stone against the body, between the genitals and the anus. With the stone
bulging against the skin, the surgeon "first maketh Incision upon the stone,
and then with his fingers thrust into the fundament, laboureth to drive it out."
If the stone was too large to pop out this way, various hooks, scoops, or
crochets would be inserted to pull it out.[81] Since healthy urine contains no
bacteria, if the cut was made so that urine could drain out freely during the
operation, it would irrigate the wound and perhaps lessen the chances of
infection.[82] The wound would be left to heal by itself, or partially sewn
together with a silver tube left in for drainage, the patient first being placed
in a warm hip bath and the wound afterward being kept warm with oiled
cotton cloth. Rochus van Dijk had performed a lithotomy successfully on
the count of Waldek and Culemborg; but unfortunately, according to Hildanus, the minor operation held great danger for the patient, especially for
males over fourteen years old.[83]

A more noted Amsterdam surgeon than Rochus van Dijk, Allardus Cyprianus, operated according to the "apparatus major," or greater section, also
called "cutting on the staff" or "cutting on the itinerarium" (the name of the
instrument used), or the "Marian" operation (after Marino Santo, who in-
vented the method in the early sixteenth century). Hildanus, who popularized
this method, described it in some detail. "The Patient being well bound, and
all things fitly disposed," the surgeon inserted a kind of probe (called the
itinerarium) through the penis into the bladder. This staff, grooved on one
side, maneuvered the stone into the neck of the bladder while the grooved
side also pressed against the perineum. Then, one finger's breadth toward
the thigh "from the seame that goeth from the Scrotum unto the fundament,"
a pointed knife sharpened on both sides was thrust into the bladder onto the
grooved itinerarium. The surgeon then inserted another instrument, called
the "conductor" (or semispeculum), "upon the Itinerarium unto the very
stone." The conductor was "an hollow instrument, and open on one side . . .
bigge in the end," and therefore had to be thrust in deeply, so that it would
"open the wound and the neck of the bladder." The surgeon could then
remove the itinerarium. Along the open side of the conductor he thrust the
"hamulus" onto the stone, which gripped it and pulled it out.[84]

Unfortunately for both Van Dijk and Cyprianus, many of their patients,
operated on in 1667 by either method, died. One source even states that

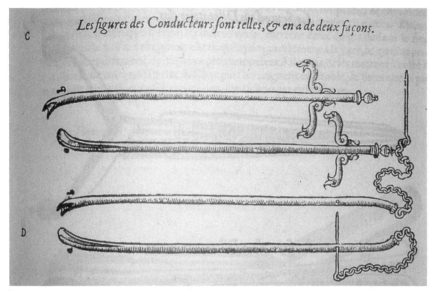

FIG. 15. *Two kinds of conductors, illustrated from both sides. From Ambroise Paré,* Dix livres de la chirurgie *(1564).*

Cyprianus had fallen into such disrepute because of his lost patients that he was sued over his surgery.[85] Since the local lithotomists were not trusted, a renowned Parisian surgeon named Philippe Colot (or Collot) came to Amsterdam at the invitation of some important people and operated on them according to a new method he developed, with great success.[86] According to Groenevelt, who learned to operate according to Colot's technique, the main difference between Colot's method of section and cutting on the staff was in the instruments. The cutting was not done on the "staff" but "upon a Catheter made sulcate [grooved], and bending, according to the form and dimensions of the cavity of the bladder into which it is to be inserted." Once the cut had been made, a "director" was inserted ("whereof there are three sorts . . . according to the largeness of the stone") to guide the "dilator." The dilators were "distinct Instruments, and also of divers sizes," which made way with the "greatest ease and expedition for the taking forth of the stone." After the surgeon had dilated the opening with the appropriate instrument, forceps were inserted to grasp and remove the stone; again, these instruments were made of various sizes and shapes ("streight, and rostrate, and round, and oval, and with other differences") and used "according as the nature and magnitude of the stone and of the orifice" required.[87] Such

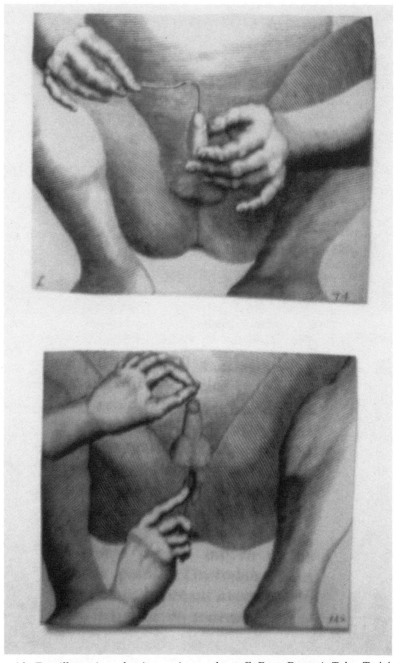

FIG. 16. *Two illustrations showing cutting on the staff. From François Tolet,* Traité de la lithotomie *(1682).*

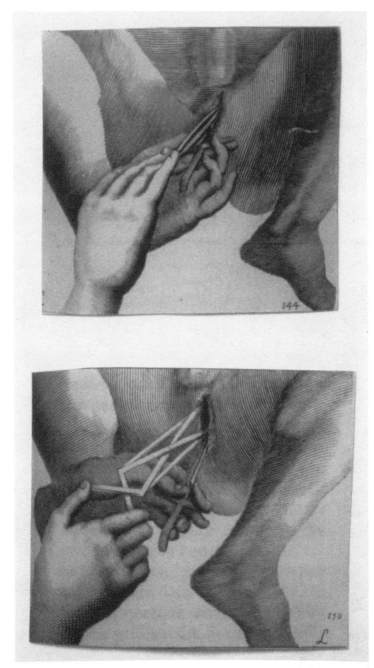

Fig. 17. *Two illustrations showing the insertion of the forceps using the conductor (above), and the forceps open to remove a stone (below).* From François Tolet, Traité de la lithotomie.

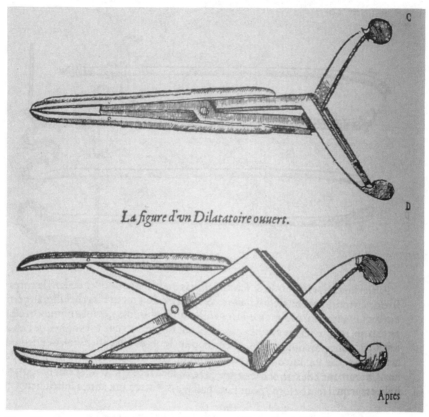

FIG. 18. *One style of dilatory, closed and open. From Paré,* Dix livres de la chirurgie.

technique created somewhat less trauma in those who were operated on, and so the reputation of the methods of the Colot family spread widely. Sir Thomas Browne wrote to his son in Paris in 1665: "take good notice of their instruments, and at least make such a draught thereof, and especially of the dilator and director, that you may hereafter well remember and have one made by it."[88]

But Colot's Amsterdam success both upset the established lithotomist Cyprianus and broke the rules governing lithotomy in Amsterdam. The local ordinances of 1552 mandated that anyone operating for stones (or ruptures or cataracts) could do so only after being examined and approved by the officers or examiners of the surgeons' guild. In the sixteenth century, the dangers of lithotomy meant that few regular surgeons undertook the operation:

having one or more of their patients die could hurt their reputations for treating other problems. Lithotomists, hernia repairers, and cataract cutters therefore made up a fair proportion of the traveling surgeons and empirics who ranged the byways of Europe. To keep the bad ones out of Amsterdam, then, the magistrates insisted that all such operators be properly examined. An amendment to the ordinance in 1621 specified that the operators who did not belong to the guild would have to be examined and pay a fee for practice, which varied depending on how long they stayed. The experienced Colot, however, had not bothered to undergo any examination by the Amsterdam surgeons' guild and presumably paid no fee, claiming that his method was and had to be kept a secret. Because he had been invited to the city by one or more influential people, and because the usual lithotomists had failed so often, the burgomasters overlooked the rules in Colot's case.[89] Needless to say, the local lithotomist Cyprianus smarted from Colot's illegal success and complained loudly.[90]

Moreover, one Noach Smaltzius used Colot's success to begin operating for stones in Amsterdam himself without undergoing examination. He had been named a city surgeon of Haarlem in May 1665 and charged a considerable sum of money for lithotomy, presumably because his patients stood a good chance of recovering.[91] Smaltzius seems to have been on good terms with Groenevelt's professor, Sylvius, for Groenevelt and a fellow student witnessed Smaltzius remove a large number of stones from a body in 1667;[92] Sylvius had been in the habit of inviting practitioners he thought well of to Leiden to demonstrate or lecture.[93] Perhaps this connection is what led Smaltzius to become one of the Leiden city surgeons in December 1672.[94] In 1667, according to Groenevelt, Smaltzius studied and "perfected" Colot's method;[95] another of Sylvius's supporters described Smaltzius as the equal of the best Paris lithotomist.[96]

The intrusion of the unregulated and innovative surgeons led to a modification of the ordinances in 1668, which created new possibilities for Groenevelt. The new rules reiterated the requirement that lithotomists be examined by the surgeons' guild but entered an exception: they could obtain the permission of at least two burgomasters directly for each operation, without having to go through the surgeons. As Groenevelt explained it, the new Amsterdam regulations required that no one be cut for stones before the lithotomist examined those who were thought to be sick from that ailment in the presence of a doctor, in order to prevent quackery. The doctor then had to reassure the magistrates that the lithotomist's diagnosis was certain before the operation could proceed.[97]

Groenevelt and Velthuis therefore worked together for several years before the latter's death in May 1674;[98] and it was through Velthuis that Groenevelt learned how to perform a lithotomy himself. In all likelihood, Groenevelt had been practicing medicine on those who suffered from stones, up to the point where he would have to recommend surgery. As he later told the story, by fortune his university disputation on stones fell into the hands of Velthuis, who then practiced as a lithotomist in Amsterdam.[99] After meeting Groenevelt, Velthuis thought that it would be a good idea to join together in practice. Velthuis therefore regularly called Groenevelt as a witness when he diagnosed those who thought they suffered from this ailment. (In effect, Groenevelt could recommend Velthuis to his patients who needed surgery, and Velthuis would return the favor by having Groenevelt confirm his diagnosis in order to fulfill the burgomaster's requirement before the operation.) During their time together, Groenevelt witnessed a great number of operations done expertly by Velthuis. When Velthuis lay dying of a hectic fever, he called his partner to him and presented him with his lithotomy instruments, urging Groenevelt to take up the use of them as a fitting memorial to him.[100]

Having an inclination to surgery (evident in the unusually detailed manner in which he covered it in his thesis), and being driven to it by circumstances, Groenevelt took Velthuis's advice and began practicing lithotomy himself,[101] following Colot's method.[102] For a physician like him to take up surgery was a very unusual step. Physicians ordinarily practiced surgery only in exceptional circumstances, even in a place like Amsterdam, where relations between physicians and surgeons were good.[103] Moreover, the Hippocratic "Oath" explicitly prohibited doctors from taking up lithotomy, swearing them to leave the operation to the practitioners of that craft.[104] Social expectations and the "Oath" both led Groenevelt to a somewhat defensive explanation of why he took up lithotomy, which he published in the preface to his major Latin treatise on the subject. He basically argued that Hippocrates' views had been appropriate for his time but that the art of lithotomy had been much better developed since, so that the oath no longer applied. Moreover, the major developments in this form of surgery had come from physicians who used their hands, like Celsus and Hildanus.[105] Consequently, practicing lithotomy as a physician contributed to the betterment of medicine.

Moreover, despite pressures against taking up lithotomy, to oversee or perform surgery for a common problem on which he had become an intellectual expert undoubtedly helped Groenevelt gain a leg up on the medical competition in Amsterdam. If we believe his statement that he had practiced with Velthuis for several years before the latter's death in 1674, their arrangement may very well have been what gave Groenevelt the security to enter into marriage early in 1672. Equally, the passing of his senior medical partner two years later must have been a blow to his practice. Established Amsterdam lithotomists like Cyprianus objected to the practice of people like Velthuis and Groenevelt as much as to Colot and Smaltzius. Many years later, in London, one of those to testify against Groenevelt would be the surgeon Cyprianus's son.

But Velthius's death was not Groenevelt's only problem in 1674. Unfortunately for Groenevelt, the years he practiced in Amsterdam coincided with the darkest days of the Republic. The year 1672 was the *rampjaar*, the disaster year for the Dutch Republic. Slightly more than a week after his marriage, on 13 March, with no warning, the English fleet attacked a homeward-bound, heavily laden Dutch merchant fleet in the channel; and following a declaration of war from the English and French kings in April, a combined fleet took to sea against the Dutch in late May. At the same time, a French army invaded from the southeast, while the forces of the bishop of Münster once again struck from a bit further north. Their troops quickly rolled over the Dutch garrisons near the borders, with resulting panic and confusion. While parts of the Dutch army fell back toward Utrecht, other parts were surrounded along the IJssel, and the eastern provinces fell almost at a blow, with all of Overijssel occupied by the bishop of Münster. Deventer held out against a French siege for less than a week.[106] On 3 July, panic caused the collapse of Utrecht almost before a shot had been fired, and only by cutting the dikes and flooding the land to create the "water line" did the army of the United Provinces manage to stop the French advance into Holland and Zeeland. French troops even came within ten miles of Amsterdam's walls, although in the end the Amsterdammers stiffened the country's resolve not to give up the fight. In this crisis, the provincial representatives elected William III of Orange as stadholder, while in August, an Orangist mob in The Hague attacked the former leader of the States Party, Johan de Witt, and his brother Cornelis, making them scapegoats for the disaster; the mob butchered them like pigs, cutting out their hearts and stringing the naked corpses up by the heels, while their fingers, eyes, and other body parts were sold in the streets. William abstained from prosecuting anyone for the violence. Even the Amsterdam burgomasters gave in to the Orangists. The overweening ambitions of Louis XIV and the duplicitous policies of Charles II not only came close to swallowing the whole Dutch nation at one gulp but transfigured the political leadership of what remained.[107]

Needless to say, the years in which Groenevelt practiced with Velthuis in Amsterdam could not have been entirely happy ones. The initial disasters in the war, including the surrender of his beloved hometown to the French, must have caused him much pain, and the initial panic that swept through Amsterdam as well as other cities must have made him fearful for the safety of himself and his new wife. Moreover, he had been raised in a city dominated by States Party supporters and taught philosophy there by one of the party's theorists, and he now practiced in the city that had previously been a bulwark of municipal and provincial liberties against Orangist aspirations. His faith might have sustained him in such disheartening circumstances. But the war-ravaged economy would not have helped.

Groenevelt had been lucky, therefore, to have been able to join in a medical partnership. When his partner Velthuis passed away, he must have seen his prospects fall into doubt. By that spring, the Republic's fortunes had improved immensely: with extraordinary leadership by Admirals De Ruyter and Tromp, the outnumbered Dutch fleet had managed to fight off the English and French at sea, while William III, in a series of brilliant moves, aided by allies from the Holy Roman Empire, had forced the French out of Utrecht and most of the major Dutch cities. By the spring of 1674, Münster had been ejected from the eastern provinces. Embattled and penuri-ous, Charles II had been forced to settle a separate peace with the Republic in February 1674 which restored the earlier status quo between the two nations, leaving the French to fight on alone.[108] But there was no question of returning to Deventer in that May of Velthuis's death despite Münster's surrender, since Overijssel had been plundered by enemy troops for almost two whole years.[109] And with the death of his senior partner, Groenevelt's medical practice undoubtedly declined.

Perhaps, then, Groenevelt sought and gained an appointment as physician to the garrison of the newly liberated Dutch city of Grave, freed from the French after a siege from July through the end of October 1674. Located on the strategic Meuse (Maas) River just south of Nijmegen, Grave had long been a contested fortress, and in 1674 the French remained there in force. Its siege and conquest by the young William III proved to be one of his most striking military achievements of this, his first war.[110] According to the dedication Groenevelt later wrote to the earl of Portland, the earl might remember how he was "by the Command of the High and Mighty States of Holland, appointed Physitian in Chief to the Garrison of that Castle" of the city of Grave about twenty-five years previously.[111] One might imagine that by calling on the earl, Willem Bentinck, who had been one of William III's closest associates, to remember an event, Groenevelt must have been telling the truth or have risked his reputation. While the young doctor is on the record neither as among the few military physicians who received a commission from the Dutch government nor as among the appointees of the municipal government of Grave,[112] the state of the Grave archives during this period leaves much to be desired.[113] He was probably telling the truth: his medical practice in Amsterdam was unlikely to be flourishing after Velthuis's death, and so the post in Grave would have looked attractive.

But if Groenevelt did in fact move to Grave after it had returned to Dutch hands at the end of October 1674, he stayed there only a month or less. By 1674, William III had time and political security enough to purge the country of States Party supporters and Coccejeans and other liberal Calvinists, something that might well have made Groenevelt uneasy if he remained a supporter of the views in which he had been educated. The economy remained weak. His friend Ten Rhijne had already shown the way, leaving for Batavia, the capital of the Dutch East Indies, in 1673. Unlike Ten Rhijne, Groenevelt had a wife, and a pregnant one at that: a long journey would not be suitable. Therefore, on 29 November, in Amsterdam, Joannes Groenevelt borrowed 100 caroli gilders[114] from one Joannis Frederick Sibmacer and took ship, leaving his books in Delft with one Dirck Woutersen, apparently as surety for the loan.[115] Delft was right next to Rotterdam, which was not only a major port but the headquarters of the English merchants in the Netherlands, with many connections by ship to London. Not long after he borrowed the money, he arrived in London, bringing the latest Dutch medical theories and surgical practices, and a taste for medical innovation, with him.

CHAPTER 5

An Immigrant Doctor in London

THE YOUNG JOANNES GROENEVELT had relocated before to seek medical opportunities. This time, in his late twenties, he made a bolder move, going to another country altogether, a place where he did not even speak the language. In many ways, the transition would have been more difficult than going from provincial Deventer to Leiden or Amsterdam. But by now he had developed the greater personal resources that came from moving several times. He now also traveled with Cristina, who would soon bear a child. He therefore had to be responsible for more than just himself, but she also undoubtedly helped make their way less difficult.

For a young doctor eager to make a success, the medical marketplace of London offered enormous potential opportunities. There Groenevelt would indeed find success as a practitioner and lithotomist, meet members of the prestigious Royal Society, join the London College of Physicians, publish a Latin treatise on bladder stones which gained him a fine European-wide reputation, and associate with a number of English and foreign physicians who were like him in believing that medical learning should be put to use by developing new and more effective remedies. Among his new acquaintances would even be the famous Thomas Sydenham. Life would have its bumps in the road, including a lawsuit from a well-established London surgeon. But on the whole, this learned medical entrepreneur finally found medical and surgical success in London, before his fortieth year.

In late 1674 or early 1675, Joannes Groenevelt arrived in London. Large numbers of Dutch-speaking people went abroad in the sixteenth and seventeenth centuries, at first primarily to avoid the religious warfare in the low countries, thereafter mainly seeking economic opportunities. The Dutch spread out not only through their colonial possessions but across Europe as well, with many traveling just across the North Sea, to England.

The Dutch helped to transform their adopted homeland. Some brought along their knowledge of how to make the latest kinds of cloth, promoting the rise of the "new draperies" in England. Others used their skills in metal founding to build a new armaments industry for their new sovereigns. Still others were engineers imported by the Stuart monarchy to drain the fens of the eastern counties. From the Netherlands came new ideas about food and agriculture—especially the cultivation and use of vegetables—and improved varieties of domesticated plants and animals. The English also learned new methods of trade and finance from their Dutch brethren and built in London a stock exchange modeled after the one in Amsterdam. Since Erasmus's time, Dutch scholars had been a model for many of their English colleagues, too, while the Dutch and Flemish dominated the fine arts. And the Dutch immigrants worshiped in their own churches under the supervision of the bishop of London, introducing Calvinist notions of theology and ritual and helping to keep alive religious alternatives to Anglicanism.[1] In short, people like Groenevelt helped to reshape the English nation.

Among the Dutch immigrants had been many medical practitioners. From the late sixteenth century, complaints by English authors about "foreign" and "traveling" empirics were frequent.[2] Whereas most of the foreigners on record in the sixteenth century came from southern Europe, by 1637 the London College of Physicians began to hear about increasing numbers of Dutch and Flemish practitioners.[3] A few Dutch-Flemish medical families made it into the English medical establishment within a generation, such as Baldwin Hamey, Jr., John King, and Assuerus Regemorter. A few others became medical practitioners to the English Crown.[4] But most Dutch medical immigrants in the seventeenth century remained ordinary practitioners who made their pitches to the general public. For instance, one handbill informed Londoners that women's diseases could be cured by "Sarah Cornelius de Heusde, Widdow of Dr. Sashout, and Grandmother of the Doctor that had his stage upon Great Tower Hill, and did so many Cures before the Fire."[5] In another, a Dutch physician "lately come from beyond Seas" informed the public that he cured dropsy, gout, agues, the king's evil (scofula), pains of the stomach, consumptions, and many other diseases; this doctor's wife also treated women for barrenness and prevented miscarriages.[6] Someone else, from Rotterdam, sold a "Universal Medicine" from the Crown and Jewell across from Exeter Exchange.[7] Still another recently arrived Dutch practitioner cured all sorts of hernias (broken navels, groins, and so on); a "Mr. C.V.P.," a recently arrived Dutchman, straightened bent bodies in Dean's Court near St. Ann's Church in So Ho; Dr. Vanforce sold his "Elixir Vitae"; and someone pronouncing himself to be a "Dutch Operator," distributing a handbill with the coat of arms of Amsterdam on the front, announced that he had especially good success in curing the French pox (syphilis): he appropriately set up shop across from the Maypole in the Strand.[8]

Like Groenevelt, these other Dutch practitioners had come over to England because of the large potential market for medical services and commodities, especially in London. With a population of around 500,000 when Groenevelt arrived (ten times the size of a century earlier), it was two and a one-half times the size of Amsterdam and growing rapidly. While Amsterdam was the largest city in a densely populated region of many cities, no other place in mainly rural England came at all close to the size and significance of London. Roughly one in ten of the English lived in London. "The" city simply dominated English urban life. Despite some foreign communities, its large immigrant population came mainly from other places in the British Isles rather than from abroad. The poor and laboring tended to live to the east, downwind and near the burgeoning docklands. The city within the walls remained an area of shops and respectable houses, while to the west, upwind in new planned developments or along the river's edge, the great houses of the gentry and aristocracy were located.

As he became accustomed to the new world around him, Groenevelt must have seen many things about the country as very old-fashioned. Unlike the Netherlands, England still had outbreaks of witch-hunting, which were supported by learned physicians like Sir Thomas Browne.[9] A monarch claimed to rule by divine right and displayed his sacred powers by using his royal touch to cure those sick from the "king's evil."[10] And to a Calvinist like Groenevelt, the English church's allowance of free will and clerical vestments must have smacked of popery. While under Henry VIII the Church of England had made the monarch rather than the pope its head, it had not dropped all vestiges of the old religion despite the urgings of "Puritans": its churches and cathedrals frequently still had their stained-glass windows and their railings separating the altar from the congregation, and their religious ceremony seemed close to the Catholic Mass. Calvinist doctrines had never been fully accepted into the Anglican church, while two years after the Restoration of 1660 the Parliament passed an Act of Uniformity that required all clergymen and schoolteachers to give their full support to everything contained in the Anglican Book of Common Prayer, making those who refused to subscribe into "dissenters"; by an act of 1664, anyone attending non-Anglican religious services could be punished, although the

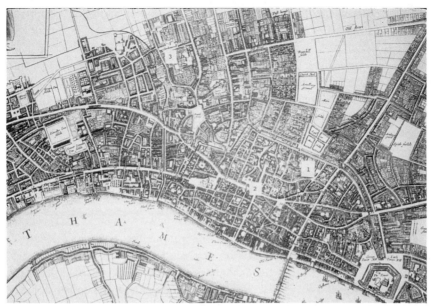

FIG. 19. *Later Seventeenth-Century Map of London. The London Tower is on the right, St. Paul's Cathedral in the open area of the center, north of the Thames. The suburban expansion beyond the old walls (which run from the tower northwest, west, southwest, and south to the Thames just east of St. Paul's) can easily be seen. The three numbered squares are at the center of the three detail maps in figs. 20, 22, and 26. From John Ogilby, "A Mapp of the Cityes of London & Westminster & Burrough of Southwark," 1677.*

two foreign churches in London, including the Dutch church, remained protected.

The burghers of the City of London did not, therefore, entirely dominate the life of the city. A powerful monarch, bishops and archbishops of a state church, and a landed aristocracy that dominated Parliament all tried to make London into a city that each preferred. While the great merchants and leading citizens controlled the government of the City proper, they had to worry, too, about an exploding population, rising poverty, unregulated trades and industries in the suburbs, religious reaction and dissent, and the overbearing rich who lived and played among them. During the fall through spring "season," the English gentry and aristocracy flocked to London to participate in the rounds of parties and gambling, to see plays, to pursue lawsuits, to work the marriage market for sons and daughters, and to attend court. Their ideas of honor, breeding, and liberality sometimes conflicted with the more utilitarian and economical values of the local burghers, occasionally causing conflict. But the combined pull of London high culture and London markets reshaped England.[11]

The wealth of both the English upper classes and the local merchants and artisans, concentrated as it was in an area of a few square miles, meant that the London medical market could yield high incomes to those who could tap into it. Those who grew up in the city could find many varieties of traditional healers and neighborly aid locally. But they and the many strangers and visitors also had a large variety of other practitioners from whom to choose. Scores of medical entrepreneurs and impresarios came to London from all over England and Europe, partly because its organized medical practitioners underserved the population compared with places like Amsterdam. The more than 200 members of the Society of Apothecaries not only operated retail shops where one could buy drugs but visited patients to diagnose and prescribe as well; but they were only about the same in number as in Amsterdam, a city two-fifths its size.[12] The 200 or so practicing members of the Barber-Surgeons' Company carried out major and minor operations and also gave medical advice; but they, too, were hardly much greater in number than the surgeons of Amsterdam.[13] The members of the London College of Physicians—organized into the fellows and candidates—and the nonvoting honorary fellows and licentiates amounted to about 122 altogether when Groenevelt arrived: about 1 to every 4,000 residents, a ratio one-fourth that in Amsterdam.[14] Like many other Dutch practitioners, then, Groenevelt saw great medical opportunities in moving to London.

Moreover, while economic opportunity provided an incentive, political events made his move possible at the end of 1674. A year before, King Charles II had been forced to abandon his ally, the king of France, and conclude a peace with the Dutch. Many leading figures in England increasingly saw not the financial might of the Dutch but the military power of Louis XIV as the greatest danger to their country and sought to support the Dutch stadholder, William III, against the French monarch. Since Charles' wars against the Dutch had led to great sacrifice for no gain, he was now trying to win friends all around, not only continuing to cultivate Louis XIV but at the same time offering his thirteen-year-old niece, Mary, in marriage to William of Orange. (The marriage eventually took place at the end of 1677). Although tensions between the English and Dutch remained, relations had improved considerably, seemingly opening new opportunities for skilled Dutch immigrants.

But Groenevelt thought he had even more specific safeguards for immigrating than generally better relations between the two countries: he had the

word of Charles II that he would be welcome. During the last war, the king
had tried to weaken the Dutch economy and morale by attracting people
from there to England. The king's Declaration of Indulgence in March 1672,
suspending all penal laws against those not within the Anglican fold, publicly
offered freedom of worship to Dutch immigrants.[15] On 15 May 1672, he had
declared that immigrants could freely come to England.[16] On 12 June he
followed this decision with a more detailed decree. This, "His Majesty's
gracious Declaration for encouraging the subjects of the United Provinces
of the Netherlands to transport themselves with their estates, and to settle in
this his Majesty's kingdom of England," was printed in three side-by-side
columns, in English, Dutch, and French. Part of the English propaganda
campaign at the start of the war, this two-and-one-half-page document circulated in the Netherlands in several versions.[17] It made six promises to the
Dutch: they could come to England free from molestation; they would have
liberty to settle wherever they liked, liberty of conscience, and freedom
from special taxes; during the next Parliament, the king would seek a bill
automatically naturalizing all such immigrants, and for the moment he would,
without charge, make them "Free Denizens"; the ships bringing immigrants
over would be treated on the seas like English ships; any sailors coming over
would be free from the press gangs seeking men for the Royal Navy; and
should they wish, His Majesty would even arrange free transportation.[18]

Groenevelt interpreted Charles' edict as granting Dutch immigrants the
same rights as English citizens. This was his claim when, three years after
his arrival, he came to the London College of Physicians to get its permission
to practice lithotomy freely. He either cited the edict precisely or brought a
copy with him, for the college registrar noted its date accurately while at
the same time misdating Groenevelt's Utrecht degree.[19] Presumably, it was
also on the basis of the edict that he made his claim of denization, which
he obtained on 24 June 1675.[20] Denization, granted by the Crown, gave
foreigners the right to lease property and to carry on their trade in England.[21]
Whether Groenevelt obtained his denization without charge, as promised in
the edict, is unknown, as is how long it took him to obtain it.

Groenevelt had therefore arrived in London sometime—probably some
months—before his denization in June 1675, and probably some time before
he first appeared in the local records, in May. It was on 5 May that he and
Cristina offered their first child for baptism, Franciscus (named after his
paternal grandfather), at the Dutch Reformed church at Austin Friars.[22] Possibly Cristina had embarked on the rough winter and spring North Sea crossing
just before giving birth. But more likely, the Groenevelts had set out for

London shortly after Joannes borrowed the 100 gilders at Amsterdam in November 1674, at a time when Cristina would be less inconvenienced by the voyage.

They found comfort and help among the Dutch-speaking, Reformed members of the church at Austin Friars, located in the heart of the city. Among the members of the Austin Friars church Groenevelt found his first patients while learning English. One of the only two openly tolerated Calvinist churches in the city (the other being the French-speaking Huguenot church), the Austin Friars church had a large membership of wealthy Dutch merchants but also included Dutch artisans and even a number of second- and third-generation Dutch, many of whom had married into English families. English Protestants who were disaffected from the Anglican church—even some of noble birth—also attended services there. The Groenevelts therefore joined a wealthy and influential community, Dutch at its core but thoroughly English at the fringes.[23] They took up lodgings on Throgmorton Street, next to the alley to Drapers' Hall (now Throgmorton Lane) and two doors from Broad Street, just around the corner from the church.[24] This neighborhood—the "East Smith field wijck" in terms of the organization of the church—had more people belonging to the Austin Friars congregation than did any other neighborhood but Westminster.[25] After a year and a half, the Groenevelts became full, contributing members of the congregation.[26] In this church they baptized not only their first son, Franciscus, but a second, Elias, and then a daughter named after her mother, Christina.[27] They remained members of the church for many decades, although Joannes did not take an active part in the consistory (dominated as it was by successful merchants) or donate money to the church.[28]

Dr. Groenevelt therefore had great ambitions for advancing his medical fortunes in London when he arrived, and by late 1676, when he became a member of the Austin Friars church, he and his wife had decided to stay. He began his medical practice among the Dutch-speaking community of London. But as wealthy as the group around Austin Friars was, he clearly felt the need to tap the larger London medical market. For this he would need to reach out to the English.

To reach the larger pool of English patients which he would need to make a true success of his practice, Groenevelt had to pick up the rudiments of their language. But he did more: the "Dr. of Physick, and Lithotomist," as he styled himself, brought out a little booklet on bladder stones printed in their tongue, Λιθολογια. *A Treatise of the Stone and Gravel; Their Causes, Signs, and*

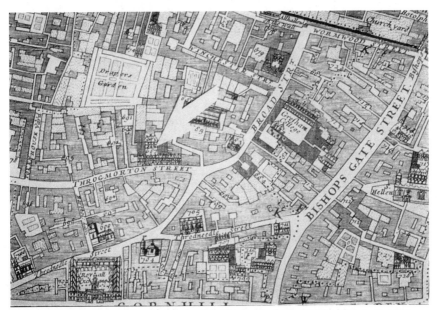

FIG. 20. *London east and a bit north of St. Paul's Cathedral (point "1" in fig. 19). The arrow points to Drapers' Hall, which stood just back from Throgmorton Street. Groenvelt's residence was on the north side of Throgmorton Street, between the entrance to Drapers' Hall and Broad Street. The Royal Exchange stood just to the south, Gresham College (where the Royal Society met) just to the east, and the Church of Austin Friars just to the north. From William Morgan's map, "London etc. Actually Survey'd," of 1682.*

Symptoms, With Methods for their Prevention and Cure. And some account also of The manner of the Collotian section. The overwhelming number of seventeenth-century medical books in English were meant either to make a polemical point or to make their authors better known to the general public. Unless commissioned to write a text, most contemporary authors received payment from the publisher in kind: that is, they received a certain number of copies of the book rather than money. Writers could sell some of these copies for money, but probably more often they gave copies away to help their reputations. Unless other arrangements pertained, then, authors wrote for reasons other than making money from the sale of their books. Their books might be intended to instruct or edify. But in the case of medical authors, certainly, many also intended to let potential patients discover them through their works. As another well-educated Dutch medical immigrant—Bernard de Mandeville—later put it in a work on his own specialty: "If a Regular Physician writing of a Distemper, the Cure of which he particularly professes, after a manner never yet attempted, be a *Quack,* because besides his Design of being instructive and doing Good to others, he has likewise an aim of making himself more known by it than he was before, then I am one."[29]

Like so many other works, then, Groenevelt's book was intended to increase his medical practice among those who spoke English. It was designed throughout to impress the readers with his knowledge and skill concerning a common complaint, in order to get the work into as many hands as possible. Printed by Henry Cruttinden, who later printed some unorthodox books,[30] it was sold at one of the largest bookstalls among the many next to St. Paul's Cathedral: at Robert Clavel's "The Peacock." It bore the date 1677 on the title page but was finished in late 1676, within two years of Groenevelt's arrival in London, about the time that he and his family became full members of the Dutch church. The text passed the royal censor on 15 November 1676 and was entered into the register of the London Stationer's Company two days later (thereby giving Cruttinden the sole right of printing the text).[31]

The book was undemanding, short, inexpensive, and illustrated. Small in size (an octavo), it was only sixty-nine pages long. Interested readers could buy a bound copy for 10d.: since books were usually bound to order by the bookseller rather than being retailed bound, perhaps half the price would have gone for the binding, making Groenevelt's unbound book among the cheapest medical books then being sold.[32] Its modest cost is especially evident when one considers that the printer incurred added expense by including several woodcuts illustrating the text, which would have attracted the attention of some of those browsing the bookstalls. (Illustrations of the surgical instruments he used are absent, however, since such pictures could have been used by competitors as the basis for designing their own instruments.) It had a patina of erudition, including the opening Greek word of the title page (a technique resorted to by other medical authors who strove for the look of learning). While the basis for his book was, in fact, Groenevelt's Utrecht medical thesis—the title page declared the book to be "Written in Latin . . . and rendered into English"—it was far from a simple translation. Among other matters, he discarded the multitude of references to other texts contained in the original, and when he did cite an author, the reference was often to a book available in English, or to someone like Jean Fernel, who had a widespread reputation for being a sound authority. Moreover, while bringing out his book in English was essential, since fewer well-to-do English people read Latin easily than was the case in the Netherlands, the fluency of the English suggests that Groenevelt had assistance in the translation.[33]

The text itself closely followed Groenevelt's Utrecht thesis, beginning with the definition of terms and a discussion of the efficient and material causes of stones in the body. His moral earnestness came through in an added reference to God's designs: "some raising their Contemplations to superior objects, derive [the cause of calculi] from the beginning of our Creation, as a punishment on mankind for our Apostacy, esteeming it not strange, that that returns to Earth, or Stone, which from Earth at first was produced."[34] But then, as in his thesis, he goes on to discard the more common opinions about stones being caused by heat, cold, a stony spirit, a petrifying *duelech*, or occult qualities. Instead, he explained that the calculi grew from part of the choler contained in the urine to which a certain salt might be added, the particles settling out because they were "unapt for motion" and being added one to another grew like an onion. He then discussed the "remote and mediate causes whereby the matter of the Stone is communicated to the mass of blood," that is, dietetics, so that the reader could prevent the occurrence of stones. For those who had become afflicted (the pathological signs were also explained), he offered some suggestions for medical treatments. In the last part of his text, Groenevelt dealt with surgical lithotomy, dividing it into six operations: the minor; the major; the use of forceps guided by a "director"; the method of Petrus Francus, who cut the perineum and then let the patient rest for several days before removing the stones at the mouth of the wound (in order to avoid damaging the bladder by the use of forceps); Francus's very dangerous method (reported by him once) of cutting above the pubic bone rather than below; and Hildanus's method of using a dilator, the method further developed by Colot. "[Colot's method] excels that of *Hildanus* and others which lately have been much in use, in respect of safety, easiness, and expedition of the performance," Groenevelt noted. After explaining Colot's method, he wrote, "The Author of this Treatise has successfully practiced, and does practice this manner of Cure." In the margin, the one paragraph of the book written in Latin gave some examples of patients he had cured through his surgery.[35]

The book's dedication also clearly pointed to Groenevelt's ambitions. It meant to suggest that he had made connections among the highest-ranking segments of London society, for he dedicated it to the elderly Henry Pierrepoint, marquess of Dorchester, one of the highest-ranking and most learned noblemen of his day.[36] Dorchester had taken up the serious study of medicine, including chemical medicine, for which he had been made a fellow of the College of Physicians.[37] Groenevelt's dedication argues that physic is the most noble of arts, since it deals with health, which is "to be preferred before all Earthly Possessions," while its subject is "the Body of Man, the

Perfection of the Universe, and the most Noble of all terrestrial creatures."
Many honorable persons and princes had therefore made medicine their study,
including the Egyptian king Ptolemy, Sabor, and Alexander the Great, to
which list Dorchester himself "added new Rayes to its lustre by [his] own
private studies, and favouring of it." It is possible that Dorchester's medical
interests had caused him to meet the new Dutch lithotomist in London, since
according to custom authors ordinarily dedicated their books to patrons they
knew, however slightly. But if Groenevelt did not know Dorchester already,
he certainly hoped to after the publication of his little book.

While Groenevelt's work seems aimed at "making himself more known
by it than he was before," as Mandeville would put it, it did not smack
of commercialism nearly as much as that of some of his eminent Dutch
contemporaries, such as Cornelis Bontekoe and Steven Blankaart. Bontekoe
had taken his medical doctorate at Leiden just before Groenevelt arrived,
followed Sylvius's ideas about acids and alkalies closely, and had gained a
reputation as one of the most vehement Cartesians of the 1670s. Blankaart
had embarked upon his medical studies at Franeker, just after Groenevelt
had earned his degree. Both became famous physicians; both published
profusely on a variety of practical and learned medical subjects, mainly in
Dutch; and both promoted their own names and views, so much so that
Bontekoe's belief in the good effects of tea earned him the epithet "the tea
doctor" and brought rumors of being in the pay of the importers of tea, the
East India Company.[38] The medical commercialism of Amsterdam caused one
surgeon-physician there, Job van Meek'ren, to urge his medical colleagues not
to dream of greatness and riches but to aspire to lighting little true flames
that would together brighten the light of the medical art and lead to a more
certain medical future.[39] Pursuing the light of knowledge in particular complaints while at the same time informing the public of one's findings went
together quite comfortably among the famous and respectable Dutch practitioners; Groenevelt simply undertook the same kind of work in London, in
a somewhat more restrained manner.

The book did indeed both edify the public and help his surgical work to
prosper. By October 1681, in reply to a letter from his old friend Casparus
Sibelius, he proudly remarked that all the copies of his book had been sold
out and that his practice had developed very well. "Prosper and be strong,"
he closed; "the former we all search after."[40] In the spring of 1682, Groenevelt
crowed to his old friend about how he had successfully lithotomized a high-
ranking person: the son of Sir John Godwin, the king's commissioner to
Chatham (in an operation at which the two ministers of the Dutch church

had been present, apparently vouching for Groenevelt's good conduct); he later did the same for Godwin's other son.[41]

But his book not only succeeded in bringing him to the attention of the English public, including knights and even lords. It brought him to the notice of the London medical establishment, too.

English physicians were to Dutch ones as London was to Amsterdam: they had many similarities but some notable differences as well. Elite English physicians ordinarily obtained their medical degrees in one of the two local universities, Oxford or Cambridge. Unlike the new and humanistically oriented Dutch universities, the English universities had long-established intellectual traditions that made curricular change more difficult to institute; they also limited their enrollment to members of the Anglican church. At them, too, relatively few students embarked upon the study of medicine. Those who did proceeded to it only after having obtained a bachelor of arts degree, and the number of years it took to get from the B.A. to an M.D. was commonly about seven. Throughout their education, English physicians acquired a fine sense of Latin and deeply immersed themselves in books, just like their Dutch colleagues, but they spent much less time in the study of chemistry and clinical cases. They might take private lessons in chemistry and spend time with an accomplished physician to learn how to observe and treat diseases, but these efforts they undertook outside the ordinary medical curriculum, which required the students to dispute in depth about various philosophical issues raised by the texts.[42] The professors stressed niceties of argument more than practical teaching. As a sign of this, instead of being examined on Hippocrates, as at Leiden, candidates for the M.D. at Oxford had to expound a passage from Galen, the prince of the philosopher-physicians.[43] To circumvent these onerous textual studies, many English medical students traveled abroad—often to Leiden—to study a more practical course of medicine and then returned to have their degrees "incorporated" in their home universities, giving them all the privileges of regular Oxford or Cambridge M.D.'s. Nevertheless, academic tradition in England remained rather defensive about requiring students to know their philosophy thoroughly, looking down on too clinical an education.

Given the scholastic and Anglican traditions of Oxford and Cambridge, the "new philosophy" could sometimes seem threatening to the medical establishment.[44] Chemical medicine, for instance, was often seen as an alternative to, rather than a component of, English university medicine. From before William Harvey's time, a knowledge of anatomy had distinguished the English learned physician from the half-learned or unlearned prac-

titioner.[45] But some of the opponents of the English medical elite turned the
tables, writing about anatomical investigations as being like a quack's show:
"In this latter Age, the great Pranks [the physicians] play now are by *mounting
the Stage of Anatomy,* (for that pass 'tis now come to) where many of them
are wont ever and anon, to make wondrous Ostentation of pretended new
Discoveries in the little World of Man; with which they have a *Mint* always
going, for coining new *Hypostheses,* out of which they start up their *Various
Dogmaticisms,* to amaze their Admirers, and amuse the World."[46] Since the
author of these words, however, was writing a preface to an English translation
of a book by Groenevelt's former teacher, Sylvius, he had to go to great
lengths to explain why Sylvius himself had spent time in anatomy, blaming
it on the fact that he held a professorship that demanded such useless things.[47]
In the Netherlands, anatomy, chemistry, botany, clinical studies, and Latinate
learning were all part of the same medical curriculum, but in England practitioners tended to be polarized into camps, with the chemists taking on
anatomists, or clinicians logicians.[48]

But the differences between learned Anglican physicians and others were
not only those of placing a different stress on various parts of medical
knowledge. Questions of personal character entered into the equation as well.
A proper English education inculcated aristocratic ideas of honor and liberality
which allowed the best students to become "scholars and gentlemen" in their
bearing. Although people of learning could never quite be treated as true
gentlemen unless they found a good and secure income, the elite physicians
did not openly charge fees, relying on "honoraria" freely offered.[49] A Cambridge or Oxford education also taught the student the use of "right reason,"
a particular kind of reason central to the moderate Anglican outlook, derived
from scholastic ideas about the connections between virtue and the knowledge
of God and nature.[50] Since the essence of a good medical practice, like
an honorable pastorate or law practice, was sound judgment, an advanced
education imparted more than mere knowledge: it gave the graduate "science,"
or what one author called "a habit" of mind, "a ready, prompt and bent
disposition to do any thynge confirmed and gotten by long study, exercise,
and use."[51] The end of an English university education was not merely to
supply the student with information, then; it was also to develop a certain
kind of character in the future physician, from which his judgment would
flow.[52] All this meant that the English medical establishment expected certain
kinds of behavior and learning from its gentleman-scholars which a Calvinist
Dutchman—or an English religious dissenter—would not possess, no matter
how learned and upright he might be in his own eyes.

Moreover, in London the Anglican medical establishment dominated the College of Physicians. It could make someone a full member of the college (a fellow, or if a vacancy was not yet open, a candidate), or an honorary fellow, or simply grant a license to practice within the college's jurisdiction (licentiate). The fellows were supposed to possess an English M.D. (or an incorporated foreign degree); the honorary fellows and licentiates might have a foreign degree or none at all. The officers of the college who decided whom to let in and whom to reject, the president and censors, often allowed nonmembers to practice quietly in London without applying for membership, as long as they did not either criticize the college, cause a great deal of harm, or try to get up a practice that might rival those of college members.

During his first few years of practice in London, then, Groenevelt had been virtually invisible to the college: he did not apply for its license, and it did not bother him. But his book, containing a fawning dedication to a viscount, caused them to take notice. Moreover, the book contained certain matters that would have offended the learned English physicians. Groenevelt had undoubtedly published the paragraph about his surgical successes in Latin so as not to appear to be advertising his practice. But although he kept the most direct testimony in Latin, Groenevelt used patients' names at one place in the text (something that many advertising practitioners did liberally as a form of testimonial), and he drew a strong connection between the best method of lithotomy (the "Collotian") and his own practice. All this clearly made the book something more than a simple contribution to medical knowledge. The association between publishing a book and seeking publicity was so strong in the minds of gentlemen and would-be gentlemen-physicians that many notable contributions to medicine, like William Harvey's work on the discovery of the circulation of the blood, begin with profuse apologies for making their ideas known through print. Many of the highest-ranking English physicians therefore never published, or went to great lengths to make sure that they could not be seen as in any way trying to expand their practices through publication. Even the much-published Thomas Sydenham (who came from a gentry family) made sure to bring out his notable studies of disease in Latin and to avoid using the names of any of the patients he had treated. Making medical pitches to the general public, and especially to the gentry and aristocracy, often drew the ire of the officers of the college.

Therefore, about a year after his book appeared, the Censors of the College of Physicians required Groenevelt to come to one of their meetings, to justify his practice without their license. They were just then suing in the law courts another unlicensed Dutch practitioner in London with aspirations among the gentry and nobility, Adriaan Huyberts.[53] Groenevelt came when summoned, on 1 February 1678, accompanied by Gerhard van Meulen, yet another Dutch practitioner. (Van Meulen may have come to the censors' attention when they made inquiries about Groenevelt, and it is just possible that he and Groenevelt had known each other previously in Amsterdam.)[54] Groenevelt told the censors about his degree and explained that he wanted to practice lithotomy among the English according to the royal edict of June 1672, which he interpreted as granting him the rights of any English person. Van Meulen, who came from Gelderland, a province neighboring Overijssel, was then living in the same neighborhood as Groenevelt in London, the Minories, and he wanted similar permission to treat anyone suffering from dropsy (an accumulation of watery fluid in the body). The censors were reluctant to accept the king's edict as making an exception to their own statutory right to prohibit all practitioners not licensed by themselves, but Groenevelt and Van Meulen seem to have held their ground, for they finally left the meeting with the matter unresolved.[55]

Groenevelt gradually made English medical friends who, like him, considered themselves "practical" doctors. Unconcerned about keeping what physicians did separate from what surgeons and apothecaries practiced, they borrowed eclectically from anyone who seemed to have a good treatment, and they energetically tried to develop new remedies. His correspondence with Sibelius illustrates that from an early period in his London days Groenevelt admired works other than those written by the English medical elite. Sibelius had initiated contact by asking Groenevelt whether a copy of an English medical book could be sent to him: George Starkey's *Pyrotechny Asserted & Illustrated* (1658). Unfortunately, the book could no longer be found in London, so Groenevelt sent him instead Starkey's *Nature's Explication and Helmont's Vindication* (1657) bound together with *An epistolar discourse* (1665). Starkey's books, especially the latter two, were highly polemical tracts in favor of Helmontian medicine, aimed against the conservative London medical elite.[56] Groenevelt also suggested that Sibelius would be interested in the "best midwives' book ever published or to be had in English," Nicholas Culpeper's *Directory for midwives* (1651, with seven subsequent editions before Groenevelt wrote): this was yet another book by a noted anticollegiate practitioner.[57] He soon informed Sibelius that "among the famous surgeons here, the edition of one Wiseman in folio is greatly admired."[58] Wiseman was a royal surgeon with previous experience in the Dutch navy and a friend of the Dutch chemical practitioner Adriaan Huyberts, having intervened with the College of Physicians in 1675 when they sued Huyberts.[59]

Groenevelt also urged Sibelius to look into the "greatly esteemed" just-published work of the doctor of theology John Jones, which he would send over if Sibelius wanted to purchase it.[60] None of these were books written by the most learned English physicians, such as Thomas Willis: far from it.

It was largely on the advice of his English friends that Groenevelt recommended such books. The titles clearly show that he had fallen in with a crowd decidedly unhappy with the medicine of the learned Oxbridge physicians. The most famous of his new acquaintances was Thomas Sydenham, whom he met in 1682. Already renowned for developing radically new methods for treating fevers, Sydenham placed himself in the Hippocratic tradition, like so many of the Dutch physicians; he even became known as "the English Hippocrates." Some members of the English medical establishment occasionally worried that his views might be subversive, so that Sydenham never rose above the rank of licentiate in the College of Physicians.[61] Sydenham himself sided with those who argued that anatomical knowledge helped not a jot in finding cures for diseases.[62] He explicitly conceived of medical knowledge as being for use, emphasizing therapy over ratiocination, and was happy to break with long-accepted methods of treatment based upon theory when he thought experience showed a better way.[63] Like Robert Boyle and other leading lights of the new science in England, Sydenham stressed observation and "matters of fact" as the basis for all knowledge. As he put it in a letter to Dr. Gould, "As I have bin very carefull to write nothing but the product of faithfull observation, soe when ye scandall of my person shall be layd aside, and I in my grave, it will appear, that I neither suffered myselfe to be decieved by indulging to idle speculations nor have decieved others by obtruding any thing upon them but downright matter of fact."[64]

Groenevelt several times urged Sibelius to read the works of this hero of the English "practical" physicians, works that were available at or printed in Amsterdam,[65] while keeping him informed of new books by Sydenham hot off the presses in London.[66] Groenevelt seems to have met Sydenham shortly before June 1682, when he noted that he was an upstanding man: "I am especially well acquainted with him," he wrote, although at the same time misspelling Sydenham's name.[67] On a later occasion, when Groenevelt passed on to his Dutch friend the recipe Sydenham used for one of his medicines, he wrote that "this formula and all the foregoing explanations have come from Heer Sydenham's own mouth."[68]

Sydenham was not the only practical physician with whom Groenevelt associated during the mid-1680s. Four others both emphasized medicine for use and took religiously dissenting views. Two were, like Groenevelt, foreigners practicing in London: Christopher Crell and Philip Guide. Christopher Crell Spinowski (who dropped his last name in England) was originally from Poland. He earned his M.D. from Leiden with a rather superficial treatise on bladder stones in 1682.[69] Given the subject of his thesis, Crell would quickly have become aware of Groenevelt's practice shortly after he arrived in London; their acquaintance began at least as early as their induction into the College of Physicians together. He seems to have been a Socinian (the Socinians followed a form of anti-Trinitarianism developed during the early seventeenth century by the Italian theologian Socinus—Fausto Paolo Sozzini—who had taken refuge in Poland).[70] The French Calvinist physician Philip Guide had been born near the eastern French border, at Châlons-sur-Saône, in the early 1640s and studied medicine at Montpellier, where he probably took his M.D. He had come to England in 1681 as a Calvinist refugee from Louis XIV's religious persecutions, after having practiced for about a dozen years in Paris. He quickly obtained denization and took the licentiate of the College of Physicians at the same time as Groenevelt and Crell.[71] The two short medical works he had published in Paris show him to be an experimentalist practitioner: one work utilized Robert Boyle's air pump to analyze drugs and the condition of the blood, carried out through experiments on animals; the other discussed venereal disease and his new methods of mercury treatment for it.[72] Once in London, he quickly published another short book in the form of two letters to Boyle, on red wine for relieving urinary complaints and on quinquina bark for fevers, while he also contributed a paper to the Royal Society.[73]

These two foreign licentiates of the College of Physicians, together with Groenevelt, were well acquainted with two English physicians. The elder of the two Englishmen was Richard Browne. Born on 15 June 1633, he attended Oxford before taking up medical practice; after serving at Port Royal in Jamaica from the late 1660s, he went on to earn an M.D. from Leiden in 1675, and he took the college licentiate in 1676.[74] He was an accomplished translator of Latin[75] and later helped edit the English in one of Groenevelt's books.[76] The younger of the two, John Pechey, was another follower of Sydenham's, the first translator of Sydenham's works into English. Born in 1654, the son of a medical and surgical practitioner in Chichester, Pechey was also well educated, having spent six years at New Inn Hall, Oxford, where he took his B.A. and M.A. (in June 1678) before taking up medical practice himself, although he appears never to have earned an M.D. He obtained his licentiate at the end of 1684 and published profusely, including a translation of many of Sydenham's works into English begun while Sydenham was still living.[77] Probably Browne, and certainly Pechey, were sympathetic to Nonconformists (those who could not subscribe to the thirty-nine articles of faith of the Anglican church) such as their three foreign associates, if they were not ones themselves.

These five practitioners took a view of medicine which irritated the leaders of the London College of Physicians. The little group stood among a long line of people who—from the late sixteenth century right through the late nineteenth—argued that the learned physicians' claims to superiority rested on book learning instead of medical experience, the latter of which was the true and original source of healing knowledge. In the introduction to one of his books, for example, Pechey wrote, "Plain Practice must expect but cold Entertainment with the speculative Physician, but such as mind and study Practice, will, I question not, patronize the Undertaking." Pechey firmly believed that "nothing has so much obstructed the Improvement of the Art of Physick, as the late unaccountable Humour of Romancing on the Nature and the Causes of Diseases." Despite the fact that "these Broachers of Whimsies [are] dignified with the Titles of Philosophers and Virtuoso's," "Reason and Argument are not the true Tests of Physick, nor indeed of any thing else, when Experience, the great Baffler of Speculation, can determine the Matter." His advice to aspiring physicians followed accordingly: "Spend not too much time upon Anatomy, Chymistry, and Herbs . . . [for] if you consume the greatest part of your time in these Preliminaries, you will be as foppish as those young Sparks that give themselves up to Dancing and Fiddling, and neglect Arm and History, the true Accomplishments of a Gentleman: But above all, be not inveigled with an Hypothesis, the bane of Art." Instead, the student should study clinical practice: "Associate with such practical Physicians as make their own Medicines, and assist in the making of Medicines, and see their Practice, [and only then] add Reading to Practice."[78] In another of his works, he scolded "the vain fictions of a sort of men, whose business it is, to make every part of [medicine] obscure and misterious."[79] Such remarks were clearly aimed straight at the leaders of the College of Physicians, who claimed medical superiority based upon the dignity and learning that came from years spent in study at an English university rather than apprenticeship in the field. Pechey even dedicated his first translation to the surgeons' company, even though the work, by Sydenham, had nothing to do with surgery.[80] In it he even declared, "That part of Physick we call Chyrurgery, is to be preferr'd before the other two, viz. Pharmacy, and the Dietetick part, if we consider the Antiquity and Use thereof."[81] After finding that the opposition of the London medical elite almost put an end to his project of translating Sydenham, Pechey openly attacked those "who arrogantly appropriate to themselves all that's excellent in Physick."[82] Pechey's colleagues shared his sentiments in favor of practice standing before theory.

They also believed that, since the goal of medicine was to find cures for diseases, the best practitioners would be people who knew all the branches of medicine. As one of Groenevelt's colleagues—perhaps Browne—diplomatically put it in a work of surgery in which an English translation of one of Groenevelt's works appeared:

> Such considerations [about the separation of medicine into the three branches of diet, pharmacy, and surgery] had once more than half persuaded me to have written only of Chirurgical Operations, without medling either with Medicine or method of Cure. But upon second Thoughts, and a review, finding Celsus of opinion, that one Man may be able to be all; a good Physician, Chirurgeon, and Apothecary; and where one Man is not all, the more of them he is, the more commendable; I thought it better to take notice of so much Medicine and Method, as fairly offered themselves in the way of Chirurgery. Since the parts of Physick are so interwoven one with another, that they cannot be well separated.[83]

Groenevelt himself became a member of a committee supporting increased privileges for the surgeons' company in 1690.[84]

But this group of practitioners went much further in their criticism of the learned physicians. None of these five practical physicians—nor Sydenham himself—had reason to be especially supportive of the officers of the College of Physicians. With the growing domestic power of the Crown in the early 1680s, the college had been hoping to increase its authority. Late in the reign of Charles II, and even more so after the accession in 1685 of his Catholic brother, James II, the Crown looked to corporations like the college to help it police the public. An irregular college committee operated efficiently behind the scenes to gain its institution the favor of the Crown, which resulted in its obtaining a new and stronger charter in the summer of 1687, accompanied by formal letters (written by the committee and signed by the king) to make sure that all government officers helped the college sort out London medical practitioners.[85] When the College of Physicians' new charter arrived, many of the honorary fellows and licentiates became fellows, including several foreigners and a large number of people with only foreign M.D.'s—but not any of the five, and not even Sydenham.

For the next ten years, Groenevelt would continue to have a mixed relationship with the London medical establishment. He and they would continue to maintain somewhat different values pertaining to medical practice and learning, with the college censors retaining their suspicions of this non-Anglican and activist physician. But Groenevelt would also do what he could to advance his career, including becoming a licentiate of the college.

At the end of the summer of 1682, Groenevelt proudly signed himself "Fellow of the London College of Physicians" in a letter to his old friend, Sibelius.[86] This might have been meant simply as a vain boast. But since he never again signed a letter using that title, it seems more likely that there had been some misunderstanding. The most probable explanation is that he had been promised by someone in the college that he would be put up for fellow, and that he stood every chance of getting it.

That Groenevelt could imagine himself entering the London medical elite in 1682 is quite possible, given his new association with the Royal Society. Founded shortly after the English Restoration of 1660, and granted a charter by the king, the "Royal Society for the Promoting of Natural Knowledge" (as it was styled in its 1663 charter) brought together a select group of gentlemen and professionals who promoted the "new philosophy."[87] Since the new philosophy included experimental natural history, chemistry, and medicine, the views of the "virtuosi," as they called themselves, sometimes exasperated learned physicians; but many of the more experimentally inclined among the English physicians joined the society and encouraged its work.[88] Clearly, being introduced to the virtuosi would be a step forward for someone like Groenevelt. His opportunity came through his old friend Willem ten Rhijne early in 1682.

In July 1681, Ten Rhijne had written to Henry Oldenburg, the secretary of the Royal Society, about a work of his on Japanese medicine. Ten Rhijne, in the service of the Dutch East India Company (VOC), had arrived in Batavia (modern Jakarta) in January 1674.[89] Six months later he left for the Dutch trading post at Deshima, in the harbor of Nagasaki, where he remained for more than two years, ministering to the needs of the Dutch embassy and picking up what medical lore he could from his Japanese hosts. After further assignments by the VOC, he returned to Batavia, where he became a member of the Council of Justice and the rector of the Latin school. He wrote up an account of some of the new methods of healing he had encountered, particularly a polished manuscript on the use of moxibustion (burning moxa on points of the body) and acupuncture, and a rough draft of one on Chinese pulse doctrine and sent copies of the manuscripts to friends in Europe, at the same time asking Oldenburg if the Royal Society wanted to examine the finished treatise for publication.[90] The virtuosi of the Royal Society thought that Ten Rhijne's views on moxibustion and acupuncture would be very interesting. The practice of moxibustion had recently come to the serious attention of the virtuosi through Constantijn Huygens, secretary to the prince of Orange, who had heard about it in turn from the son of one Hermann Busschoff, a minister in Batavia and an acquaintance of Ten Rhijne's.[91] The elder Busschoff had found relief from his gout through allowing a local "Indian doctress" to burn moxa on his toe. He described the moxa as "a very soft and woolly substance, made by a very skilful preparation out of a certain dried Herb," formed into "a little pellet . . . which is scarce of the bigness of a small white pea, at one end somewhat sharp, and at the other end flat," placed with the flat end on the skin and then set alight. It quickly burned, leaving only a bit of oil on the skin.[92] A translation of Busschoff's treatise had been published in 1676 by the Royal Society, while on Huygens' recommendation the English ambassador in The Hague, Sir William Temple, tried moxibustion on his gout and also experienced relief from it.[93] Consequently, both because interest in moxibustion had already been piqued and because acupuncture had hardly been heard of, Ten Rhijne's letter elicited considerable discussion, resulting in widespread enthusiasm for encouraging Ten Rhijne to publish his manuscript under the auspices of the Royal Society.

A delegation therefore paid a visit to the contact Ten Rhijne had mentioned in London—his boyhood friend Joannes Groenevelt—asking Groenevelt to arrange to have Ten Rhijne's manuscript sent over, which they undertook to publish at their own expense.[94] Groenevelt immediately wrote to his old friend Sibelius in Amsterdam to make the arrangements.[95] After beginning in theology like his father and grandfather before him, Sibelius had taken up the study of medicine, graduating from Leiden with an M.D. in June 1678; like Groenevelt before him, he was now living in Amsterdam as he tried to break into practice.[96] Sibelius and his friend, the noted Frederik Ruysch, had been handling Ten Rhijne's affairs in the Netherlands during his absence in the East Indies,[97] and so it was to them that Ten Rhijne had sent his manuscript. After some prying, Groenevelt got the manuscript sent over and put into the hands of the Royal Society; by the end of June, Groenevelt could report to Sibelius that the Royal Society planned to print Ten Rhijne's treatise in quarto, and asked Sibelius to have Ten Rhijne's picture sent over, so that it could be engraved for the frontispiece.[98]

The manuscript may have been more than the society had bargained for: the final printed Latin and Dutch text took up 334 pages. It contained several essays: an introduction by Busschoff; a general discussion of the gout (includ-

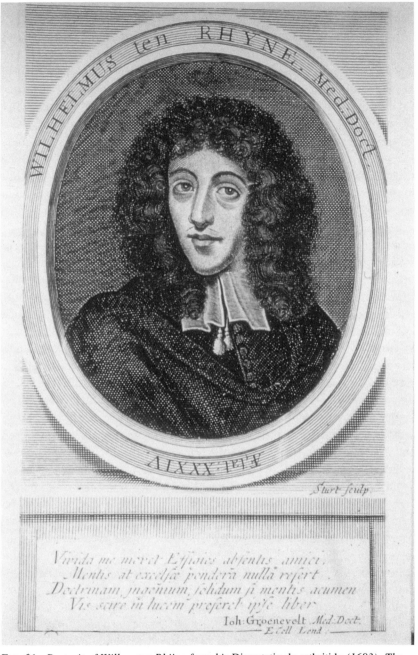

FIG. 21. *Portrait of Willem ten Rhijne from his* Dissertatio de arthritide *(1683). The Latin verse beneath by Groenevelt translates as: "The living portrait of my absent friend stirs me, though it does not show the depth of his high mind. If you wish to know the learning, genius, and pithy sharpness of his mind, this book itself will bring it to light."*

ing a section on its cure by caustics, among them moxibustion); four Japanese diagrams showing the points to which the moxa and the acupuncture needles ought to be applied, together with a short description of Japanese medical practice; a discussion of acupuncture; an account of a pestilential fever that had struck a ship he was aboard; and three assorted essays (on the antiquity and dignity of chemistry and botany, on physiognomy—the reading of a person's character by his or her face—and on monsters). Japanese and Chinese doctrines were interpreted in light of pneuma circulating in the blood.[99] About a year after Aston had written Sibelius that the Royal Society would publish the book, it finally appeared (with the engraved portrait and a little Latin motto by Groenevelt), and Groenevelt forwarded to Sibelius sixty-six of the sixty-eight copies intended for Ten Rhijne (keeping two for himself).[100] A long account of the work quickly appeared in the Royal Society's *Philosophical Transactions,* and a Dutch translation was published not long after.[101] The interest among the virtuosi in moxibustion also soon led Sydenham to mention it favorably in his book on the gout as well, although without acknowledging Ten Rhijne,[102] while the book also caused physicians in Germany to use it with apparent success.[103]

Groenevelt continued to serve as an occasional intermediary in exchanges between Aston and Ten Rhijne. Since Groenevelt was neither an English gentleman nor an important foreign investigator, he had to keep in touch with the Royal Society through Aston and Houghton rather than being asked to join the group. As one of the society's secretaries, Aston was charged with keeping up a correspondence with possibly interesting people like Ten Rhijne, while Houghton had many friends among the less exalted followers of the new philosophy.[104] Through them, Groenevelt communicated to the Royal Society Ten Rhijne's reminder that he had written an essay on the Chinese doctrine of touching the pulse much superior to Cleyer's (who he believed had simply paid someone to translate a Chinese book into Latin rather than studying the subject himself). Ten Rhijne offered to polish it for publication if the society desired.[105] Having already invested much in Ten Rhijne's first book, however, the members of the Royal Society let this last request go unanswered.

It may have been these various contacts with members of the Royal Society which led someone to suggest that Groenevelt would make a fine fellow of the College of Physicians. Unfortunately for him, this was impossible without an Oxford or Cambridge M.D. (or the incorporation of his Utrecht M.D. at one of the two English universities).

During 1682, however, the College of Physicians was trying to expand its authority. One of the fellows, George Rogers, had used the occasion of the annual Harveian Oration to suggest that the college needed to better police the multitude of unlicensed practitioners in the metropolis.[106] Groenevelt remained one of them. A Jewish doctor by the name of Jacobus Sylvius, who had studied medicine at Leiden during Groenevelt's years there and had recently come to London and visited with Groenevelt, was among those sued by the college for unlicensed practice, although a fellow, Dr. Humphrey Brooke, finally persuaded the censors to drop their suit on the condition that Sylvius pay all the legal fees and no longer practice in London.[107] During the spring of 1682, too, the person with whom Groenevelt had come to the college in 1678, Gerhard van Meulen, was sued by the college for practicing without its license for twenty months (amounting to a fine of £100). Van Meulen managed to find someone at court to take up this matter with the king, who allowed Edward, Viscount Conway, to issue a letter to the college in his name asking it to drop the suit. Conway had been a friend of empirical physicians before, and he wrote that the king had taken Van Meulen into his protection "for his eminent skill" in treating dropsy and gout because of the "good testimony" that had been received about his successful practice in these two diseases.[108] But the College of Physicians humbly stuck to its guns, stating "[We are] bound by solemne Oath by law, and by the duty we owe both to your Majestie and to the safety of your subjects, by the due course of Law to prosecute all Empiricks, and other illegal Practicioners of Physick whatsoever in London." The college also claimed that it had heard many complaints from people of "good quality and credit" against "several dangerous and fatal effects" of Van Meulen's practice. It therefore humbly beseeched His Majesty to leave this matter to the law courts.[109] Nothing more was heard about Van Meulen's lawsuit, although Thomas Novell, a fellow, was given a warning (after being threatened with a fine of £10) for consulting with Van Meulen in April 1683.[110]

The growing threat of lawsuits and virtual excommunication from the community of physicians for unlicensed practice therefore caused a number of London practitioners to come to the College of Physicians and apply for their license, including Groenevelt. He arranged to undergo the usual three-part oral Latin examination in physiology, pathology, and therapy at the beginning of January, February, and March 1683, respectively. Although he passed to the censors' satisfaction, it must have been a humbling experience to be at the mercy of the approval of the London physicians, despite his university degree and years of successful practice. But it was probably better than being sued. That the several people who underwent examination during the same time did so under threat is suggested by the fact that the college soon decided that no one would be admitted to the examinations on the pretext of being prosecuted unless he showed a letter of testimony to that effect. Groenevelt must have felt some relief when he stood as one among six physicians who were inducted as licentiates ("as long as they conduct[ed] themselves properly") at one of the large quarterly meetings of the college on 2 April 1683, paying £10 for the privilege.[111]

Groenevelt continued to pursue his medical and surgical interests in stones with vigor. He had successfully operated on Sir John Godwin's elder son in 1682, and in 1684 Godwin was seeking further help from Groenevelt. Godwin wrote a letter to "the most famous, and certainly erudite and experienced," Groenevelt on 2 March. In the case of his elder son, Godwin had tried all sorts of lithontriptics offered by impudent empirics, but his hopes had been dashed, leaving his son tortured by stones until he had been freed of them by surgery. He hoped that Groenevelt knew of some medicine that would gently free his younger son of the ailment. Groenevelt replied (citing Galen) that unfortunately, despite his sympathy for Godwin's younger son, there was no medicine he could recommend.[112] But he did try to find out more about a Dutch empiric who had practiced in London for a year, "even though it is against" the statutes of the college. This Captain Rijbeeck gave out blue powders as a lithontriptic, which Godwin thought to be completely fraudulent; Groenevelt was certain that Rijbeeck's son-in-law, Hendrijck ten Toorn, who had been "a special friend" of his when Groenevelt lived in Amsterdam, knew the recipe. Over the course of several letters, Groenevelt wheedled Sibelius into seeking out Ten Toorn for him. Groenevelt had "seen great effects from the medicines of the Captain," although he noted that such a view went "against the feelings of the doctors" who governed the college as well as Godwin's. In the end, however, Rijbeeck's recipe turned out to be nothing but calcified mussel shells with spirit of juniper added, a remedy good for gravel but not effective in breaking urinary calculi, Groenevelt thought.[113]

Without a new breakthrough on lithontriptics, lithotomists like Groenevelt had plenty to do. Perhaps as a kind of reply to Groenevelt's English work on calculi, an English translation of a French work on lithotomy was published in late 1682, dedicated to Thomas Hobbs, the lithotomist of St. Bartholomew's Hospital. The original French work had been published by François Tolet earlier in 1682. Another person who had learned Colot's surgical methods,[114] Tolet wasted few words on the causes or medical treatments for stones, spending almost the whole of the text describing the various forms of the operation to remove them. This he did clearly, and with illustrations.[115] Given the public interest in lithotomy, a London publisher almost immediately brought out an English edition, which exactly followed Tolet's French and also reproduced his illustrations.[116] The dedication to Hobbs reminded the public of the most visible native English lithotomist.[117]

Now that he had finished seeing Ten Rhijne's work through the press, Groenevelt replied to the English edition of Tolet with yet another book on the subject, this one meant to keep his reputation high among his new colleagues of the college. His *Dissertatio Lithologica,* an octavo of 137 pages in large type, was again based on his Utrecht dissertation but with a few new points and, like Tolet, including several illustrations. One of the illustrations, that of the lithotomist's knife, was clearly based on the same illustration in Tolet, and others, such as the picture of various stones, or the way in which a child would be held for the Celsian operation, had their inspiration in Tolet's pictures, although they were not as well executed.[118]

The preface to Groenevelt's new book told the story of how Groenevelt had fallen in with Velthuis and so had taken up the practice of a matter he had first investigated as a student and physician. In it, too, he praised physicians who engaged in surgery to further the art, like the Roman Celsus and the Swiss Hildanus, while he also tried to make the Hippocratic injunction again cutting for the stone into a mere historical artifact. He also noted that the statutes of the London college allowed physicians to exercise the whole of medicine, in all its parts, including surgery. He therefore pursued lithotomy out of both Christian love and pity for the weak patients.[119] The text reassembled his original twenty-three theses into twenty-six "articles" and added further examples to illustrate his points. As before, he discussed the disease, its causes and preventive regimens, and the possible treatments. These medical aspects of the subject had been largely ignored by Tolet. On the question of lithontriptics, Groenevelt was fair-minded but clearly a bit suspicious by now. If the bladder stones were loosely concreted from sand and mucus, they might be broken up by a medicine made from millipedes, he wrote; in other cases, spirit of niter—a potential lithontriptic recommended by his teacher Sylvius—occasionally worked.[120] But given the common need to have the stones removed surgically, he concluded with a description of the various methods of lithotomy. Although he detailed these methods more briefly than Tolet, he also provided descriptions of methods not used by the French surgeon, arranged as before into six kinds. The book combined the medical and surgical aspects of treating calculi better than Tolet. Groenevelt sent Sibelius copies of his book with a request that he pass them on to various old friends.[121]

The new book was a success. A second edition appeared within three years.[122] An English translation also soon appeared in a general work of surgery edited by one of Groenevelt's new English friends.[123] The editor might have used Tolet, but instead he took the trouble to make Groenevelt available in English. "An thô several have writ on this subject [of lithotomy,] yet I shall only make use of what one of my Colleagues, Dr. Groenevelt (of whose lithotomical administrations I have been an Eye-Witness, and of whose success therein, not only I, but multitudes are witnesses) has made publick on this subject."[124] Very quickly, too, Groenevelt's work became the new authority on lithotomy cited by Mangeti in editing the works of the Dutch surgeon Paulus Barbette; Mangeti praised Groenevelt's book highly and used it heavily in adding footnotes to bring Barbette up to date.[125]

Groenevelt sent Sibelius not only copies of his new book but also other information about English medical books and authors and about drugs being used in London, even forwarding quantities of medicines themselves—as long as Sibelius paid for them.[126] He hosted a number of Dutch friends of Sibelius's in London and obtained letters of introduction for them.[127] But in return for passing on books and information, and for helping to get out their friend Ten Rhijne's book, Groenevelt asked Sibelius to undertake many and various favors for him in the Netherlands. He asked him to send over the new edition of Van Beverwijck's work on stones when it came out. He referred a London apothecary, Israel Wormall, to Sibelius, when Wormall wanted to be put in contact with an Amsterdam apothecary who could supply him with various drugs.[128] He managed to persuade Sibelius to pay off the loan Groenevelt had taken out in Amsterdam in 1674.[129] He even got Sibelius to travel several times to Delft to have his library packed up and sent over; and to look into getting the books returned which the family he had left them with had kept (or sold) for themselves.[130] An inheritance from his father-in-law brought him enough money to pay off his loans and underwrite the costs of shipping his books, but he needed Sibelius to spend a considerable amount of time and effort actually extracting the books from their keepers and arranging shipment.[131] For this favor Groenevelt offered his profuse thanks and a present for Sibelius's wife "which people here wear on their forearm [called] a bracelett." He also noted, "I would have sent you a dozen pewter plates for yourself, but I thought you would not accept them thus"; he later offered to send Sibelius the twelve plates, but for 14s.[132] Of course, Groenevelt wheedled Sibelius into investigating Captain Rijbeeck's lithontriptic for him, too.

It would appear that Groenevelt's constant demands on Sibelius, like his constant promises to settle up any debts he owed Sibelius because of his efforts, wore thin. Sibelius eventually broke off the correspondence. Two years after he did Groenevelt the favor of pestering Ten Toorn for his father-in-law's lithontriptic, Sibelius received a further missive from Groenevelt in which the latter pleaded: "I have been very unfortunate in not having heard from you for so long. In case I have given you any 'discontent' at me because of 'neglect' or anything else, I pray to be excused. Or if I still owe you anything for what you have sent over to me, you shall be fully thanked."[133]

That Groenevelt could be difficult became clear, too, in a lawsuit against him lodged by John Browne, surgeon of St. Thomas's Hospital. Groenevelt's reputation as a lithotomist had become great enough that Browne studied with him for a time to learn his technique. But Browne came to be quite unhappy with the treatment he received from Groenevelt. We only know about their relationship because of a lawsuit brought by Browne against Groenevelt in 1687.[134] Browne was a very successful self-promoter: he took the title of "royal surgeon," which, one contemporary wrote, "was procur'd him" by his sister, who managed it because she was "of private use to some Courtiers"; he had obtained a position as surgeon to St. Thomas's Hospital through court favor over the objections of the governors; and he wrote several books, the *Compleat Treatise of the Muscles* being largely plagiarized from William Molins but underwritten by a subscription to which a great many peers gave money.[135] The surgeons who had a competence in lithotomy had recently retired from St. Thomas's Hospital, but the hospital statutes still provided for an extra fee for operations for stones performed on the poor inmates.[136] Browne would therefore have benefited from learning the procedure from Groenevelt. For his part, Groenevelt may well have seen going into business with Browne as a way to increase his connections with the highest levels of English society.

The contract drawn up between the two is revealing about Groenevelt's surgical practice. Browne and Groenevelt set down their agreement in 1686.[137] For the first year of their arrangement, Groenevelt agreed to notify Browne at least two days in advance of each operation he was to perform; Groenevelt would do the cutting and allow Browne to observe his technique, while Browne himself took care of the patients postoperatively. For the care Browne provided, Groenevelt would pay him 5s. on every pound he earned (that is, one-quarter of the amount) over and above the first £5, unless the patient objected to having Browne involved. (From a later report, it would appear that patients paid Groenevelt at least £20 for a successful lithotomy; if he regularly kept the first £5 for himself, and paid a quarter to one-half of the rest to his assistants, Groenevelt would have been clearing between £12 and £15 per operation, a tidy sum.)[138] After May 1687, Browne had the option of delegating the postoperative dressing of the wounds to a servant or to another surgeon employed by him; at the same time, Browne would also call in Groenevelt for all the lithotomies he performed except those done at St. Thomas's. In return for Groenevelt's teaching, Browne would pay him "one full Moyety [i.e., half] of the Reward" earned by Browne from his own lithotomies. The agreement was to be in effect for seven years, and if either party failed to live up to it, he would forfeit £100.

Frictions soon developed, however: Groenevelt argued that Browne was not taking care of the patients as promised, and Browne stated that Groenevelt did not notify him of all his operations. They differed particularly about the postoperative care of one Mr. Champion, a minister. Groenevelt claimed that Browne had been so negligent in dressing Champion's wounds that he, Groenevelt, had been forced to call in others to save the patient; Browne claimed that Groenevelt had said his own servants would take care of Champion but then left town with them to perform another lithotomy, so that Browne had to nurse Champion back from a dangerous infection of his scrotum. Groenevelt further stated that after Browne had failed to live up to his side of the bargain in caring for Champion, he would have nothing more to do with Browne, and that he and Browne agreed to waive their former contract. But Browne brought an action of debt against Groenevelt after Groenevelt operated on one Thomas Wright without calling Browne in. Groenevelt therefore pled in Chancery for relief from Browne's suit, believing that Browne had been the first to break their agreement. Browne argued that they had not legally voided their contract and that he had demanded his £100 from Groenevelt for failing to live up to their agreement only after he heard from a friend of Groenevelt's that another surgeon had promised Groenevelt £100 to take Browne's place.[139] Whatever the merits of either side's claims, the case clearly shows that during the mid- and late 1680s Groenevelt was in demand by English patients who wanted to be cut for the stone, that he earned a good livelihood from it, and that influential English surgeons thought so highly of his methods that they offered to pay very large sums to learn it themselves.

The doctor also began training his son to carry on in his footsteps. Beginning in the late 1680s or early 1690s, as Franciscus Groenevelt reached his early teens, Groenevelt began to fill a notebook with detailed instructions for lithotomy, together with recipes for medicines of use in the practice, in

order to pass his knowledge on. Being a dissenter, he could not send Francis
to an English university, and he either could not or would not send him
abroad to a place like Leiden, bringing him up as his own apprentice instead.
But apparently in the mid-1690s, when he had reached his late teens, Francis
died.[140] Groenevelt therefore inserted a short "admonition" before his notes
using the past tense: "In writing notes (wch are of dayly use ffor a Lithotomist)
to this booke of myn i have writt course ordinary Latin, as boys use at
School; i writt it ffor my son Francis onely, considering his capacity, ffor
he never had university learning; God give his blessing to these, is with
Paternall Wish."[141]

Within ten years of his move to London, when still in his mid-thirties,
Groenevelt had obtained modest success. Now a lithotomist in demand, he
had established a good reputation for his work among the public, and English
surgeons were offering to pay him large fees to learn his surgical method.
He had published a Latin treatise on bladder stones which impressed surgeons
and physicians in England and Europe, had helped to see an old friend's
important work through the presses, and had met a number of members of
the Royal Society. He had earned the licentiate of the College of Physicians.
He had done all this without any dishonesty. But in London, Groenevelt and
his confreres remained a step below the medical establishment, even though
they had M.D.'s and wide experience. In the turmoil of the late 1680s, which
brought William III of Orange to the English throne in 1688, he and several
of his acquaintances would try to transform the medical arrangements in
London. They tried to expand their medical practices greatly among the
London public, not aways using methods accepted by the local medical
establishment. When the leaders of the College of Physicians heard of a
complaint against Groenevelt from Mrs. Withall, therefore, they would do
their best to make him pay for his insolence.

CHAPTER 6

The Troubles with Withall

BY THE END OF the 1680s, Joannes Groenevelt had established a successful surgical practice in London and had entered into a joint medical practice as well. He remained at the fringes of the London College of Physicians, although as a licentiate he had a right to practice freely no matter what the opinion of the more exalted fellows. Following the Glorious Revolution of 1688, however, licentiates like Groenevelt supported what amounted to a virtual revolt among some of the fellows against the continuing attempts of the president and censors to impose their own medical views on all London practitioners. At the same time, Groenevelt developed his medical practice well beyond cutting for the stone. He joined with his four licentiate friends—two English and two foreign—in a joint practice called the "repository," setting up an office in a good part of town to diagnose and treat large numbers of Londoners. The officers of the College of Physicians were outraged and did what they could to break up this joint practice, eventually succeeding. Groenevelt therefore took other steps to extend his medical practice, offering new treatments for cases of gout and other chronic diseases based on the latest Dutch medical theory. As when he first brought his knowledge of treating calculi to the attention of the public, so he again published a little book on the subject. He was trying to become much more than a surgical lithotomist; he wanted to be a very successful London physician.

The Censors of the College of Physicians correctly perceived that this foreigner, with his different notions of medical theory and medical virtue, a troublemaker and a friend of troublemakers, was trying to become one of the leading London experts in the treatment of chronic diseases. Thus, when one of the treatments he developed for his new practice seemed to cause an Englishwoman, Mrs. Withall, harm, the censors spent enormous time and energy trying to make him an example of their intention to bring their discipline to London practitioners, sending him to prison. Groenevelt would fight back, justifying his treatment of Withall and rallying his allies within the college. His reputation and livelihood stood in jeopardy.

By the late 1680s, with the help of his dissenting medical friends, Groenevelt presented himself to the London public not only as a surgeon but as a physician. Despite changes in college policy which were intended to limit the practice of people like himself, Groenevelt and four other licentiates— Crell, Guide, Browne, and Pechey—entered upon a bold and very unusual experiment: a joint practice, in which they could pool their expertise. No other example of a joint practice among English physicians from the seventeenth century is known, although Groenevelt had earlier worked with Velthuis. The practice seems to have begun with Browne and Crell, probably in March 1687.[1] They had taken out a five-year lease on a property "commonly known by the name of the Golden Angel and Crown" in King's Street, next to the alley that led to Ironmonger Lane. The Angel and Crown was situated not far from St. Paul's Cathedral, in the center of the city, and contained several rooms, suggesting the latest in medical offices. While physicians had previously visited the sick in their homes, by the late seventeenth century some practitioners had begun to see patients in the coffeehouses (which served as places for all kinds of public business), and still others had begun to see patients in private rooms leased for the purpose. Such rooms allowed patients to be more anonymous to their practitioners than if the practitioners visited them at home, where their advice could not be given without the knowledge of close friends, family, or even servants. For example, one Dutch practitioner who advertised being able to treat venereal diseases (which often brought a moral taint to the sufferer) notified the public that those desiring privacy could come to see him—without being seen—"through the Red Lyon-Inn . . . which is directly against my Back Door."[2] Presumably Browne and Crell joined forces to share the cost of a lease on consulting rooms (£32 per year, payable in quarterly installments) and the costs of furnishing the rooms in a suitable manner, which would bring advantages to their practices. There, each one saw the sick once a week, while they continued to visit their private patients during the other days of the week. Browne and Crell drew up a document bringing Guide, Groenevelt, and Pechey into the practice on 12 August 1687; on the same date, they transmitted the lease to the other three as well.[3] At the Golden Angel and Crown the group now collected a stock of drugs (the "repository"), saw patients by turns, and held a weekly meeting to divide the profits. At the same time, each continued his private practice.

The members of the repository practice let people know about their work by printing a handbill for distribution around the metropolis. "The Physitians of the Colledge, that us'd to consult twice a week, for the benefit of the Sick, at the Consultation-house, at the carv'd Angel and Crown in King-street," would now see patients there on Mondays, Wednesdays, Thursdays, and Fridays from two until six in the afternoon. As for their fees, "the known poor, and meaner familes" would have their advice for free, and people "from the middle rank" would be expected to pay only something moderate; "but as for the rich, and noble, liberality is inseparable from their quality and breeding." A later advertisement notified the public that the group gave advice in the morning as well as afternoon to people of all ranks, charging what was "suitable to their abilities," while the poor would get advice for free and the prescribed medicines "at very low rates."[4]

Because they knew that their practice would be viewed unfavorably by many other physicians, they took some trouble to explain what they were doing in a little book called *The Oracle for the Sick*.[5] The preface says that the group had been set up to oppose the "plague" of empirics ("for, take it from Us, every Disease undertaken by a Quack is altogether as dangerous as the Plague"). But in doing this they foresaw that "Empiricism, like Infection, [would be] falsely imputed" to them. The College of Physicians, of which the five were members, "ha[d], to a Man of them, been affected by the dying Groans of Persons Murdered by Intruders into Physick," who were now appearing in London in very large numbers. The college had justly used the law against such persons and considered other steps that might be taken. The physicians had decided that "Some Undertaking like this of Ours would prove the most effectual." The five had been encouraged "by several of the Society," to join together "for the Publick Good, and . . . not to the Discredit of [their] Profession." They therefore would see anyone at the Angel and Crown at announced days and times,[6] they would consult the poor for free (even at the five's own homes), and they would give medicines to the poor at low rates. They followed with a defense of how important it was for physicians to make their own medicines: only physicians like themselves, used to study-ing the practical aspects of treatment rather than theory and books alone, could give effectual cures.[7] The preface concluded by giving the names of the five members of the group and their home addresses. They reiterated their view that other physicians would think that they despised them, but in fact they honored them and stood ready to consult with them at any time;[8]

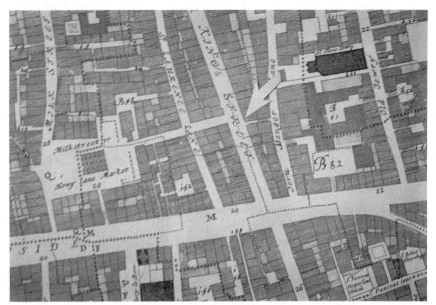

FIG. 22. *London immediately east of St. Paul's Cathedral (point "2" in fig. 19). The arrow points to the alley joining [New] King's Street and Ironmonger Lane, next to which the "Oracle Men" set up their business. From John Ogilby's "Large and Accurate Map of the City of London" of 1676.*

an "Advertisement" at the end also notified the surgeons that they wished to cooperate with, not replace, them. *The Oracle* also played up the fact that members of the college were now required to give free medical advice to the poor, by a college order of 27 July—just days before the agreement bringing Guide, Groenevelt, and Pechey into business with Browne and Crell.[9]

But *The Oracle for the Sick* was far more than an advertisement and justification for the joint practice; it was quite innovative in bringing any patient in England within the reach of the group. The body of the work was made up of questions that a physician would ask a patient in order to diagnosis an illness, and the possible answers that a patient might give. The patient was supposed to underline appropriate answers. He or she was also to make marks on the three included woodcuts (a frontal view of a man, a frontal view of a woman, and a rear view) to point out where various problems appeared. The handbook had eight "chapters" of questions: general problems, male complaints, female complaints, swellings, wounds, ulcers on the body, broken bones, and dislocated bones. With the book filled out, the patient

cil, or draw a flight line with a Pen upon the number, or on that part of the Figure which one would denote: With this
diftinction in reference to the Figures re-
prefenting the Body of Man or the parts
thereof, that to mark a pain or any external ail, the line ends on the Skin or
the outfide of the Figure, without being
continued with Points: but to fignifie an
internal pain or ail of the fame Part, one
muft continue the line with Points.

As, to figni-
fie a fuperficial
wound on the
right Cheek I
muft reprefent
it by the line
[A,] which fim-
ply ends on that
part, without
being continu-

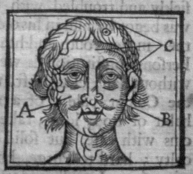

ed by Points. But to fhew a deep wound
or pain in the left Cheek, beyond the line
[B,] which ends there, this line muft be
yet continued with more or lefs Points,
accordingly as the Ail fhall lye deep. And
when the pain or other grievance is any
way extended, the line muft divide it
felf into two, three or more Rays,
which

FIG. 23. *Directions for making the figures. From* The Oracle for the Sick *(1687).*

could come to the repository for a quick diagnosis and prescription. Or more to the point, he or she could send it to them through the newly developed penny-post system for a diagnosis, with the medicines sent back to the patient through the mail, too.[10] Whether a bill followed or preceded the sending of the medicines is unknown. While literate patients often consulted physicians by letter, *The Oracle for the Sick* was something else again: mail-order medicine for anyone who knew someone who could read.

The five probably believed what they wrote: that they would be the enemies of quacks by serving the public cheaply. As already noted, the population of London had fewer regular practitioners than Amsterdam, and it was undoubtedly true that the poor had the fewest opportunities to get the advice of knowledgeable practitioners, a point made by many adversaries of the college.[11] Moreover, Groenevelt, Browne, and Crell certainly had no compunctions about helping the censors to condemn the practice of quacks. Together with the surgeon John English, they wrote out an account of one Russell's treatment of a child named John Theobald. Immediately after Theobald's death, the four had performed a postmortem and found the stomach "corroded and inflamed, and a gangrene begun about the orifice of the same, which [they judged] was occasioned by taking deleterious medicine inwardly." It turned out that Russell had paid the college's beadle 2 or 3 guineas, being persuaded that he had been made a licentiate thereby. The beadle was dismissed; Russell was first warned and then found guilty of malpractice and fined £10.[12]

But, as anticipated, the censors were not happy with the members of the repository. They first attacked Browne for advertising his pills, accusing him of acting like an empiric and so casting aspersions on the faculty of physicians. At their meeting of 28 September 1687 (at which Browne had been present), the college had passed a statute requiring all members to obtain the permission of the censors before publishing anything. Browne tried to argue that he had printed his handbills before the statute had been passed and only distributed them after the fact and therefore that he had not "published" after the end of September. But he finally had to agree that this is not what the statutes said. When he continued to distribute advertisements for his London Pills, he was told to remove his "bills" within a month or face being locked up in debtors' prison. He apparently obeyed, since the censors did not take up this case afterward.[13] But other physicians soon brought charges against Browne (and against Francis Bernard, a fellow) for frequently disobeying the new statute that required members not to consult with unlicensed practitioners, for which Browne was fined 10s.[14] One of his accusers soon charged him

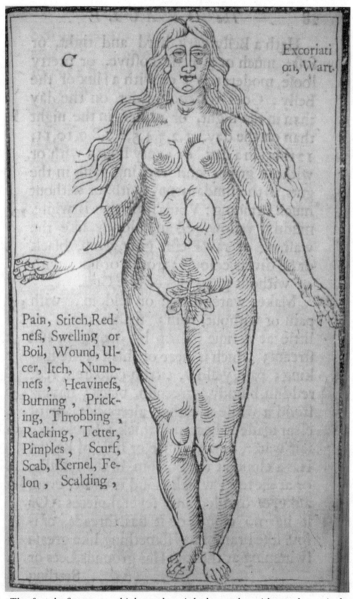

C

Excoriati on, Wart.

Pain, Stitch, Redneſs, Swelling or Boil, Wound, Ulcer, Itch, Numbneſs, Heavineſs, Burning, Pricking, Throbbing, Racking, Tetter, Pimples, Scurf, Scab, Kernel, Felon, Scalding,

FIG. 24. *The female figure on which marks might be made, with words to circle on the left, from* The Oracle for the Sick.

with further breaking the statutes by stealing a patient through visiting her ahead of the hour appointed for their joint consultation.[15] A year later, Browne complained in his turn that a fellow, Edward Tyson, had refused to consult with him, calling him a quack because he gave out his own medicines, which led to a fine for Tyson.[16] When Crell asked permission to print a certain tract (probably *The Oracle*), the censors refused.[17]

But despite problems for its participants, the *Oracle* practice continued: someone even proposed a similar repository for the College of Physicians as a whole, although nothing would come of it for some years yet.[18] By the end of October 1688, Browne had dropped out of the joint practice, perhaps because of the trouble it caused him with the college. With Browne gone, the distinctly Nonconformist group of Guide, Groenevelt, Crell, and Pechey had to draw up "articles . . . for the better management of the business of the Repository." They agreed on seven points: (1) each would take a week-long turn visiting the sick in their homes within twelve hours of being called; (2) on every Monday, the "Steward" would examine the repository and deliver a list of drugs that needed to be replenished to the meeting of the group that afternoon; (3) each member had to take a turn preparing the medicines needed for restocking; (4) each member would take turns providing a servant to wait on them at their Monday meetings; (5) anyone absent from the Monday meeting without a good excuse would forfeit his share of the profits; (6) the Steward was to notify the group every two weeks of the debts owed and to send out bills to recover them; and (7) each member would have liberty to take two weeks off "to recreat himself in the country or to mind his business there." Failure to live up to any of these conditions would result in a specified fine.[19]

By the late 1680s, then, Groenevelt had become identified as a member of a group of licentiates who were trying to increase their medical practices by using methods not liked by the censors of the college. His lithotomy practice had become quite well known and lucrative, but Groenevelt wanted to develop a solid medical practice in addition. Then the political world changed in late 1688 and early 1689, when a Dutchman, William III, seized the English throne. At first, the changes seemed to favor Groenevelt's ambitions by undermining the old guard of the College of Physicians and encouraging a large Dutch immigration. But by the early to mid-1690s, owing in part to the disobedience of his colleague Pechey, in part because of rising xenophobia on the part of the English, and in part by a politically conservative backlash, many practitioners in London, like Groenevelt, found themselves struggling to retain their practices. Not only Groenevelt's association with the repository practice, then, but the politics of the nation and the College of Physicians made the censors anxious to use Withall's case to make an example of Groenevelt.

The Glorious Revolution of late 1688 and early 1689 which made the stadholder William III and his English bride Mary Stuart king and queen of England brought much institutional and legal confusion in its wake. For William, his enormously successful invasion of England, toppling his father-in-law James II, meant that England would at least be neutralized in his ongoing struggles with His Most Catholic Majesty, Louis XIV: there would be no repetition of 1672, in which England and France combined to overrun the United Provinces. As he consolidated his power with the help of his queen, he soon found that he could even bring England into his wars against France as an ally of the Dutch.

In the wake of William's coup, a wave of Dutch medical practitioners soon flooded into England. The new king naturally employed Dutch physicians in the royal household: Abraham Rottermondt as a royal apothecary and William Van Loon as serjeant surgeon (that is, the personal surgeon of the king) as well as surgeon general to the army and navy. William also often relied very heavily for medical advice upon the services of the physician Goverd Bidloo, who was called to England to attend the king many times and perhaps become a royal physician.[20] Some Dutch physicians made the journey across the North Sea, such as the later notorious Bernard de Mandeville.[21] Plenty of empirics also came over. One of the best-known ordinary practitioners in London at the end of the seventeenth century, for example, was Cornelius à Tilburg, who obtained the favor of someone in the government of William and Mary. On 20 May 1689, the king's Warrant Book noted that Tilburg had "made experiment of the virtue of his antidote against poison and other distempers, to the general satisfaction" of the court. Consequently, the Crown granted Tilburg a royal license "to sell the said antidote, and other medicines, from a stage in any city or town, he first acquainting the chief magistrate with his intention to do so."[22] The handbills Tilburg distributed as advertisements therefore often have the English royal coat of arms at the top, and underneath the slogan: "By His Majesty's Special License and Authority."[23] Despite attempts by the learned physicians in the London College of Physicians to make Tilburg quit his practice, Tilburg simply ignored the college and continued. Another Dutch physician took to advertising in London newspapers: a paid news item "from The Hague" announced, "[Dr. Herwig,] Physician to the Princesses of Walduk living with them at Cuylenburg near Utrecht in

Holland gives notice, that he hath found out an infallible method to cure all Mad and distracted Persons. . . . He cures likewise all Lunaticks and Hypocondriacks, in seven or eight weeks."[24]

Among the new group of Dutch practitioners trying to tap the London market was Groenevelt's old friend from Deventer Casparus Sibelius, who used his acquaintance with the English physician and philosopher John Locke to help him set up a practice. Locke had been forced to leave England for the Netherlands in September 1683 after his complicity in a plot against the government.[25] During the six years he spent away, he became acquainted with a number of Dutch physicians, including Sibelius, who was living in Amsterdam when Locke moved there at the beginning of his exile.[26] Sibelius showed him a copy of Ten Rhijne's new book—which had been out for just a few months—and within ten days was entertaining the Englishman in his home.[27] In the spring or summer of 1684, Sibelius returned to Deventer, and in September Locke spent almost two weeks with him there.[28] Locke returned to England in 1689, and by the end of January 1692, perhaps inspired by his friend Groenevelt's example, Sibelius too had decided that pastures would be greener in England.[29] He stayed in London with his old friend. But in the early 1690s the college officers were cracking down on unlicensed practitioners, and Sibelius did not know English well (if at all), so that matters became difficult for him. Some of his friends in London—perhaps including Groenevelt—suggested that he move on to Dublin, since, Sibelius explained, it did not have so many physicians or cost so much to live.[30] (Moreover, Irish resistance to William's rule had been crushed by the end of 1691; the French that Sibelius spoke was more common among the affluent there. Sibelius and Groenevelt's mutual friend, Jacobus Sylvius, had made the move to Ireland successfully in 1683, and many of the Dublin physicians had also been educated at Leiden.) In early April, therefore, Sibelius explained his predicament to Locke and begged his old acquaintance for letters of reference—he got at least one.[31] Sibelius quickly developed hopes of becoming the physician to William's new Lord Lieutenant of Ireland, Henry Sidney. Sidney had been one of the chief architects of the design to bring William to the English throne, and Locke may have known him as a fellow plotter in 1687.[32] Sidney had received his new appointment in March 1692 and apparently needed a physician to attend him. Unfortunately, Sibelius's hopes failed.[33] Sibelius's chances at a career beyond the confines of Deventer ended up virtually ruining him: he quickly passed back through London again in May or early June 1693, presumably stopping at Groenevelt's again for a time, and died not long after in his hometown.[34]

But William's seizure of power indirectly brought on even greater changes in Groenevelt's life than opening the floodgates to more Dutch practitioners. The structure of the English constitution became quite confused, causing anxiety among the officers of the College of Physicians and eventually bringing them to try to discipline people like Groenevelt. Many members of the new Parliament objected to various laws that had been made during the reign of James II. Eventually, a number of statutes were abrogated, including many of those enacting the new charters from James' government. The charter that the College of Physicians had obtained in 1687, granting its officers much greater powers to control medical practitioners in the metropolis, came to nothing, as did the royal letters expanding upon those powers. Finding its charter null and void, the College of Physicians entered a period of great confusion. The abrogation of the college charter not only undercut the censors' ability to carry on prosecuting others as before but even brought into question the issue of whether the great numbers of new fellows created by virtue of the new charter would remain members. The college finally emerged from this confusion led by a group of officers determined to reassert their authority even without James' charter. Opposed to them was a group that included Edward Tyson.[35]

Tyson engaged in a series of obstinate disobediences, even refusing to acknowledge the authority of the censors' board. One member of the college named Browne—either Groenevelt's colleague Richard Browne or Edward Browne—complained that Tyson had refused to consult with him. When Tyson refused to come before the censors to answer the charges, he was heavily fined both for breaking the new college statutes governing consultations between members and for contempt of the censors.[36] Moreover, Tyson was among those opposed to writing directions to patients in English for taking their prescriptions, as the new statutes required. The new statute was meant to prevent the apothecaries from altering the course of treatment when they interpreted an abbreviated Latin prescription to the patient.[37] Several fellows of the college opposed this plan.[38] The censors fined Tyson most heavily of all those who were disobeying the statute, partly because he disobeyed it often, partly because he refused to acknowledge their authority to enforce it.[39] When he refused to pay the £8 he owed in fines, the censors ordered him to be taken to court to recover the money. But President Rogers, who by this time had joined with Tyson and others in opposing the college charter issued under King James, on his own authority ordered the college's attorney to stop the suit against Tyson.[40] Off the hook for the moment, Tyson then benefited from the period of quiescence which followed under the presidency of Walter Charleton, before in September 1692 the college officers returned to their former attempts to restore internal and external discipline.

But it was the conflict between Groenevelt's colleague John Pechey and the censors which triggered the events leading to the emergence of a strongly disciplinary group within the college in 1692. The censors disliked the fact that Pechey was distributing handbills advertising his new place of residence and fees.[41] The censors first warned him; when he continued to publish his announcements and refused to take down the sign over his door advertising his practice, he was fined £4. But in the legal confusion following the fall of the old government, Pechey simply refused to pay the fine.[42] As the officers of the college tried to sort out their affairs and to gather money to finance their petitions to Crown and Parliament, a long list of licentiates—including Groenevelt, Guide, Crell, and Pechey—were ordered to pay arrears in their dues.[43] The licentiates, who worried about what their money might help to bring about, delayed paying. The censors therefore decided to make an example of the "Oracle men," who were summoned to appear before the censors in mid-January 1690. There Crell still refused to pay his dues without consulting his "friends," although he had by then left "his partnership in the Oracle with which this Boarde [of Censors] was not displeased." Pechey still refused to pay his £4 fine, whereupon the censors doubled the amount and ordered their attorney to sue him for it in court.[44] But Pechey eventually got off on a legal technicality: the College of Physicians could not fine him for nonpayment of dues because the college book in which its statutes had been entered had no date on it, and so no legally binding evidence existed of the statutes having been approved before he was sued for breaking them.

What followed was a new round of disciplining members of the college, especially the licentiates. In handing down his decision in Pechey's case, Lord Chief Justice Holt had recommended to the college that its statutes be voted affirmatively yet again, dated, and marked with the college seal— which was done during the summer months of 1692.[45] Then, at the next annual meeting of the whole College of Physicians, the fellows went even further and chose an entirely new slate of officers who initiated a crackdown on unlicensed practitioners and on those candidates and licentiates who had dealings with empirics.[46] For the next two years—until the officers were changed again—the president and censors met more often, heard a greater number of complaints, and imposed more penalties than at any other time but one in the late seventeenth century.[47] They also warned the candidates and licentiates that whether they liked it or not they had to come to meetings

of the college and to give information against "unskillful, and illicit prac-
tisers," as well as to hear the statutes read to them—statutes that were to
regulate their conduct and prevent them from associating with outsiders.[48]
The new censors soon also entered upon a new set of lawsuits against Pechey
for the dues he continued to refuse, despite the new vote on the statutes.[49]

Unlike his colleague Pechey, Joannes Groenevelt did his best to abide by
the wishes of the new officers. At the same time that the censors entered upon
a new set of lawsuits against Pechey, when none of his former colleagues in
the repository practice would attend the revived college anatomy lectures as
required, Groenevelt took the time to come to the first two of the three days of
the lectures.[50] Then, too, soon after their warning that the licentiates had to
give evidence against empirics, Groenevelt testified against one Charles Carter,
a cooper who practiced medicine. Perhaps Groenevelt wanted to distance himself from true empirics and to show the new officers how obedient he was, or
perhaps he came only because the censors required it of him. Whatever his
feelings, his testimony brought no results, since the patients on whom Carter
had practiced would not say that he had been a public nuisance: in fact, they
"rather appeared on his behalf, declaring the Great Good he had done, without
giving further evidence."[51] The kind of testimony brought to them by Groenevelt would not have endeared him to the new censors.

During these disputatious days, Groenevelt published a little pamphlet advertising his ability to cure the gout with a new remedy. It amounted to a public
declaration that Groenevelt intended to acquire an important medical practice
on his own, despite the views of the censors. A disease in which the joints
(most commonly in the big toe) became swollen and very painful, gout
periodically struck many of Groenevelt's contemporaries, especially the affluent. A number of people therefore published on gout, including Groenevelt's friend Ten Rhijne, who had recommended moxibustion for it.[52] Had
Groenevelt successfully moved from treating bladder stones to treating the
gout, he would have considerably extended his medical practice. The secret
remedy alluded to in Groenevelt's pamphlet could be used in many chronic
diseases, including urinary complaints. It would be this new remedy of
Groenevelt's which brought Mrs. Withall to him.

A small and cheap booklet, Groenevelt's pamphlet had all the marks
of self-promotion and was published by Groenevelt himself rather than a
bookseller.[53] Originally written in Latin, it was translated into good English
for him by his colleague Richard Browne.[54] It began with remarks common
to such pamphlets. All improvements in the arts, he wrote, are at first frowned

on "by the censorious" until they were "crown'd with success," physic being "more than the rest capable of improvement." While the many daily "vain pretences of the ignorant" made even judicious people suspicious of medical innovations, not "every thing that seems new" or is "beyond the common method of practise" ought to be rejected, for some novelties could be good and true and "verified by experience." Groenevelt hoped in this regard that both his M.D. and his license from the College of Physicians would keep him from being "accounted only a pretender" to what he professed. Then, after he had thus distanced himself from empirics and quacks, Groenevelt went on to claim that he had indeed found a new and useful remedy. In the course of treating the ailment of stones successfully "both by inward remedies and manual operation," he had found gout to be a disease equally tormenting and "altogether of the same origin." As he investigated the gout, "by the blessing of God" he had discovered "a seldom failing method for the cure of, and preservation from that disease."[55]

The pamphlet went on to explain his theory of the cause and cure of gout based upon Sylvius's notions of a thick, salty serum breeding "nodes" and stones in the body.[56] He was extending the theories he had first learned in Leiden about disease causation to account both for the stones in the body and for a host of other chronic diseases, including gout. The book concluded with an advertisement for a special remedy of his own, which brought off the salty serum in the urine gently but in large amounts, without the necessity of bleeding. Since the best remedies for gout scoured the joints and brought off the thick salt, he believed, his cleansing astringent was just the thing needed. Like empirics, or like his colleague Pechey, Groenevelt did not give away the composition of his remedy. He included several pages of examples of people whom he had successfully treated. And the tract concluded with "A Pindarick Ode on the Discourse of the Gout" by "F.F.T.," which ended: "From these great Evils when thou sets us free, / Greenfield, thou shalt our Guardian-Angel be."[57]

Thus, when Mrs. Withall came to complain to the censors about Dr. Groenevelt, he had begun to move from surgery into medicine publicly, reaching out to the many people who suffered from chronic diseases, especially gout. By the early 1690s, the repository practice was suffering strains, with Browne having left and Crell about to. If he was to maintain and extend his medical practice, Groenevelt would again need to strike out on his own. He had developed a proprietary remedy to bring off urine gently, in large amounts: in retrospect, it can be seen that this was his mixture of cantharides and camphor, from which he hoped to cure various diseases and develop his medical custom. Sylvius and his students believed that diuretics provided an important, perhaps the most important, treatment for chronic diseases, which were caused by an accumulation of serum in the body, which had to be removed through urination or other means.

Groenevelt had solid reasons for using cantharides as a diuretic. Since physicians used diuretics in attempts to purge the bladder of stones, Groenevelt had much incentive to investigate various compositions of diuretics as much as of lithontriptics. Since the ancients, cantharides beetles had been collected, dried, and powdered; they were one of the few animals left in some contemporary pharmacopoeias—although not in the London one authorized by the college.[58] Physicians had long noted the usefulness of cantharides in diuretics and in lithontriptics and emmenagogics (remedies to bring on stopped menstrual discharges);[59] even the famous Amsterdam physician Nicolaes Tulp apparently used a lithontriptic composed in part of cantharides.[60] Steven Blankaart had mentioned cantharides as a excellent but dangerous diuretic—Groenevelt probably knew of Blankaart's work, since he had hosted in London Jacob van de Velde, Blankaart's friend and Amsterdam publisher.[61] But such notions went back a long way: one late fifteenth- or early sixteenth-century English manuscript stated simply: "for the gowt. Take a grene flye called cantaridis."[62] By rectifying with camphor this long-used treatment for chronic disease, Groenevelt had found an excellent remedy against a number of chronic diseases, certainly including diseases of the urinary tract. He had been using cantharides rectified with camphor for well over ten years.[63]

Therefore, when about a year after his pamphlet appeared Mrs. Withall was suffering from pains in her "lower parts," someone recommended that she send for this expert in treating chronic complaints, especially those involving the bladder. He examined her with a catheter (something he had long been using in the diagnosis of calculi) and determined that she had an ulcer of the bladder but no stones. He decided to treat her with his secret remedy, making up the pills himself (so that no apothecary would find out his method) and sending them to her, with directions. She began to take the pills he had sent alone; he claimed that he had explained in his directions that she was to take pills containing camphor as well (which she could have obtained from an apothecary). He thought her hurts had been caused by her own misbehavior in not taking the camphor; she believed they had been caused by his remedy.

Withall's husband had taken the remaining pill to the doctors and surgeons at St. Thomas's Hospital, where one of the physicians, Richard Torlesse, took a dim view of Groenevelt's practice. Torlesse happened to be one of the most important people within the College of Physicians' movement to enforce medical discipline among both members and outsiders, soon encouraging the college to establish a public dispensary to attack the Society of Apothecaries. Torlesse may have been personally prejudiced toward Groenevelt as well, because of John Browne's views—the St. Thomas's surgeon who sued Groenevelt for breach of contract. Quite possibly, then, Torlesse encouraged Withall to bring her problems to the college censors: Groenevelt later blamed his problems on a personal grievance Torlesse had toward him because of some "hard words" Groenevelt used to Torlesse's face.[64] A year after he sent Withall the pills, then, in July 1694, she finally brought her complaint to the censors.

A few months after Withall's initial complaint, Torlesse became one of the censors. Following the revolution of 1688–89, Groenevelt seems to have had no politically well-connected patrons who could have intervened with the college on his behalf, making him vulnerable to becoming an example for others. The majority of the censors placed no faith in Groenevelt's version of events and mistrusted his reasoning, shaped as it was by a medical theory they did not accept. Thanks only to Tyson's recalcitrance, Groenevelt had gotten off during late 1694 and most of 1695. But now, in November and December of the latter year, the censors had taken up the case again, with Torlesse but without Tyson sitting among them. The moment coincided with a steep decline in the popularity of William III (now sole ruler, since Mary had died at the end of December 1694) and his Dutch advisers.

The new censors proceeded cautiously. At the beginning of December they heard Groenevelt's statement that he had ordered Withall to take cantharides in conjunction with camphor. As in the year before, they thought of the administration of large doses of cantharides, whether in conjunction with another ingredient or not, highly dangerous. But punishing Groenevelt for his deeds could not be done immediately because the officers of the college feared a countersuit. The president and censors therefore began by trying to put an end to the internal differences within the college which made it vulnerable to outside pressure. Because of Tyson, the Groenevelt matter had already become a source of deep divisions within the college. Without the full support of the fellows, the censors would not be able to act as forcefully as they might wish. The president and censors therefore asked the fellows to subscribe to a document obliging the signatories to stand by the officers of the college to the amount of £50 per person. The document stated that "divers good and wholesome lawes and statutes of the College" had been made both for "the good and Welfare of the Subjects of this Kingdome" and for "the maintainance and Supporte of the honour and Reputation of the said Colledge and the Fellows and members thereof." But the statutes had not been enforced because the president and censors "were apprehensive [that] divers suits and controversies might arise and be prosecuted" against them, the "costs and damages as well as the trouble whereof they might in their owne particular persons be subject to and yet not sufficiently indempnified by the said Colledge." In order to allow the president and censors to "doe theire respective dutyes without the danger of suffering for the same in theire owne persons or estates," the subscribers to the document pledged to "assist, support and maintain" the president and censors or else pay a fine of £50.[65] In other words, if someone like Groenevelt brought suit against the officers of the college for the actions they took on behalf of the corporation, the fellows would pay the costs of the officers' defense out of their own pockets.

But the document also proved divisive, since it made clear who supported the officers and who did not. At the first meeting of the fellows after the latest testimony in the Groenevelt affair, just before Christmas, the president showed the document to the whole college, with the signatures of twenty-six fellows. He asked the remaining fellows to sign their names. Fourteen "refused to do it." Heading the list of the dissenters was Tyson.[66] This group of dissidents constituted a large and vocal minority of fellows. The attempt of the officers to reinforce their authority would certainly not heal the divisions in the college.

The splits within the ranks of the fellows over college policy had emerged not only from the Groenevelt case. About the same time that the censors were first hearing his side about Withall's case, in the middle of December 1694, Torlesse alerted the college officers to a bill of the Society of Apothecaries pending in Parliament which would allow apothecaries to avoid serving in lower-ranking London public offices. These precinct duties, such as supervising the removal of night soil from the streets, or staying up all night serving on the watch, were troublesome for men constantly serving the public by visiting the sick, the apothecaries argued. Without legal relief from these offices, they would have to keep paying fines for not serving. The physicians were understandably suspicious about the apothecaries' motives in introducing their bill, for in exempting them from lower-level public duties, the bill declared them the equal of other professionals, like the attorneys and physicians. In fact, when the bill passed the Parliament in February, it did indeed call the apothecaries "professionals." The counterstrategy the officers of the college hit upon was to attack the apothecaries by establishing the Dispensary for the Sick Poor, which took up much of their energy over the next few years. The dispensary scheme resembled in some way the joint repository of Groenevelt and his colleagues: physicians would regularly be on duty to diagnose and to prescribe medicines from a stock of drugs kept up by servants of the college. But the college would also post the base price of the drugs, which would allow the public to see how much they were being overcharged by the apothecaries. This counterattack by the college on the Society of Apothecaries stirred up violent opposition among a group of fellows, who were supported by many licentiates, including Groenevelt.[67]

Nevertheless, the opponents of strong college authority could be outvoted by the others. The late December 1695 meeting of the fellows therefore did obtain some results: not only had more than twenty-five of the fellows agreed to stand by the officers, but two new statutes were proposed, read, and affirmed for the first time; and the college agreed to an order "that the four Censors be joined with the President to discharge and release those that shall be committed for Mala Praxis."[68] Thus, not the president alone but the president and four censors would sign any warrant of committal to or release from prison for malpractice; five people instead of one would have to agree to let someone back on the street after being locked up, and five would have to be sued by someone upset at his or her treatment.[69] They now seemed fully armed to make an example of Groenevelt.

But again, delay ensued. The regular monthly meetings of the censors in January and February had to be canceled because of the "indisposition" of the president.[70] The business of setting up the dispensary continued apace.[71] Time also had to be taken to change the college statutes. Counsel for the college advised that the potential problems the courts would have with interpreting the Latin words of its statutes mandated that they be translated into English and voted on again and approved.[72] The censors took this opportunity to change some of them (especially by increasing the fines) and to add some new rules. At the end of September, the new statutes were read and approved twice, although on the third occasion, "a debate and Controversie arising among some of the Fellowes[,] it was omitted."[73] At a special meeting at the beginning of November, the new statutes were voted on a third time and approved, and the president formally attached the seal to them.[74] Among the new provisions were two to prevent anyone like Tyson from undermining the other censors again: a penalty of 40s. would be imposed on any censor who differed in opinion from the rest and so refused to sign a judgment against him; moreover, "any Censor after declaring any person guilty of mala praxis, refusing to fine the person so declared guilty and to sign a warrant for committment" to prison would be "forthwith expelled."[75]

On 21 November 1696, a meeting of all the members of the college was called, in order to have the new statutes read out to all the fellows, honorary fellows, candidates, and licentiates. Groenevelt attended. The meeting exploded in controversy. Josiah Clerk, a fellow, rose to tell the president that the new statutes had been "illegally made." "Some other of the Fellowes with great heat and passion, for the same reason expressed themselves against them, [and] the Licentiates being thus encouraged did in a very rude and tumultuous manner pretend to a Right in the making of the statutes." The president, Sir Thomas Millington, explained ("with great moderation," Registrar Gill added) that he and the college's lawyers thought otherwise. The college statutes had always been made the way they had been made this time. Millington proceeded to order Registrar Gill to read them out. Upon this, Tyson led twenty-six members in a walk-out, despite being "comanded" by Millington to stay to hear the statutes read. Groenevelt was among those who turned their backs on the president.[76]

Thereafter, fellows like Sir Richard Blackmore took the line that the new statutes were invalid because they had not yet been promulgated to the whole group. They also petitioned the government "visitors" listed in the charter of Charles II to inspect the doings of the college.[77] Much the same group continued to oppose the establishment of the dispensary.[78] The censors tried to get the statutes promulgated by calling another meeting a month later, and Groenevelt was among those who took their places to hear the first part of the statutes read to all the members.

Finally, after all this quarreling and maneuvering, more than a year after the last hearing on the matter, the censors—Torlesse still among them—felt strong enough to think yet again about disciplining Groenevelt for malpractice. On 5 February 1697, "there was a Complaint" made by someone unnamed "against Dr. John Groenvelt for Mala Praxis upon the body of Mrs. Susanna Withall." The censors ordered that the witnesses should attend the next meeting and bring with them the depositions they had given under oath. At the next meeting, on 5 March, Groenevelt appeared, but Torlesse had not come because of sickness, and another censor, William Dawes, was simply absent; the meeting had to be canceled.[79]

Then, at the April meeting of the censors in 1697, well over four years after his administration of cantharides to Mrs. Withall, the censors heard the testimony from all parties all over again and finally acted. The witnesses against Groenevelt appeared before the college on the afternoon of Friday, 9 April (the first Friday in the month having been Good Friday, no meeting had been held on 2 April). They brought with them depositions that they had given upon oath to the Lord Mayor's Court. Among the legal powers of the college called into question at the end of the century was the ability of the censors to put witnesses to an oath. But if they were to punish someone for malpractice, it would be well to pay attention to legal niceties and have the testimony given according to the oaths necessary in a court of law. On 5 February, the censors had therefore ordered that the testimony on the case be brought before them in the form of formal depositions, in which the witnesses took an oath as to the validity of their words. They gave their depositions under oath to a notary two weeks later, on 19 February. Thus, when the Groenevelt affair came up again, the censors examined the depositions (which were transcribed into the Annals), read them aloud, asked the witnesses if they stood by their testimony, and proceeded accordingly.

The depositions repeated most of what had been laid before the censors three years earlier—so close to the words in the Annals that one imagines the depositions to have been drawn up by the college's lawyer from the Annals beforehand—although a few additional details were added. After their sworn statements had been read to the witnesses and to Groenevelt, and the witnesses had agreed to the veracity of their words, Groenevelt was asked for his statement. The registrar simply noted that Groenevelt said he had been summoned by Mrs. Withall about four years previously, diagnosed her as having an ulcer in her bladder, and had given her his pills of cantharides and camphor. Rather than plea for mercy, Groenevelt told the censors that it was "his Common Practice" to prescribe "that quantity of Cantharides or greater, with some Pills of Camphire, & Crums of bread." The witnesses against Groenevelt were called upon in final rebuttal, the main points being that Groenevelt had given Withall only eighteen pills, "which were those made up with Cantharides"; that the doctor "was not present at the taking of any of them neither did he give any of them to her himselfe"; and that Groenevelt did not return to see how his patient was doing "till after she had taken fifteen of the eighteen Pills, and then he was sent for to Mrs. Withall about four of the clock in the afternoon, by reason of the great pain and torment that she was in and the great quantity of blood which she had made."[80]

The censors discussed matters privately and drew up their own record of what they thought had occurred. On the crucial matter of the pills, they believed the witnesses rather than the doctor: that Groenevelt had given only cantharides. Such a practice they "unanimously and utterly" considered to be "unfit, improper, and very pernicious." They declared Groenevelt "guilty of the evil practice aforesaid." As a penalty, they sentenced him to pay "a fine of Twenty pounds of Lawfull money of England" to be given to the college treasurer "within two days." But they also ordered him "committed to his Majesties Goale of Newgate & have & suffer Imprisonment therin at his own Costs & Charges without Baile or Mainprice [i.e., release on surety]" for the duration of the "Twelve weeks next ensuing unless he [was] sooner discharged by the President of the said Colledge & by such persons as by the Colledge shall be thereunto lawfully authorized."[81] A week later, the college beadle deposited him in the notorious Newgate prison.[82]

The censors had tried hard to make Groenevelt an example for other licentiates, persisting over many years and through serious difficulties. They wished to impose discipline among the members of the college and to wield authority against unqualified outsiders. Groenevelt happened to be a foreigner without an influential English patron, making him vulnerable to attacks by the censors. He possessed troublemaking friends among his former colleagues of the repository practice, advertised his practice, and gave out new proprietary medicines rooted in Dutch theory. In his wrangles with other London surgeons and physicians, he had made enemies. He also advocated medical ideas that had not been widely accepted among the English establishment. When the censors, probably Censor Torlesse in particular, heard of a case in which Groenevelt's remedies seemed to be the substance that had caused an Englishwoman grave harm, they seized upon the case, prosecuting it doggedly over a period of three years, even undertaking controversial revisions of the college statutes to do so. They finally imprisoned him for malpractice. The issue had almost from the beginning been caught up in the medical politics of the mid-1690s.

It would continue to be; but now Groenevelt's very livelihood was at stake. Groenevelt had tried to move from a largely surgical practice into a medical practice that treated chronic diseases, especially gout. If he allowed the charges against him to go unchallenged, the publicity surrounding the case would surely end all hopes he might have for extending his medical practice. It might even damage his reputation enough to dry up his surgical practice as well. This stubborn, self-confident man from the Dutch provinces had survived many threats before and prospered despite them. But now he faced a more difficult task: he was no longer an up-and-coming young man who could freely seize on new opportunities or go elsewhere. He had been put on the defensive: he had lived in London for twenty years and had his family to consider, too. Almost fifty years old, at the peak of his abilities, he would have to save his reputation. If he did not, the elite London physicians might succeed in ending his practice and driving him from London, forcing him to start his life over again. But defending his reputation against what he saw as half-truths would be no easy task. Perhaps it could not be done. For the moment, he pondered his predicament as he sat in Newgate.

CHAPTER 7

Becoming a Cause Célèbre

AN EXPLOSION OF popular anger followed Groenevelt's imprisonment, which he helped to orchestrate. Imprisonment deeply threatened Groenevelt's reputation as a person and as a practitioner. With the inner resources of the righteous, however, he fought back. He refused to think that he had done anything wrong. Rather than kowtow to the officers of the College of Physicians, he used the law courts to defend himself, and with the help of others he turned all the means of publicity at his disposal against his opponents. He made sure that his imprisonment brought to the attention of the public what had previously been an issue for discussion mainly in the medical community alone: the objectionable behavior of the college censors. Many opponents of the college censors, from inside the college, from within the Society of Apothecaries, and from among the many unlicensed empirics in London, came to Groenevelt's assistance or held his case up as an example of the malicious behavior of the censors. Within a short period, the publicity about the Groenevelt affair merged with several other medical brush fires to become part of a general conflagration threatening the whole edifice of establishment medicine in London.

The Groenevelt matter triggered a series of public debates and court cases, although the legal battles ended in a draw. Chief Justice Holt, of the Court of King's Bench, managed to uphold all the powers of the college censors: Groenevelt got out of prison on habeas corpus but eventually lost a case against the censors for false imprisonment, both in Holt's courtroom. A civil suit for enormous damages brought by Mrs. Withall against Groenevelt failed, while Groenevelt in turn harassed the Censors of the College of Physicians for not taking the proper oaths of allegiance and supremacy. The question of whether Groenevelt had practiced wrongly was never legally resolved;

nevertheless, the many pointed attacks on the college which were sparked by the public controversy over Groenevelt's practice helped to shake public confidence in the college censors and to undermine their authority over others. In the 1690s, when public opinion counted for a great deal more than ever before, the Groenevelt affair and its consequences provided grist for the gossip mills of coffeehouse and newspaper for several years. Yet, while battling his enemies to a stalemate might have kept Groenevelt's surgical career alive, it damaged his reputation, too, ending his hopes for improving his medical practice. At the height of the doctor's career, a respectable future evaporated in the fierce heat of publicity.

Groenevelt's case had been heard by the censors on Friday, 9 April 1697. After taking the few days he was given to think things over, Groenevelt had been hauled off by the college beadle to prison on the following Thursday, the fifteenth.[1] On the Sunday after his conviction by the censors, before the college beadle forcibly put him in prison, Groenevelt sought out the senior censor, Dr. Burwell, after church, begging him not to send him to Newgate, but Burwell refused. In denying Groenevelt's petition after church, Burwell seemed especially hardhearted.[2]

His confinement in Newgate could not have been a pleasant experience for Groenevelt. To begin, it cost him a lot of money: the conditions of his imprisonment meant that he had to pay the warden and keepers for food, fuel, and other necessaries out of his own pocket. Naturally, too, he lost money during his imprisonment because he could not see his patients. But the financial costs of his imprisonment were the least of his worries. Newgate was a place of infamy, and many of the doctor's fellow prisoners were highwaymen, rapists, and murderers. As Groenevelt later put it in the dedication to a book giving his side of the matter, the censors sent him to live among "a Den of Thieves, a gang of Rogues, Villains, and Parricides" in "the most infamous Gaol for Rogues and Villains of all sorts in the whole Kingdom, NEWGATE."[3] Within the confines of the prison, gangs of inmates took matters into their own hands, demanding money from newcomers on threat of stripping them naked to shiver and sometimes die. The place itself was cold, filthy, and ridden with disease; its stench could be overpowering on the clothes of visitors for hours afterward.[4] Even a day confined to such a prison, living among the worst criminals in utter filth, would have been unpleasant, to say the least, for a person brought up as one of the elect.

Groenevelt's imprisonment had the potential to damage his living quite seriously. It certainly cut him off from caring for his patients. According to one story, Groenevelt had cut a young boy for the stone earlier on the day he was imprisoned, whose recovery he could not now oversee.[5] Even if the report exaggerated the life-and-death issue, it remains a reminder that the absence of a surgeon-physician who practiced among a large number of Londoners would be quickly noticed, and people would begin to ask questions about him. Upon inquiry, they would easily have heard rumors about the doctor being imprisoned for malpractice in a jail used to confine the very worst criminals; and all this would have brought questions to their minds about ever consulting him again. Thus, the most important consequence of being imprisoned was the potential loss of his personal reputation.

Facing the ruin of his livelihood and reputation, Groenevelt fought back with everything in his power. His first move was to get out of Newgate. To do this, he retained a group of excellent lawyers.[6] On the first day of the new law term, 21 April,[7] they entered a plea of habeas corpus on his behalf in the Court of King's Bench, the court that had the duty of investigating whether prisoners of His Majesty had been locked up for good reason. Groenevelt's lawyers advanced eight arguments for his release.[8] The first argument made a general plea; the others struck at legal technicalities about the form of the warrant committing him to Newgate. The first and most general argument claimed that the crime for which Groenevelt had been committed had occurred "before his Majesties pardon," and so he should not have been locked up for it. English monarchs had been in the habit of granting a general pardon once during their reign: to commemorate the death of Queen Mary in the winter of 1694–95, William III had granted a pardon for all those who had committed offenses before 29 April 1695, excepting certain very grievous crimes.[9] The other points took up the result of the lawyers' detailed study of the warrant.[10] For instance, they argued in point two that the warrant did not spell out what Groenevelt's "evil practice" had been: the claim of "undue practice" was too vague. A further argument had it that since the court could not determine from the warrant whether he had been locked up for good reason or not, it should presume his innocence and let him out. They made six other arguments about what they thought were problems in the warrant. Groenevelt's lawyers probably had little idea that the warrant confining him to Newgate had been made out according to the formula of Chief Justice Holt himself, the chief of the judges before whom they made these arguments.[11]

Fortunately for Groenevelt and his lawyers, although Holt had no problem with the body of the warrant, the more general plea still needed discussion by the justices. According to the college registrar, Thomas Gill, "whether the Crime was within the Kings Pardon or no was the matter singly debated."[12] Since the "crime" had been committed before April 1695, the only question could have been about whether the act came within the list of exempted offenses or not. Groenevelt's lawyers also brought in Dr. Francis Bernard— one of the college dissidents—to tell the chief justice that Hippocrates had prescribed a similar amount of cantharides in the same kinds of cases and in many others and that Dr. Martin Lister "had avowed it to be good practise in a booke he had lately printed."[13] Arguing on the other side were several other powerful men. The attorney general himself, Sir Thomas Powys, to- gether with Sir Bartholomew Shore and Serjeant Levinz argued the college's case.[14] They presented a Latin declaration signed by William Withall and his wife, Susanna, concerning Groenevelt's treatment, which restated their testimony before the college.[15] After hearing arguments on both sides, the justices finally decided that "the Crime was within the pardon, and so ordered the Prisoner to be discharged." Nevertheless, Chief Justice Holt tried to save matters for the college by making a statement, "to which the Judges agreed," that "the Colledge might Comitt without Baile for a Mala Praxis and might also impose a reasonable fine and Comitt the offender till the fine be paid."[16] Had King William not coincidentally declared a general pardon for crimes committed before Withall had brought her case to the college, the doctor might well have remained in prison.

Released after almost a week in Newgate, Groenevelt initiated a series of moves centered upon defending and restoring his reputation for, although he again walked the streets of London, his imprisonment had brought the charges against him to the attention of his patients and friends: his imprison- ment had even been publicized in one of the London newspapers, the *Post Boy*, one of the channels used by the College of Physicians to explain its positions to the public. Published by Abel Roper, the *Post Boy* became the principal Tory paper; and among Tories, foreign dissenters like Groenevelt— especially Dutchmen—were not well liked. The *Post Boy* circulated well beyond Tory circles, however. While some private people subscribed to the London papers, and while they were also hawked about the streets and shipped to the provinces, the mainstay of newspaper circulation was among the coffeehouses of London. There were an estimated three thousand coffee- houses in London at the beginning of the eighteenth century. They were places of public business and vigorous discussion, being "attended by the male sex only," with women present only behind the bar as coffee servers. Since at these coffeehouses men met to hear and exchange the news, coffee- house proprietors subscribed to one or more of the several newspapers that circulated in London after the lapse of the licensing act in 1695. Although the proprietors of inns and taverns also subscribed to newspapers for their clientele—and even small alehouses and brandy shops, and tradesmen such as barbers and chandlers, provided a paper or two for their customers—some coffeehouses even composed their own newsheets. Medical people were acutely aware of the influence of the newspapers, and empirics took advantage of them through frequently placing advertisements, especially in the last five years of the seventeenth century. Moreover, the newspapers and coffeehouses increasingly became places where political opinion was shaped—and this in an era when popular politics could greatly affect the city and nation.[17] Consequently, the Groenevelt affair would be fiercely debated in public.

For both personal and professional reasons, then, becoming the subject of a newspaper notice, and hence becoming the butt of coffeehouse chatter, could not have been a pleasant experience for Groenevelt, especially given the words used by Roper. "Last *Thursday* the Censors of the College of Physicians committed Dr. *Gronfeld*, one of their Members, to *Newgate*, without Bail or Mainprize, for refusing to pay 20*l*. in which they had fined him for Evil Practices."[18] This notice appeared not among the advertisements but as a regular item of news. The matter-of-fact report that Groenevelt had been imprisoned not merely for refusing to pay a fine but for "evil practices" made the story all the worse for him in the rumor mills. Among those who saw his name was someone in the Dutch church at Austin Friars. This person brought a copy of the *Post Boy* to the consistory meeting on the Sunday before Groenevelt's release, apparently wanting the criminal thrown out of the congregation. Had it not been for one of the ministers, Emilius van Cuilemborgh, who thought of himself as the "greatest bosom friend [Groenevelt] ever had in this world," such a move might have succeeded. Fortunately for Groenevelt, Van Cuilemborgh took his side and, in order to prove his point, on the Sunday following showed a newspaper to the congregation which favored Groenevelt.[19]

This second notice, countering the one in the *Post Boy*, appeared in the advertising section of the *Protestant Mercury*, immediately after Groenevelt's release and a couple of days before the Sunday service.[20] While the coffeehouses gossiped about Groenevelt's release,[21] this newspaper notice spread the word more widely and told his side of the case. The *Protestant Mercury*, published between 1696 and 1700, made a bid for wide circulation in London, although it never quite became one of the major papers.[22] The title itself suggested an affiliation with strong Protestantism: whoever placed the ad could assume that it would reach many people in the congregation at Austin Friars. The advertisement certainly minimized Groenevelt's troubles. Perhaps Groenevelt himself placed the notice and bent the facts; internal evidence suggests that he at least discussed the case with someone who wrote it up for him, somewhat straining the facts in the process.

The account began by praising Groenevelt's surgical skills, at the same time portraying the charges against him as malicious. "Three or four sports of the Warwick-lane Colledge" had confined "Dr. Gronfeld (who Cuts admirably for the Stone in the Bladder)" to Newgate on 15 April. The reason for his confinement was "prescribing about five years agone (to a Woman who recovered, and is yet alive) two grains of a Medicament (calling it Mala Praxis)." In other words, the patient was said to be well, and the amount of cantharides Groenevelt had prescribed was reduced to what only one of the eighteen pills contained. "The same Medicine" had been prescribed by "Sir Tho. Witherly (sometime President of the same Society)" as early as "the 27th of December 1686" to "one Mrs. Folks without the least Blame." Having justified Groenevelt's practice, the account continued: "The Question now arising here from is, how that can be Mala Praxis and deserve Newgate without Bail or Mainprize in the One, which was without Censure in the other? Or whether to squeeze £20 or it may be a much lesser sum out of the sufferer, was not the main inducement of this barbarous Prosecution?"

Having made his practice seem good, and the prosecution seem wholly pecuniary, the advertisement went on to say that the law had been entirely on Groenevelt's side.

> On Wednesday the 21st Instant, the Cause came to a Hearing at the King's Bench-Bar, before the Lord Chief Justice Holt, and the other judges of that Honourable Court, where upon the Pleading of Mr. Serjeant Wright, and Mr. Northey, who were for the Defendant Dr. Greenfield, it appeared by their Defence, he was illegally and Maliciously Prosecuted, against the Privileges of English Men; and accordingly the Judges, as with one joint voice and Consent, did honourably Acquit and Discharge him, leaving him to the farther Justice of the Law, to exact a full satisfaction for that his False Imprisonment.[23]

The newspaper story thus anticipated Groenevelt's next move: he tried to restore his reputation not only by public stories but by exacting his own punishment on the censors. While the justices of the King's Bench probably did not encourage Groenevelt to sue for false imprisonment—far from it, if the Annals are correct—his lawyers apparently thought he had a case. As the advertisement predicted, at the end of April he launched a lawsuit for false imprisonment against the censors of the college, the college beadle,

and the warden of Newgate prison. The case took several years to come to
an end but in the meantime caused much trouble to the censors.

In response to Groenevelt's suit, the officers of the college called a special
meeting of all the fellows on 4 May in order to explain their position and
to drum up support for themselves. President Millington explained what had
happened over the last few weeks and that Groenevelt had now brought suit.
He asked the college to hold its beadle and the warden of Newgate "harmless."
The fellows agreed to pay the defense of these two out of college funds. The
president then "discoursed the matter of fact as it appeared before him."
He reported that false rumors were circulating around London about what
Groenevelt had done (perhaps in part rooted in the advertisement in the
Protestant Mercury). He also told them about stories that some in the college
"did seem to avow and justify such practice." Millington then went on to
inform the whole college of what the censors had done: they had imprisoned
Groenevelt for the administration of thirty-six grains of cantharides to be
taken over the course of twelve or fifteen hours for an ulcer in the bladder.
He asked each and every fellow, one by one, in public, whether they agreed
that what Groenevelt had done constituted malpractice or not. According to
the registrar, "some did suspend their opinion, but none did attempt to justifie
the giving so great a quantity of Cantharides in that disease, nor in any other,
in so short a time."[24] We may assume that Tyson, Bernard, Blackmore,
How, and other of Groenevelt's supporters within the college were among
those who "suspended their opinions," since once again the college officers
had refused to suggest that his practice might have been something other
than the administration of cantharides alone. But any fellow who defended
Groenevelt now, after not supporting his administration of cantharides in a
college meeting, could easily be portrayed as a hypocrite.

This victory within the college behind them, the censors took the next
step of placing a further notice in another of the major London newspapers.
The censors quickly set the record straight for the public in the Whig *Post
Man*, with a circulation of perhaps four thousand.[25] "A Paper called the
Protestant Mercury, having falsely, Scandlaously [*sic*] and maliciously represented the case of Dr John Groenvelt," the censors wrote, public justice
required a correction. Groenevelt had not been sent to Newgate for prescribing
two grains of a medicament to a woman who afterward recovered. Instead,
he had given thirty-six grains of Spanish fly to cure an ulcer in a bladder,
with consequent painful effects and a continued bedridden state for the patient.
"For this practice, and to deter him from the like again he was by the said
Censors committed." When he brought his habeas corpus, he had been

discharged from Newgate "by pleading the Kings General Pardon, as a Criminal, and upon no other account."[26] In a fury at this last charge, Groenevelt threatened to sue not only the censors but the publisher of the newspaper.[27]

The censors not only continued their attack on Groenevelt in public, they also found a vehicle for further harassing him legally. They helped Mrs. Withall bring a civil suit against Groenevelt for £2,000; or rather, they used Withall as a foil for their own further legal maneuvers, since they and their attorney Mr. Swift handled her suit themselves.[28] A later petition to the Parliament noted that the costs of Withall's case against Groenevelt were too high to have been borne by Withall herself, and it remarked that the college beadle had admitted before his death that the censors had "encouraged" her suit.[29] Precisely when the suit was brought is unclear, but it must have been done in Trinity term (roughly June). Civil suits against medical practitioners seem to have been relatively uncommon in the period; certainly there is no example yet known other than Withall's of a contemporary suit for such a huge amount of money. It is hard to imagine that Groenevelt would have been able to pay such an amount if found guilty, which would have sent him to debtors' prison, perhaps for the rest of his days.

In short, neither Groenevelt nor the censors would let the matter rest. Each considered their public reputations to be at stake. If the censors won Withall's civil suit, Groenevelt's livelihood would be greatly damaged, perhaps beyond repair. If Groenevelt succeeded in breaking the censors' punitive abilities by winning his suit for false imprisonment, then the censors would be virtually powerless to control what they considered to be malpractice. A bitter public battle therefore soon raged on several fronts: in the law courts; in papers, pamphlets, and books; and in and among the medical corporations of London.

The continuing suits by and against Groenevelt had become just one aspect of a broad policy of the college officers to crack down on what they conceived to be medical misbehavior. At the time, the officers were not only continuing to make life difficult for Groenevelt, they were beginning to launch a public condemnation of the medical ideas and practices of the apothecary-doctor John Colbatch.[30] Samuel Garth's Latin Harveian Oration—soon published in English translation—made a vigorous plea to the Crown for increased support for the new college policy of cracking down on illicit and bad practitioners.[31] The college officers continued with the dispensary scheme against the apothecaries, while many of Groenevelt's allies, including Tyson, Bernard, and Blackmore, "positively refused to subscribe" to the project.

The censors in turn continued to remind the many fellows (and virtually all licentiates) who were in open revolt against the leadership that they had to obey the new college statutes.[32]

As an indication of the deep divisions in the College of Physicians, one or more fellows tried to block the election to the censorship of one of the most vigorous defenders of the hard line, Charles Goodall, at the September 1697 meeting. Goodall had become the strongest defender of the rights of the college to control medical practice in London: for some years he had headed the special committee governing affairs behind the scenes,[33] and the apothecaries were convinced that the dispensary project—which they took to be an assult on their business—was Charles Goodall's idea.[34] At the September meeting, Goodall for the first time agreed to stand for the public office of college censor. Voting was done by having the fellows place a black or white bean in a jar: on this occasion, the fellows appeared to refuse Goodall the censorship by one vote until it was discovered that more beans had been put into the jar than there were fellows: someone or some group had resorted to ballot-box stuffing. Only on a second vote, after a stern lecture by the president and a check to make sure that each fellow took only one bean, did Goodall become one of the new censors.[35]

Goodall, Samuel Collins, Edward Hulse, and Richard Morton replaced Groenevelt's adversaries on the censors' committee but continued their policies. Goodall set about gathering information in support of Withall's suit against Groenevelt.[36] By the autumn of 1697, then, it was clear to all that the college officers would neither change their policies nor stop their support for Withall's civil suit against one of their own licentiates.

Groenevelt had already brought suit against them for false imprisonment; now he launched a further attack on the censors—presumably with inside information from one or more of the fellows. He thought he had a chance not just to embarrass the censors but to break their power with yet another lawsuit against them in the Court of King's Bench. This time, he charged them with not having formally taken the oaths of allegiance and supremacy to the government, as required of all public officials. In this, Groenevelt imitated proceedings being brought against the Commissioners of the Excise for the same offense. During the parliamentary debate over the religious framework of England in the early 1670s, the Test Act had been passed renewing the requirement of James I that all governmental officers had to "take the severall Oathes of Supremacy and Allegiance" (together with "the Sacrament of the Lords Supper according to the Usage of the Church of England"). Those neglecting or refusing the oaths were to be "ipso facto adjudged uncapeable and disabled in Law to all intents and purposes whatsoever to have occupy or enjoy the said office."[37] Groenevelt therefore argued that since the censors had not taken the oaths, they could not hold their offices of public trust. On 29 October, the college officers delegated former censors Dawes and Gill—two of the victims of the action—to "manage the Law suite with Groenvelt, and the information brought against the Late Censors."[38]

A few weeks after Groenevelt brought his second suit against the censors, Withall's suit against him finally came to trial. The case was heard at London Guildhall on Tuesday, 7 December 1697, taking six hours to hear, and pitted about twenty fellows who testified against Groenevelt's practice against three others who were self-confident enough to testify on his behalf.[39] Owing to the preservation of a remarkable document, we know precisely how the college lawyer intended to present the case to the jury.[40]

Since a few other sources suggest that the case went much as Attorney Swift expected, this, then, seems to have been the way in which the trial proceeded. Swift opened the case on behalf of "William Withall and Susan his Wife" with a short recital of Mrs. Withall's sufferings over the last four and one-half years, the pains and evil consequences of Groenevelt's bad medical treatment still causing her to languish in danger of her life. The case centered on William Withall's claim that he had paid out £2,000 to try to care for and treat his wife, he demanding that amount from the offending doctor, Joannes Groenevelt. (It seems incredible that a chapbook salesman could have obtained cash and credit worth such a huge amount.) Groenevelt responded with a plea of not guilty. Then began the business of putting people in the witness box to testify on Withall's behalf.

Swift's strategy was first to call the same witnesses who had testified before the college on several earlier occasions. Jane Daylight, Prunella Beckett, Barbara Curtis, Hannah Walding, and Jane Butterfield would all give or verify the same statements that they had given previously to the college. Hannah Walding would also give further testimony as well, telling the court two things: that when Groenevelt was first accused of using Spanish fly he had denied it, and that his directions were exactly followed. To prove that before she took the pills Mrs. Withall had been in good health, Swift prepared to call Mrs. Withall herself and two others. To prove how much had been spent on her recovery and how greatly she still suffered, six other people would testify. To show that Groenevelt had admitted that he used Spanish fly in pills to cure some complaints, including ulcers in the bladder, the president and three of the censors of 1694 to 1695 were to be put on the stand.[41] To prove that this practice was "exceeding dangerous" and properly condemned as malpractice, Swift could count on seven physicians, including a Dutchman new to London, Dr. Abraham Cyprianus, the son of one of Velthuis's former rivals in Amsterdam, a person now trying to become a high-flying lithotomist and physician in London. Then Groenevelt would have a chance to give evidence justifying his treatment. Swift could count on nineteen surgeons and physicians to rebutt Groenevelt.

Swift anticipated that the argument of Groenevelt would be that he had prescribed not the eighteen pills of cantharides alone but eighteen pills of camphor as well, to be taken with the cantharides. Groenevelt would argue that his pills "were not given as he directed." To this, Swift prepared two counterattacks: first, Mr. and Mrs. Withall and the other women would "positively denye it"; second, even if Groenevelt had prescribed camphor and the patient had taken it, Swift would try to show that camphor was "noe corrective" for the cantharides. To prove this second point he had a dozen distinguished physicians ready to testify. But Groenevelt could produce other physicians in his defense, testifying that giving thirty-six grains of corrected cantharides in cases of an ulcer in the bladder was good practice. Consequently, the case against Groenevelt might have to enter upon the shifting sands of a complex medical debate. For this, Attorney Swift had been extensively advised by the officers of the college. He would first ask about how the cantharides had been prepared, on the assumption that he could show Groenevelt's to be plain Spanish fly. He noted to himself: ask the witnesses on Groenevelt's behalf "strictly whether they ever did or would give 36 graines of plaine . . . Cantharides. . . . They will evade it by burneing or calcineing it into powder which quite alters the Nature of the Cantharides." As a final general reminder about the medical debate, Swift made a note to "insist throughout that such a quantity [of cantharides was] utterly improper in any case and the least quantity in this case."

But Swift had to prepare himself even more precisely for the specific testimony on Groenevelt's behalf from Sir Richard Blackmore (recently knighted and made one of King William's physicians in ordinary) and Dr. William Gibbons, a society doctor.[42] They would testify that such a quantity of cantharides as Groenevelt had used had been successful in other, similar cases. Such testimony would force Swift to give some ground on the medical issue, since one witness against another in such debates tended to show that the defendant had had good medical reasons for doing what he did, even if others disagreed. Thus Swift expected to have to establish that Groenevelt's prescription could not have produced any good in a case like Withall's.

"Suppose it was proper, which is not granted, yett aske them how they could direct the medicine soe that it should not touch the other soundness of the bladder," he noted to himself. In short, Swift's medical argument set out to show that in Withall's case the "horney lipps" of the ulcer had been eaten down by the cantharides, causing her bladder to bleed and leading to other problems: he had six people (Cyprianus and five surgeons) who would testify to this probability. If the doctor "or surgeons for the defendant" testified that they had given cantharides without harm, Swift would insist that not harming was different from curing.

Anticipating being forced to argue this much weaker line about medical probabilities, differing judgments, and not curing rather than harming, Swift had to prepare for an even greater problem for his case: Dr. Francis Bernard would testify not only that giving cantharides might have done Withall no harm but that it was a positively good practice. To counter such testimony, Swift prepared to attack Bernard's veracity by calling on Dr. Edward Hulse. Hulse would state that he had once heard Bernard say "he would not have done" what Groenevelt had. Swift had a final counterargument:

> If Dr. Bernard or any other Physitians insinuate to the Court and Jury as some of them did to my Lord Chief Justice [during the habeas corpus hearing] . . . that Hypocrates prescribes it in the same case and in many others the like quantities & that Dr. Lyster himselfe in one of his bookes (notwithstanding when he was Censor [in 1694] he had condemned this verry case for evill practice . . .) had avowed it to be good practise . . .: Aske which Cantharides these were Hypocrates gave; they were a quite different sort from those now in use.

Swift prepared himself to bring into court Hippocrates' books to show that nowhere could anyone find a passage in which Hippocrates had ever used more than six grains of plain cantharides, and never in such a case. To top off this part of the case, Swift would try to prove that cantharides were absolutely forbidden "in all ulcers of the bladder" and that they were "onely to be ventured in desperate dropsies & stranguaries." Five distinguished fellows would testify to this. Swift would also attack Bernard's motives, asking him if he was not a member of the Society of Apothecaries and a member of its Court of Assistants (the apothecaries just then feeling very threatened by the college's dispensary, thus having an interest in attacking the censors).[43] If Tyson testified for Groenevelt, then Swift would try to make him seem hypocritical, too, by asking him if he had not found Groenevelt guilty of malpractice at the beginning of Tyson's censorship.

Swift also prepared to assault Groenevelt's practice of using cantharides more generally. He could summon witnesses to testify to Groenevelt's having caused the death of patients through the use of his remedy. In one case Groenevelt gave a woman a liquid, and she went out of this life "in flames"; in another case Mrs. Mary Thorneton "dyed in the same manner by Canthari-des given her by ye Defendant after her Lyeing in"; Nurse Bale "dyed in the same manner by Cantharides given her by the Defendant." And there were also the fatal examples of Mrs. Whites and Mrs. Weilder; Mrs. Wooton, who took five years to recover from Groenevelt's cantharides; and the serious damage he had done to Mrs. Peirez. There were other examples. Swift could also bring forth witnesses to tell how Groenevelt had done various "mischiefs" in cutting for the stone. And Swift would show that Groenevelt's way of practice was "Quack-like": "halfe in hand, and haveing that[, he] cares not what becomes of the patient." He ended his brief with a recital of the laws empowering the College of Physicians to arrest for malpractice and the reasons why the apothecaries were opposed to the college: the officers seem to have told Swift that the reason some fellows would testify for Groenevelt was because they opposed the dispensary.

The lineup of witnesses for and against Groenevelt suggests that those who advised their attorney thought that the issue of dispensary doctors against the others was the crucial dispute dividing the physicians. Swift noted the names of sixteen ordinary people, included Suzanna Withall, who would testify against Groenevelt. But to establish a case of medical malpractice against a defendant who would accuse the witnesses of not understanding his medical directions, the testimony of knowledgeable physicians would be crucial. Each of the twen-ty-three physicians willing to testify against Groenevelt had been an original subscriber to the dispensary, including one of the few licentiates who had sub-scribed, Dr. Hamilton.[44] Aside from Hamilton, the other twenty-two physicians against Groenevelt were fellows. Twelve of them served or had served as offi-cers,[45] two had gained knighthoods,[46] three served as royal physicians,[47] and the others were up-and-coming Whigs.[48] Of the eight surgeons and apothecaries prepared to testify against Groenevelt, all had good personal relationships with the establishment physicians.[49] One of them, Dr. Abraham Cyprianus, whose father had been opposed to Groenevelt's partner Velthuis in Amsterdam and who was now Groenevelt's rival London lithotomist, had recently given up his professorship at Franeker University and, with John Locke's help, settled in London to practice medicine and surgery.[50] There he had cut Sir Thomas Mil-lington (now president of the College of Physicans) for a bladder stone: Milling-ton clearly had no wish to use Groenevelt for the operation. Cyprianus would stay on in London until his death.[51]

On Groenevelt's side were three important opponents of the college officers. Francis Bernard was a wealthy and learned apothecary as well as a physician; he had collected one of the largest libraries in London, although "for use, and not for ostentation or ornament."[52] Another, William Gibbons, like Bernard, had been one of the most vigorous opponents of the "new College" that appeared after the revolution of 1688–89, refusing to subscribe to the dispensary and signing petitions to have the college reformed by the government. He and Bernard had also been passing along information about college policy to the Society of Apothecaries.[53] Sir Richard Blackmore, too, had refused to support the dispensary while signing petitions against the "new College." For his poetry he had also been recently made one of the king's personal physicians. While his art has been found too earnest for the taste of modern critics, he stood in the forefront of those who were trying to instigate a reformation of manners in England.[54]

Moreover, Groenevelt had a very different version of the facts of the case than his accusers. According to a pamphlet published after the trial, Groenevelt had been sent for because he had developed a cure for previously incurable ulcers of the bladder. He had found Withall suffering not only from an ulcerated bladder but also from "a scyrrhus" (a hard swelling without pain) "in the Vagina Uteri, and Cancerous Piles." When he sent her his pills, he also sent her instructions telling her not to commence her treatment until he had arrived. She nevertheless took the pills of cantharides without the "corrector" of camphor, consequently suffering pains and bloody water, and thereupon sent for the doctor in haste. He chided her for not waiting for him, but he still "took off" the pains and bloody urine "immediately" and then sent her to the country, attending her almost daily to cure her of the ulcerated bladder, in which he succeeded. But her other medical problems remained. Withall had first tried to blame her remaining troubles on the midwife Mrs. Salloway, who cleared herself only by calling in Drs. Coatesworth and Gibson, who found the source of Withall's pains to be the cancerous piles, Groenevelt having cured the ulcer by then. Two years later, Groenevelt had been "thought on at the Instigation of one of the Censors [Torlesse], whom the Doctor had exasperated, as he easily [would] be." The idea of Withall herself suing Groenevelt had also been put into her head by the censors: Dr. Burwell's servant John Cole had been sent by the college lawyer to another solicitor, Mr. Ambrose, who took Cole to Withall's house to deliver a message. Shortly after the visit, she had brought suit. In short, Mrs. Withall was a sick and dishonest woman who had brought her complaint against Groenevelt only in an attempt to recover the 40s. she had already paid him, and when she got no redress from the college, she tried to "jump into an Estate" by suing for £2,000.[55]

Thus, Groenevelt had a different explanation for what had happened than the college censors, and while fewer physicians would testify in favor of his use of cantharides, they were no less distinguished than his medical opponents. If the jury decided against judging the medical theory and practice of the day in the face of two equally learned opposing parties, all that remained of the case against Groenevelt was his word about thirty-six pills against ordinary witnesses to there being only eighteen of cantharides alone. Again, each side could advance arguments to show that the other had reasons for twisting the evidence: on Groenevelt's side Mrs. Withall could be shown to be the tool of the malicious and monopolistic censors, on their side the college officers could show that he practiced a risky method and had the support of the college's enemies for it. Given the contradictory nature of the testimony, in a kind of medical "she said, he said," the trial took a very long time to be heard. But in the end, "after a debate of 6 hours, a verdict was given on his side."[56] Groenevelt had been found not guilty.

In the immediate aftermath of Withall's trial against Groenevelt, his affair became the subject of renewed coffeehouse discussion. Narcissus Luttrell noted the outcome of the trial in his diary, although the newspapers were silent.[57] The fact that a public jury had let Groenevelt go free also augured ill for the future of college authority. The more its officers had to explain defensively why their powers were good and necessary, the more their adversaries had opportunities to persuade the public that these learned men should not be trusted, portraying them as wishing only to restrict trade. As long as some of the fellows supported those who tried to break the censors' powers, splitting the authority of the college, making war by public suit and pamphlet did not favor the officers.

Groenevelt immediately published his own version of events after the trial, in the form of a preface to a book he wrote on the safe internal use of cantharides.[58] Because it appeared in Latin and cost a fairly high price, the book clearly aimed to impress the learned rather than the general English reading public. He was therefore trying to restore his reputation among the educated without doing the physicians themselves public damage: he still tried to defend himself rather than to bring down his opponents. (The work had a second Latin edition in 1703 with some additional case reports of his remedy,[59] and an English edition only in 1710, which included a new dedication, a Latin poem to the author, and some additions by the translator.)[60]

Groenevelt dedicated his book to the three physicians who had testified on his behalf in the recent trial, Sir Richard Blackmore, Francis Bernard, and William Gibbons. No one could accuse him of quackish behavior for publishing a learned treatise in Latin on his method of practice.

Groenevelt's account of the case for his Latin readers began straightforwardly enough. He had found it necessary to go public to vindicate himself from "a most impious Ignominy" caused by his being sent to Newgate; in order to fully vindicate himself, he found it necessary to "expose the Arrogance as well as Ignorance of [his] Detractors." He had practiced medicine successfully for more than twenty-seven years, paying special attention to diseases of the kidneys and bladder. His work in this area had led him to the discovery of the use of cantharides corrected by camphor, "a most noble and safe Remedy" in ischuries (the suppression of urine in the bladder), dysuries (trouble in making water due to some obstruction of the organs by stone, gravel, or thick slime, together with warmth in the urine), stranguries, ulcers of the bladder, "etc." The remedy worked especially well in women, who had a larger and shorter ureter than men; he had cured more than one hundred women with his remedy, he claimed. He had prescribed this same remedy to Suzanna Withall in early 1693, who did not obey his written orders but took only stimulating pills made up of cantharides rather than all the pills brought by him. She had been bedridden for some time previously because of a difficult childbirth; but even taking only the pills of cantharides she found herself feeling better. Since one of the censors in 1692–93, Josiah Clerk, had seen for himself the beneficial effects of Groenevelt's remedy, the censors dismissed the original complaint of Withall in that year "without any manner of Censure at all" for Groenevelt. But in 1697, "the bitterness of Gall appeared and speedy Vengeance was designed."[61]

He skipped over completely the other events and hearings before the spring of 1697. Then, he wrote, the matter had been revived because of "some sharp Words that had pass'd between [him] and one of the Censors for [that] Year, viz. R[ichar]d T[orle]sse."[62] Because of Torlesse's personal animosity toward Groenevelt, the censors called him before them once again. Groenevelt offered not only to explain his method of practice but to demonstrate on two dogs, then and there, the difference in the effects of cantharides given alone or together with camphor. He also offered to bring in as witnesses to his practice some of the many women whom he had cured using his pills, as well as "Physitians of our own College who were Eye Witnesses of the same; but it was Preaching to a dead Wall, all was to no purpose, they refuse[d], reject[ed], and distain[ed], all that could be offered in my Defence."

Instead, the censors "gave a particular and pleasing Attention and Credit to the Railings and Calumnies of three Women, Sworn clandestinely and privately in my absence, and deny'd me the liberty to hear their Examination, or to make any reply thereto, tho' often requested, but sent me away wholly Ignorant of what was done." Fourteen days later, the censors committed him—not a mountebank or quack but a doctor of physic and member of their own college—to Newgate, "the common Gaol for Thieves and Rogues." Such a thing had never been "heard of or seen by any Body before, since the foundation of either College or Gaol."[63]

In conclusion, Groenevelt, like the other adversaries of a stronger college, asked, "Must none but three or four judge of the Medicinal Art? Certainly unless such would be accounted omniscient or Infallible, Remedies may be administered which they understand not, since many things are daily found out by the curious Enquirers into Nature, for the benefit of Mankind, which was condemn'd as hurtful by the Antients." As an example, Groenevelt mentioned the new discovery of Edward Baynard of very cold baths as a cure for palsies and other diseases of the limbs. Most of the members of the college—except those "of lesser note" who had to fear the censors to get ahead—agreed with Groenevelt that new experimental medicines ought to be developed, he wrote. He ended by appealing "to the Throne, [and] to the great Council of the Nation, the Parliament, the living Oracles and Founders of our Laws," to declare that the power of the censors to throw physicians into jail at their pleasure was "an unaccountable Grievance."[64] After this, he explained the reasons for his practice at length. The local issue remained clear and uncompromising: should the college officers have the support of the law and government to regulate practitioners in London as they liked, or not?

Groenevelt also used this book to try to obtain the private support of at least one grand personage: William Bentinck, the earl of Portland. Bentinck had been a boyhood friend—and probably a lover—of William of Orange and remained the king's most trusted adviser. The English edition of Groenevelt's work contains a dedication to Portland; in it, Groenevelt also mentioned having been appointed a physician at Grave about twenty-five years previously.[65] Taken together with the fact that Grave had been retaken in 1673, it seems clear that the dedication to Portland was written for the first Latin edition of Groenevelt's book, although only printed with the English edition. It seems therefore to have been a private dedication, sent to Portland along with a copy of the Latin treatise. In it, he appealed to Portland as a former fellow student of Portland's brother-in-law and as a fellow countryman. This dedication was full of righteous indignation at the college's behavior. "I am convict only upon the Railery or Clamour of three old women about the more abstruse Practice of Physick; and condemned without so much as being hear'd, or any Witnesses examined, and Sentenced to perpetual Imprisonment, had their Wills past for Law." The "Sacred Authority of our Constitution" had saved him, but the college certainly seemed to be a body that had little to do with defending good medicine, and everything to do with arbitrary government.

But the College of Physicians, too, made its appeals to the throne. President Millington made a December 1697 address to the king after His Majesty's safe return to England in November from making peace with the French. The college was among the many corporations presenting their congratulations, meeting to vote the address on 3 December (just four days before Withall's trial against Groenevelt), with Groenevelt among them.[66] Millington, later one of the king's physicians-in-ordinary,[67] made the oration before William a week later, taking the opportunity to solicit the king's support for the college: "[The College of Physicians] owes its being to Your Royal Predecessors, and the Privileges it enjoys to Your Majesty's Favour."[68] Appealing to the Crown for support had been the subject, too, of Samuel Garth's oration to the college in September and would be the solution to the college's troubles suggested in his mock epic *The Dispensary*.[69] Without the support of the monarchy itself, the college could only wage its war through the courts, where results were not always to its liking, or through public pamphleting, which so often backfired. But King William himself remained silent on the subject of the college, even when he had an easy opportunity to lend the censors assistance.[70]

The king could have given the censors a helping hand in January but chose not to do so, perhaps because Portland had listened to Groenevelt. The suit Groenevelt had launched against the censors before Withall's trial was due to come before the courts in Hilary term (from c. 20 January) of 1698. The censors had been charged with not having taken the oaths of allegiance and supremacy as required of those holding public office. In January, the censors therefore asked the king for a nolle prosequi: a writ that the king could issue to stop any suit in the common law courts. In theory, breaking the king's law first and foremost damaged the monarch himself, so he could in turn choose to overlook the offense and stop the case from coming to trial. The censors petitioned for such a writ of nolle prosequi on the grounds that "noe Censor ever did or ever thought themselves obliged to take the said oathes as not themselves to have an office or employment within the words and meaning of the said Act." Moreover, no censors had ever before "been questioned for refusing or neglecting the same till now that an Information was proferred against" them. In short, they had not taken the oaths simply because they never had thought it necessary, "not out of any Aversion to the government or dislike to the Oathes."[71] Even before the king heard the petitions, the censors had given up on their earlier agreement to stand by one another. William Dawes petitioned the king first, leaving the others to follow the procedure on their own two weeks later. Dawes's petition was referred to the attorney general, that of the others to both the attorney and solicitor generals.[72] Apparently the attorney and solicitor generals reported in favor of the censors.[73] But despite such legal advice, William himself refused to stop the lawsuit.

In the trial against three of the censors in the Court of King's Bench, the jury turned matters over to a special verdict: that is, the question at issue involved an interpretation of law the jury could not decide itself, and so it placed the matter back in the hands of the justices themselves for a resolution.[74] Dawes expected to come to trial during the next term.[75] By April, the various matters concerning public officials who had not taken the oaths (including the Commissioners of the Excise) came before the House of Lords. The Lords rejected the bill to allow these officials more time to take the oaths.[76] But two weeks later the House of Lords accepted the substitution of a much more specifically worded bill and gave it a reading.[77] Perhaps the reason for the first rejection had been that the vagueness of the wording allowed the college censors to be included. Certainly now the college officers lobbied the Lord Chancellor to be included in the second bill, although without apparent success.[78] After the second reading on 10 May, the college petitioned the houses of Parliament to allow the president, censors, and other officers to be included in this bill to allow more time for the officers to qualify themselves.[79] Typical of the parliamentary lobbying of the period,[80] the censors printed up a short summary of their argument for advanced distribution to their supporters and to members of the House of Lords as they came into their chamber for debate.[81] But in alliance with the Society of Apothecaries, Groenevelt used the same tactics to keep the censors from being included with the Commissioners of the Excise. Thus, when the House of Lords decided in June that the Commissioners of the Excise had not broken the law, it helped the censors not one jot.[82]

The decision in the House of Lords to leave the censors to the courts had been fought for not only by Groenevelt but by the apothecaries as well. The apothecaries were deeply concerned about the college officers' attempts to control practitioners—including themselves—in London. The college's attorney Swift had already noted in the fall of 1697 that Groenevelt "and Gardener the Apothecary who [was a] Kinsman" of his had been in practice together.[83] Thomas Gardener then served as deputy warden of the Society of Apothecaries and, in 1702, became its master.[84] Perhaps because of this personal connection, the society had paid Groenevelt £16 10s. to help with the costs of his suit against the censors.[85] But more was at stake than personal connections between Groenevelt and an influential apothecary. Just as the censors used Withall as an instrument for their own attacks on Groenevelt, so the Society of Apothecaries used Groenevelt as a foil for their own attacks on the college. The Groenevelt affair mushroomed not because Groenevelt himself was so important but because the issues were important for many others in London, too. He had become a pawn in a battle for the control of medical practice in London, in which the Society of Apothecaries had a deep interest.

Just before the case of the censors had come before the House of Lords, the college officers had finally opened the doors of their dispensary despite internal opposition from some of the fellows.[86] This constituted a sharp attack on the Society of Apothecaries. The officers of the society therefore not only gave Groenevelt moral and financial assistance in his lawsuit, they also lent him their legal aid in an attempt to break the power of the censors. They helped to plan how he could keep the censors from being included in the bill to exempt the Commissioners of the Excise from their oaths. Serjeant Thomas Adamson wrote one of the society's liverymen, Mr. Samuel Doody: "Sr: This day the Commissioners of the Excise have brought in ye bill to the house of Lords, in a day or two the Censors desire to peticion to be included, for Sir Tho. Midington [*sic*] labours might and maine to engage severall of the peers for them, so that you will do a great piece of service to get the Case of Dr. Greenfield delivered as fast as can be." The letter went on to include a list of members of both houses of Parliament who as "men of Justice" could be counted on to hear sympathetically the argument being made by the Society of Apothecaries and Groenevelt.[87]

The "Case of Dr. Greenfield" mentioned to Doody was a single-sheet handbill designed to be distributed to Their Lordships beforehand or as they entered their chamber, bearing the name of "J. Groenevelt" as author. Groenevelt and the apothecaries argued, first, that the power exercised by the censors clearly bore on the "Liberty and Property of the Subject," although the censors had not "qualified themselves" with the proper oaths. Despite not having the proper qualifications, the censors had executed their powers "with utmost violence against an innocent Person, as may more plainly appear in their Proceedings against Dr. John Greenfield." The handbill then briefly reported that the judges of King's Bench had discharged him from Newgate, where the censors had put him. Second, the censors had not been "satisfied with the designed Ruin of the Doctor and [his] family" but also proceeded to try to effect his ruin "by stirring up and assisting the aforesaid turbulent Woman to bring an Action of 2000 Pounds against the said Doctor," although he had been acquitted by Chief Justice Holt. Third, "the said Censors having thus notoriously acted like ill Men, Informations, by order of the King's Bench, were brought severally against them . . . for not having qualified themselves for a place of high Trust and Judicial Authority" by taking the oaths. The suits were costing the censors a lot of money, and so they were trying to slip away from the suit by getting the Parliament to excuse them. Finally, one of the censors, Dr. Burwell, had been "tried at the sitting after the last Term upon the Information aforesaid," and a special verdict had gone against him. The rest of the censors had joined together and were to be tried in the next judicial term. Groenevelt concluded by begging the Lords not to "suffer the Prosecutor to lose the Benefit of the Penalty [given to informants against lawbreakers], as by the law allowed against such Offenders, or otherwise indempnifie the Prosecutor aforesaid."[88] The members of the House of Lords indeed did not stop the prosecution against the censors.

To accompany Groenevelt's plea, someone at the same time also printed the text of the oaths the censors spoke upon taking office. The oaths only concerned the censors' duties toward the admission of members into the College of Physicians: "You will not consent to admit any Person into the College, but such, whom without any favour or affection you shall judge to be sufficiently qualified, both for learning and Morals." As for taking an oath to allow them to interfere in the lives and property of practitioners, the censors' oath merely included a vague "in all things else you will diligently do your duty, as God shall help you, and the Holy Gospels." Beneath the oath, this one-sheet handbill also included a copy of the college statute on the admission of licentiates, giving them the right to practice in London: "For We judge it reasonable that the College should admit all Persons to Practice, whom upon Examination they shall find duly qualify'd; lest our College should be lookt upon as a Monopoly." Anyone reading the censors' oath and statute on licentiates would presume that as a licentiate Groenevelt had been learned and moral—again raising grave doubts about whether the censors had the right to fine and imprison him.[89]

The college in turn presented Their Lordships with another handbill of their own, presenting fourteen objections to Groenevelt's four points.[90] Groenevelt quickly counterattacked with yet another sheet for the Lords, printed in two forms. One, printed on three of the four sides of a large sheet of paper folded in half, repeated the objections of the censors to his petition and then refuted each of their fourteen points in turn.[91] The other document took the form of a large, closely printed one-sheet folio with three columns: in the left-hand column was Groenevelt's four-point case; in the center column was a shortened version of the censors' fourteen-point objections; and in the right-hand column were the fourteen replies to the objections.[92] Among the points made in this reply to the censors were that Dr. Briggs and Dr. Clerk were ready to testify that Groenevelt had been acquitted by them of charges against him in 1693; Registrar Gill's record in the Annals could not be trusted; several physicians, surgeons, apothecaries, and midwives had testified in court in favor of Groenevelt's practice; and the apothecaries Speers, Dare, and Boucher could show by the bills in their possession that Drs. Burwell and Torlesse had prescribed cantharides in their own practices. But perhaps the most damning language came in the charge that the "court" of censors resembled "something of the nature of an Inquisition, and Matters transacted in private." What late seventeenth-century English Lord could like the idea of an inquisition operating in London?

At the same time that Groenevelt kept the pressure on the censors through his lawsuit and parliamentary petitioning about their oaths, he also cooperated with the Society of Apothecaries in launching further public attacks on the college. He willingly became an intermediary between the apothecaries and Dr. John Badger. A few years earlier, Badger had taken up his pen on behalf of the Society of Apothecaries at its request during the dispute between the College of Physicians and the Society of Apothecaries over the 1695 act allowing the London apothecaries to be exempt from certain public duties. When the college had lost that battle in Parliament, it had decided on setting up the dispensary, which now in the spring of 1698 the apothecaries were battling energetically. In 1695, Badger had been very angry at the college, having been refused admission despite his M.D. from Cambridge,[93] and he had worked together with the officers of the Society of Apothecaries and Dr. Francis Bernard (soon to be one of Groenevelt's most important supporters) to subvert the officers. Bernard had fed Badger information about the strategies of the college elite and had given him copies of the new statutes, so that Badger could publicize the monopolistic behavior of what he and others were calling the "new College." Badger's pen work had been very important in making the college appear to be a repressive institution that was bad for all Londoners, although he also ended up feeling that he had not been paid enough for his services by the Society of Apothecaries.[94]

In the spring of 1698, therefore, when the Society of Apothecaries again needed a literate front man, Badger had been approached—this time via Groenevelt. The society needed to respond to the college's flood of publicity in favor of the dispensary, which the physicians were portraying as a solution to the medical problems of the metropolis. The apothecaries were especially concerned about a recent pamphlet published at the end of April by two of the censors, Thomas Gill and Richard Morton.[95] According to Badger's later account, "by the sly and secret Intreague" of some of the apothecaries, he was "again requested by the mouth of Dr. Greenfield to answer that Paper." Groenevelt told Badger that "Mr. Deputy [Warden] Gardner had wrote something in Answer to it" and that he had read Gardener's response. In order to make Badger's job easier, Groenevelt would pass Gardener's response along to Badger to help him compose the reply to Gill and Morton. Badger communicated this message to the master of the Society of Apothecaries, Thomas Elton, and "he appointed to meet [Badger] and Dr. Greenfield, at Leonard's Coffee-House in Finch-Lane." The three of them met there and to complete the plot decided to have Gardener joint them, but he was not at home when sent for. After staying at Leonard's for a while, Groenevelt and Badger walked over to Gardener's house in Leaden-Hall Street. Since he was still not at home, Groenevelt left a message for Gardener to send his reply to Groenevelt's house.[96] Although in the end Badger did not undertake the reply to Gill and Morton (perhaps because of what he thought to be his earlier ill-treatment from the officers of the society), he helped Groenevelt get William Salmon to write it.[97]

William Salmon happened to be one of the best-known empirics in London. Salmon rivaled Pechey for the place of the most prolific medical author and translator of the late seventeenth century. He also advertised his remedies widely in handbills and in the newspapers, so that to some his name had become a watchword for quackery.[98] Salmon had been among those warned not to practice without the college's license in the autumn of 1689 and had been taken to court by the college censors in 1693;[99] when the college's case against him was lost on a demurrer in 1694, the censors ordered their attorney to start the suit over again. As partial protection, Salmon joined the surgeons' company in September.[100] The censors would exert new efforts in the Salmon case shortly after Groenevelt's loss in 1700 and eventually win against him.[101] Groenevelt found in Salmon—a fluent author and despiser of the college censors—an excellent ally.

Salmon had been recruited to respond to *The State of Physick in London.* That tract by the censors had argued several points. First, given the advances

in medicine since the days of Hippocrates, it was right to divide practice into
three branches (physic, surgery, and pharmacy), since no single person could
understand all three in all their detail. The practice of physic, though, required
"not only sound Judgment, but likewise great learning and suitable Experience": hence, physic had become a branch of university study, with its practice
being limited to those with university degrees. To further control the practice
of medicine, Henry VIII had established the College of Physicians of London.
Organized in their college, the London physicians had gone on to make a number
of great discoveries in nature and improvements in physic. But the number of
apothecaries had been increasing in London beyond all necessity and without
control, which not only increased the prices of the medicines they sold and the
danger of their practice but also discredited surgery. The Parliament was urged
to do something to restore the earlier status quo by supporting the college. In
the meantime, the college had established the dispensary, which sold well-
made medicines at one-quarter the cost to be found in the apothecaries's shops.
The authors concluded by noting that in the last two months since the dispensary
had been open, the poor—for whose relief the scheme was entirely intended—
were beginning to flock to it.[102] The apothecaries might have added: so were
the affluent, who saw no reason not to buy their medicines there if they could
be had more cheaply.[103]

   The State of Physick in London aroused the anger of the apothecaries to
such an extent that the apparent authors, Drs. Gill and Morton, tried to
distance themselves from it. Shortly after it appeared, the *Post Man* published
a notice: "The subscribers, whose names begins [*sic*] with those Letters
[Th.G. and R.M.] disown it, nor was there any such Pamphlet writ by the
Colledge or Subscribers, or ordered to be published or Printed by them."[104]
This notice provided Salmon with a beginning point for his reply. He could
call it a "little penny Quack-book" which was "only a Fardle or Bundle of
Lies" designed to "decry, abuse, scandalize, and undoe, if possible, the
honest and skilful Apothecaries, and Ruine the whole Trade." The notice in
the "*Post Boy*" [*sic*] had been a trick designed to "prevent an Answer thereto."
If Gill and Morton had not written it themselves, they knew who did, for it
represented the views of the censors. But Salmon claimed that the publisher
himself had told him that Morton's servant had brought in the manuscript
to be printed.[105] The rest of the book refuted *The State of Physick* line for
line, arguing above all that the combination of physic, surgery, and pharmacy
in one person had been the cause of the advances in the medicine of Hippocrates' time and would continue to be so in the present. It was the apothecary
who best represented the combination of necessary medical skills in the

modern period. The censors were simply trying to monopolize physic for those who had enough money to join to the college: the largest part "of the Warwick-Lane sparks" were "Mandamus Doctors, Grace Doctors, [and] Proxy Doctors" who had not gone through a long English medical education according to the university statutes.[106]

To prove that the college was a tyrannical monopoly, Salmon turned to the example of Groenevelt. When "three or four of them [thought] fit, to Prejudge a Man a Criminal, and guilty of male Practise in the Art of Physick," they could simply do it. In case of the "learned and Worthy Dr. Groenevelt," it was "a very great question whether they themselves [understood] what the true practise thereof [was]." They had committed him to Newgate as "a Criminal only of their own making," while "many others more Learned and Skilful then they, had formerly declared the same to be good and true Practise."[107] In short, for those opposed to a stronger College of Physicians, Groenevelt's case provided a perfect example of malicious, monopolistic, and ignorant medical behavior on the part of the censors. Defending themselves from Groenevelt's handbill and Salmon's pamphlet, the censors in their turn appealed to the public with a little tract of their own.[108]

By this time, a pamphlet war over medicine burned everywhere, with the public being subjected to constant bombardment from the various parties. The next barrage apparently came from Groenevelt himself, who publicly rebutted the censors with a pseudonymously published little pamphlet that appeared early in the autumn of 1698.[109] As usual, the author argued against the control of medicine by a few censors of the college, this time by reprinting Groenevelt's *Humble Petition*, the parts of the censors' tract rebutting it, and his own rebuttal to the censors' account. Because the censors had found no refuge in the king, the House of Lords, or the courts, they "at last, as their utmost Effort, bethought themselves of the late Expedient of Popularity." The tract reviewed yet again the proceedings against Groenevelt and what he conceived to be their illegal imprisonment of him, stressing that the censors had all along willfully misrepresented the case he had been called to treat and the medicines he had given. The author even reported that Groenevelt had gone to Dr. Burwell as he came from church, begging him to stop the censors' proceedings against him, but was refused even on such an occasion: "This last it was, first caus'd my Blood to boile." Torlesse took the blame for wanting to get at Groenevelt, while Goodall seemed to be the mastermind behind the college's general policy. The most "violent" opponent of Groenevelt had been Cyprianus, because he was trying to jump into Groenevelt's lithotomy practice.[110]

But because they had promoted a woman's civil suit, the censors had

"open'd the Eyes of the Mob, and the Flood-gates of the law against [them]":
anyone now might sue any physician for money, even if he belonged to the
college. In the whole affair, Groenevelt had stood above the storm, only publishing a reply in Latin: the handbill to the House of Lords had been written by
the "prosecutor" rather than Groenevelt himself, and he had had nothing to
do with the recent scandalous tract published against the censors by Salmon,
"Celer" averred. On their side, however, the censors had resorted to publishing
their version of the affair in a newspaper as soon as Groenevelt had been imprisoned. Who now behaved as a quack? By imprisoning one of their own, the
censors were destroying the respectability of physic in London. Why? Because
Groenevelt had opposed the dispensary and seemed to be an easy target and an
example to other licentiates. What the college censors were really up to these
days would be "unriddled" when "Mr. Bolton's book against Dr. Greenfield
[came] out, under the auspicious Conduct and Influence of Dr. Goodale."[111]

Indeed, people were becoming aware of a series of attacks launched against
the censors' adversaries by Charles Goodall. Goodall had recruited Richard
Boulton, a poor student of Brasenose College, Oxford, to write medical tracts
against Groenevelt and John Colbatch in return for the promise of his medical
patronage. Boulton had previously written some learned medical books in English, which attracted positive notice among the learned physicians of London,[112] and shortly after the House of Lords had rejected the plea of the censors
to get the suit against them dropped, Goodall decided to employ Boulton's pen
on behalf of the college.[113] In a letter of 26 May 1698, Goodall asked Boulton
to come to London to help him with a work of natural history, but when Boulton
arrived, Goodall immediately set him to work translating into English and writing a reply to Groenevelt's book.[114] At the same time, Goodall urged Boulton
on against Colbatch. Goodall corrected the proofs of Boulton's book against
Colbatch, kept him at work against Groenevelt, and also commissioned the
surgeon James Yonge to write an attack on Salmon's recent pamphlet against the
censors.[115] Yonge's book against Salmon had begun with sentiments obviously
close to Goodall's heart: the law had been changed to allow apothecaries to be
exempt from being scavengers in London when instead new laws were needed
to keep empirical practitioners obedient to their medical superiors, the Censors
of the College of Physicians.[116] But Boulton could not resist making some nasty
remarks of his own about the Manchester physician Charles Leigh, which Goodall soon had to deny having anything to do with; this in turn caused Boulton
to confront Goodall as a turncoat and make the whole affair public, revealing
the machinations behind the several attacks on opponents of the college and
calling Goodall's own reputation into question.[117] By 11 December 1698,

Goodall was forced to write his friends to stop them from continuing to help Boulton with his project against Groenevelt.[118]

Thus, the public turmoil surrounding the Groenevelt affair slowly became diverted into other attacks in a general medical war. Salmon (or one of his friends) replied to Yonge with a newspaper advertisement for his own *Rebuke* by saying that it was a reply to "All the Works of a Couple of Coxcombs: Written by the stupendious Critick, Crackbrain [James] Young of Plymouth, and Rattlehead Good Ale of London."[119] One of Goodall's defenders replied in turn with a newspaper notice asking that two quacks be brought to the madhouse of Bedlam for treatment: the first being William Salmon ("a Wit without Sense, and Scurrilous without Wit, Gentle without Breeding"), the second being Boulton ("pale Faced, of a down grining, flearing look; wears his own hair; late of *Brazen Nose* and still of *Brazen Face*").[120]

The London coffee houses now echoed with gossip about the argument among the medical practitioners in town. As 1698 turned to 1699, the medical community in London became the butt of many poetical satires and comedies.[121] Tom Brown's play *Physick Lies a Bleeding, or the Apothecary turned Doctor* pitted John Badger and John Colbatch against Charles Goodall.[122] Doctor Samuel Garth made jokes about the defenders but lambasted the opponents of the college dispensary in his mock-heroic poem.[123] Ned Ward continued to use the case of Groenevelt as an example of the slanderous behavior of the college censors. When he published part 6 of his witty *The London Spy* at the end of April 1699,[124] he had his hick visitor to London introduced to the pompous College of Physicians. In describing the privileges of the fellows, Ward made the following point:

> They lately committed a more able physician than themselves without bail or main prize, for malpractice in curing a woman of a dangerous ulcer in her bladder by the use of Cantharides, which they affirm not fit for internal application, tho' the patients life was saved by taking it; which shows they hold it a greater crime to cure out of the common method, than it is to kill in it. And in persecuting their antagonist for the contempt of Gallen and Hippocrates, they charg'd him for the doing that good which themselves wanted either will or knowledge to perform, and thus made themselves all fools in attempting to prove the other a knave, who procur'd his discharge at the King's Bench Bar, without a trial, and now sues them for false imprisonment; having also inform'd against 'em in the Crown Office, as common disturbers.

Ward then went on to describe the dispensary as a device for making money through quackish promises of good medicine at low cost, showing the physicians to be no better than the worst empirics.

In short, the Groenevelt affair helped to bring down the reputation of the College of Physicians. In trying to prosecute him without the support of the government, the censors had subjected themselves to public ridicule. Some meetings at the College of Physicians had to be canceled because many fellows now refused to come, so that quorums could not be mustered.[125] The Groenevelt affair was slowly drawing to a close in the midst of a general collapse of the college's reputation.

One last major episode remained: Groenevelt's suit against the censors in the Court of King's Bench on charges of false imprisonment, which resulted in an important ruling creating new legal precedent. He had brought the charges against the censors in the spring of 1697, very soon after getting out of Newgate on habeas corpus. The decision in the case went in favor of the censors, but in doing so it placed them under the direct supervision of the common-law courts. The immediate question that had to be decided was whether the censors had the authority to imprison Groenevelt for malpractice. But to answer the question, the judges found that they had to be clear about what constituted good medical practice by a physician.

Groenevelt's lawyers argued four points.[126] The first two concerned the warrant of commitment to Newgate, both as to its form and substance. The general point of this argument stated that the censors had not made clear the reason why Groenevelt's medicines had not been liked, with the result that the higher courts could not judge for themselves whether the practice had been good or not. Groenevelt's lawyers also argued two other matters: first, the censors had no right to both fine and imprison; and second, the censors only had the right to fine people for illicit practice if they were not licentiates of the college. Since the censors had not shown that Groenevelt had not been licensed by the college, they had not proved that they could do anything other than fine him.[127] The central points of these last two arguments arose from the distinctions made by Chief Justice Coke in Bonham's case of 1610.[128] In their own defense, the censors argued that they were judges of malpractice in London, and as judges they could not be sued for judging as they did; moreover, the writ they had made out had been good in both form and substance.[129]

As for the first two arguments, Holt and the other justices decided that the form of the writ imprisoning Groenevelt had been good[130]—this probably came as no surprise, since Holt himself had recommended its formula. As for the other two arguments deriving from the objections arising from Bonham's case, Holt thought that the declaration of Chief Justice Coke in that

case did not provide a precedent. Coke had found the college not to be a
court of record but a kind of medical fraternity; while it could govern its
own members' behavior toward one another, it had no right to govern medical
practice in London. Holt, however, declared that Coke's words only constituted an opinion rather than "a resolution" that carried the force of legal
precedent. He thought rather that the college was indeed a court of record.
Holt made a further distinction, too: in Bonham's case, Coke had found that
the censors did not have the right to imprison (only to fine) for cases of illicit
practice, but Groenevelt's case concerned malpractice, not illicit practice.
Holt thought the charter of Henry VIII confirmed by act of Parliament sufficiently clear to allow the censors to punish for malpractice. In such matters,
the person imprisoned might make a plea by certiorari to King's Bench for
the court to determine whether the censors had sufficient reason to imprison
or not.[131] But Groenevelt could not sue the censors for carrying out their
duty; no one could sue judges for exercising judgment. If Groenevelt could
sue the censors for their decision, a slippery slope would follow: the precedent
would "expose the justice of the nation" so that "no man would execute the
office" of judge "upon peril of being arraigned by action or indictment for
every judgment he pronounce[d]."[132] Instead, the Court of King's Bench
ought to oversee lower courts like the college and so bring such bodies into
the framework of English common law.[133] This declaration has rightly been
seen by legal historians as creating very important precedent in English
administrative law. Without it, it would be possible for some courts to remain
outside the system of review by courts of common law such as King's
Bench.[134]

But Holt and his colleagues had to probe even deeper into the matter.
Once a case like Groenevelt's came before the Court of King's Bench on a
certiorari, what then? Would the justices then be judges of good and bad
medical practice? Holt did not much like this idea. Instead, he thought that
the court only had to determine whether the censors had good reason to do
as they did. After that, the justices would not (indeed, they could not) reverse
the decision of the censors as to whether the practice had been good or bad,
"for this Court [could] make no judgment, whether they were wholesome
[medicines] or not."[135]

What the justices were deciding here went to the heart of the medical
issues of the century, in Bonham's case of 1610 as well as in Groenevelt's
of 1700. Would "experts" be left to determine for themselves what was good
practice? In Bonham's case, Chief Justice Coke had worried about this in
his opinion against the college. But Holt's court decided that the censors of

the college could indeed judge questions of both malpractice and illicit practice and simply leave it to the courts to determine whether their procedures in doing so were good. Underlying the issue was a question about what it was that physicians did. If physicians had to exercise judgment about unique cases that varied not only from place to place and person to person but even from moment to moment, then no one could second-guess learned physicians, since only they had inculcated in themselves the excellent medical judgment to know what constituted good practice in one case and not in another.[136] Holt's court noted on this question that "none but physicians [could] judge" whether a practice had been good or not; "for that which is good physick for one person may not be so for another, according to their different constitutions, or according to certain seasons of the year."[137] In short, only learned physicians could judge whether Groenevelt's practice had been good or bad, and they had the right by their charter of Henry VIII to imprison for bad practice. No one could overturn the decision of the censors, unless their procedures had been flawed.[138] The right of the censors to judge medical practice in London had been reestablished in the courts.

But the situation was only temporary, for Holt's words reflected a now old-fashioned view of medicine. The future clearly lay with people like Groenevelt and his friends, who were developing medical specifics for particular diseases rather than treating unique patients with protean imbalances. Other people had strong opinions on this question of whether medicine should be controlled by one group or allowed to flourish in a free market in which anyone could decide for themselves the propriety of a treatment. The Lords of the Admiralty and the generals of the army, and soon the House of Lords itself in the Rose case of 1704, would decide differently than Holt and his confreres.[139] They thought of medicine as specific treatments for specific diseases, acting the same way in all persons, in any climate or circumstance. The majority of the Lords of England disagreed with Holt and the other justices, allowing a free medical market to develop without supervision by people like the censors of the college. Groenevelt's case had helped them to see the point.

Outside the courtroom, then, public opinion had been turned against the college censors. The publicity surrounding Groenevelt had much to do with that change. He had been found not guilty of malpractice by an English jury, even if the judges sided with the censors; and his case had been a contributing cause to a rash of vigorous attacks on the censors as nothing better than monopolists. The army and Admiralty, too, had had their fill of learned and bewigged physicians lording it over useful practitioners like apothecaries and surgeons. Given such views, the House of Lords itself decided to restore the earlier status quo with their reversal of Holt's decision in Rose's case in February 1704, which allowed for relatively free medical practice in London.[140]

To save his own reputation, then, Groenevelt had contributed to a violent assault on the forces of the London medical establishment. But at what a cost! Groenevelt's personal reputation had also been publicly attacked, and despite damaging the college's good name, he could do little to restore his own. While the censors could not extract from him the punishment they desired, his reputation remained under suspicion. He would never fully recover from the blows the censors had dealt him.

CHAPTER 8

One Life's Shipwreck and Its Ghosts

IN THE YEARS following Groenevelt's celebrity, his practice declined. His hopes for a medical practice had been reduced by the charges against him, forcing him to rely almost entirely on his surgical practice for his livelihood. But this, too, began to suffer, as rival lithotomists made their own reputations among the social and medical elite, and as Groenevelt's age began to catch up with him. He was not yet fifty when Mrs. Withall had first brought charges against him, but he had almost reached his next decade by the time his case against the censors had come to naught. As he approached his sixtieth year, rumors about his declining surgical skill began to trouble him; by his mid-sixties, his enemies, he believed, had virtually destroyed him with rumors of his failing sight and shaking hands. As his practice declined, without family to support him, he fell into financial ruin. He came to know the inside of debtors' prison, while his wife had to leave him and stay with relatives in Amsterdam. He was forced to move, taking up residence in a cheaper suburb and renting out some of his rooms. He sought refuge in making a few pounds from the market for books—but Grub Street was hardly a path to fortune. In the cold winter months of 1716, just short of his sixty-eighth birthday, probably lacking enough of either coal or food, bereft of family, the doctor breathed his last. Some of his works continued to be praised through the eighteenth century, but the last two hundred years have been less kind to his memory. Only the faintest traces of his life and work remained, buried under increasingly thick layers of misinformation and misunderstanding.

Echoes of the controversy over Groenevelt's use of cantharides could be heard for many years. Gossip hit the coffeehouses for a final time after Holt's June 1700 verdict. "This day the court of Kings bench delivered their opinion in the case of an action brought by Dr. Greenvelt against the colledge of physitians for fining and imprisoning him for unskilfully practising physick, and gave judgment for the defendants," wrote Narcissus Luttrell in his diary.[1] The news that he had lost his suit could not have helped Groenevelt's medical reputation. Moreover, by the time the case had reached its conclusion, English xenophobia against the Dutch had worsened. Now that the admired Queen Mary was dead, local suspicions of the Dutch had little check. William III and his Dutch friends became very unpopular, despite their forcing a peace on France: given feelings in Parliament, William even had to disband his Dutch guards, while his close friend, Portland, had to decline some of the honors the king had offered him. Groenevelt, too, felt some of this. As he wrote to Portland about the censors' attacks on him: "the most inveterate enemies could not have done more, had they been implacable to a Foreigner, hateful to a Hollander, and resolv'd utterly to destroy a Man void of all Help, Patronage, or Protection."[2] Circumstances certainly did not favor the doctor's situation.

The case had cost Groenevelt not only a substantial amount of money but several years of trouble. Only someone with a righteous sense of having been gravely wronged could have fought on for so long, even with the encouragement of his friends and the financial help of the Society of Apothecaries. Once his ground had been lost, Groenevelt's uncompromising stand would make an orderly retreat very difficult. It must have been terribly hard for him to accept the authority of the censors after he lost his case against them. He refused to attend the meeting of the whole College of Physicians called for about two weeks after the court's decision in 1700, at which the president warned all the candidates and licentiates that the statutes governing their behavior would be enforced.[3] Because he had refused to come to a required meeting, the censors summoned Groenevelt to appear before them to explain why. He had no choice but to pay a 2s. fine for his nonattendance and to promise that "for the future . . . he would be obedient to the Statutes of the Colledge."[4] But there was no mention of an apology from Groenevelt, and he showed signs of further recalcitrance. When the censors set about trying to force the members of the college into signing a bond requiring observance of all the statutes, they called in all those who did not to come before them in small groups either to sign or defy them openly. Those who had supported Groenevelt—and many more—refused to sign, as did Groenevelt himself.[5] Divisions in the college remained irreconcilable.[6] Not until well into the eighteenth century would tempers in the college cool down.

Given the benefits of hindsight, we can see how general political sentiment was turning against the censors. But for the moment, the censors interpreted the result of Groenevelt's lawsuit not as bringing matters to a legal draw but as a mark of support by the courts. The censors launched attacks in the courts on a large number of illicit practitioners. Within five months of Groenevelt's case, the censors had also been alerted to several physicians practicing in London without their permission, and a few months later they decided to make an example of one of them, Dr. Levett.[7] Levett was prosecuted before Chief Justice Holt for £25 (for five months' illicit practice), and the censors won their case.[8] The censors pressed ahead with their case against William Salmon in November 1700.[9] They also mounted their attack on the apothecary William Rose in February 1701; Rose was defended in turn by the Society of Apothecaries. The Rose case resulted in further legal victories for the college in the court of Chief Justice Holt before finally being overturned in the House of Lords in 1704.[10]

The Latin treatise published by Groenevelt in 1698 to defend his practice of prescribing cantharides internally also led to further debate in the medical community. A correspondent of Hans Sloane's added a postscript to one of his letters in the spring: "Next week I intend [to send] you the paper [I have written] about Cantharides."[11] William Cockburn, a military physician and follower of Sydenham's as well as Isaac Newton's, and also a member of both the College of Physicians and the Royal Society, published a long discussion of his investigations into the constitution of cantharides. These beetles had "set all the Physick in [the] Town in a Combustion, or Ferment (to use the universal and common word)," to such an extent that Cockburn felt obliged to comment on their internal use even when his main concern was with the way they caused blisters and cured fevers when applied externally. He tried applying cantharides topically by themselves and also mixed with camphor ("the most unfit correcter so far as I can expect in reason") and found both applications to produce the same kind of blister. This he thought proved that camphor did not correct the effects of cantharides, although he left "these particulars to be spoke to at greater length, by those who [were] Concerned."[12]

Gradually, however, Groenevelt's views gained acceptance. James Yonge, a military surgeon, soon came to follow Groenevelt's practice, despite having written a tract against William Salmon, who had attacked the college partly on behalf of Groenevelt. "You know the controversy which happened lately concerning the Internal use of Cantharides, occasioned by Dr. Groenevelt's giving them to cure Ulcers of the Bladder," he wrote to his friend John Houghton in the summer of 1702, "and I have read his Learned defence of that Practice, and must acknowledge that by what I found . . . of that Ingenious

Apology, . . . I became encouraged to use it." Yonge administered five
cantharides (without the heads, wings, or legs) via two pills, to a gentlewoman
suffering from a total suppression of urine. In less than twenty-four hours,
a "flood" of urine resulted, "and continued above 48 hours," much relieving
the patient. "Some Gravel, and Sabulous [i.e., sandy] matter" came away
in the urine, but no hurt was given to "the Stomach, Bladder or other Bowels."
In fact, the cantharides "operated so quietly, as if nothing but two doses of
Lapis Prunellae had been administered." Yonge had also given it in several
other cases without any painful effects, even though he did not mix it with
camphor but only gave it with large amounts of something to drink.[13] The
continuing interest in Groenevelt's remedy caused a second edition of Groenevelt's book to be published in 1703, to which the author added further cases
illustrating the successful use of cantharides.[14] Three years later, in December
1706, Yonge sent "the Honored Dr. Groenveldt" a personal letter recounting
another successful use of cantharides—this time mixed with camphor—to
treat a stoppage of urine with pains in the kidneys.[15] He also allowed an
account of this case to be published in the *Philosophical Transactions* of the
Royal Society.[16]

But it was the publication of an English edition of Groenevelt's treatise
which brought his use of cantharides to widespread attention. The translation,
which now earned the imprimatur of the president and censors of the college,
followed the Latin very exactly—earning Groenevelt's endorsement—and
added further material in marked passages.[17] The surgeon John Marten probably did the translation as claimed on the title page, although one of Marten's
enemies published an affidavit stating that a lawyer, Mr. Joshua Stephens,
had in fact been the translator of it.[18] Marten had developed a reputation for
treating venereal diseases and had published a kind of bestseller on the
subject, his *Treatise of all the degrees and symptoms of the venereal disease,
in both sexes*, which went through a number of editions at the turn of the
century. (The sixth edition, published three years after his translation of
Groenevelt, contained by way of appendix a medical manual on sexual
relations which veered into pornography.[19] On this basis, his enemies brought
a legal indictment against Marten for "being evil disposed and wickedly
intending to corrupt the subjects of the Lady the Queene and seduced by
cupidity.")[20] Since Groenevelt's use of cantharides was said to be a good
remedy for the effects of gonorrhea, Marten had a professional interest in
the new treatment. He therefore took the liberty of adding large numbers of
his own observations and case histories—many having to do with the use of
cantharides in venereal diseases, some being quite racy accounts—to the

translation of Groenevelt, almost doubling its size. Groenevelt's old ally, Edward Tyson, suggested further medical precedents for using cantharides for the new edition.[21]

Despite Marten's self-advertising and discussion of sexually transmitted diseases, the translation brought Groenevelt further renown. One letter that came his way from an unknown correspondent almost immediately after the book's publication addressed itself to the "Worthy Dr." Groenevelt because he had "been an Eye and Ear witness off the advantageous internal use of Cantharides in the practice of Physick." The author flattered Groenevelt effusively: "You are like to be ye head of us all." He detailed how three London apothecaries were now making up medicines using cantharides for himself, who administered them with excellent results—although the edge of competition entered his language: "I am much made on abroad by persons of learning, who move their difficulties to me in ye use of that insect, and they have my answer as far as I am capable."[22] William Smyth of Dublin wrote to Groenevelt at about the same time. He had read Groenevelt's book with an open mind and was grateful that envy among the former censors had caused him to put his practice in writing, revealing the best method ever for curing ulcers in the bladder. He wondered about Groenevelt's use of this remedy only in women because their urinary passage was shorter and wider than in men, and what the reasons were for his giving different doses in different cases.[23] Groenevelt wrote back explaining his reasons and urging Smyth to keep investigating.[24] Physicians on the Continent came to know the English version as well as the Latin original of Groenevelt's treatise, apparently because of the interest in using cantharides to treat venereal disease.[25]

By the mid-eighteenth century, partly because of Groenevelt's work, the internal use of cantharides had become widely accepted. The famous medical professor Herman Boerhaave recommended their use when large quantities of urine needed to be flushed from a patient. He warned that they seemed to augment rather than diminish the underlying inflammation of many diseases, so that they had to be used only in people of a cold and watery temperament. Used to treat gonorrhea in men, they could also cause swelling of the testicles. But carefully employed, they could be an excellent treatment.[26] The edited lecture notes of an English student of Boerhaave's further say, "The great Use [of cantharides] is in Blisters; but People who know how to manage powerful Medicines, give them internally with great Success, in Tinctures."[27] Boerhaave cited a few of Groenevelt's authorities, rather than citing Groenevelt himself; but one of Boerhaave's English students was clear about the connection between the modern use of cantharides and Groenevelt's practice. Henry Bracken thought that although the use of cantharides could damage a patient's "fertility," it was a useful treatment for women who needed cleansing of the "viscid Foulnesses" of the womb (which "viscidities" protected against "any Erosions from the Flies"), a treatment he attributed to Groenevelt.[28] In the late eighteenth century, Dr. Andrew Duncan, Sr., still prescribed the internal use of cantharides in cases of diabetes, leucorrhea, and gonorrhea at the Edinburgh infirmary.[29]

Groenevelt may eventually have won his point about the internal use of cantharides with many in the medical community at large. Yet "Dr. Greenvelt . . . suffered much by a Prosecution for giving them so. . . . The Issue ruined the unhappy Doctor," Henry Bracken remembered.[30]

Indeed, Groenevelt's life was gradually falling apart. Because the college had so publicly attacked him for malpractice, Groenevelt was never able to develop a good medical practice apart from his surgery. His little pamphlet on the gout was his last on a strictly medical complaint, and there is no hint that his use of cantharides became a widespread treatment for the gout. He seems to have remained aloof himself from the somewhat suspect practice of treating venereal diseases (although a neighbor of Groenevelt's on Throgmorton Street marketed a "pleasant drink" that purged the urine and was especially good in cases of French pox—syphilis—perhaps getting the recipe from Groenevelt).[31] And because his reputation as a physician had been called into question so widely and publicly by the censors, there is no evidence that he ever was able to develop a good general practice. His hopes never recovered from the blows of the 1690s.

Groenevelt therefore had to fall back on his lithotomy practice for his livelihood. But his Dutch rival, Abraham Cyprianus, was becoming the darling London lithotomist of the moment. One of the last English notices of Groenevelt's ideas concerning bladder stones came in a reference in the *Philosophical Transactions* of the Royal Society in 1698.[32] But Cyprianus became a member of the Royal Society itself (in 1700), as Groenevelt never did; in the year following, he was invited to teach the surgeons of St. Thomas's Hospital how to operate for stones.[33] Cyprianus had also become a licentiate of the College of Physicians in 1699 and successfully lithotomized the royal physician and president of the college, Sir Thomas Millington. To publicize his success further, Cyprianus published a Latin account of this operation, while Millington himself talked up Cyprianus to all and sundry.[34] For instance, when James Yonge came to London in 1702, the "genteel and civil . . . old

I N

Frogmorton-Street,

AT the *Golden Ball* over againſt *Draper*'s Hall, betweeñ *Bartholomew* Lane and *Broad.ſtreet*, near the *Royal Exchange*, May be had of *T. C.* an approved Phyſician of long Practice, A pleaſant Drink which purges by Urine, at two ſhillings ſix pence the Bottle, with my Anti-Venerial Pills, which purge by Stool, at three ſhillings the Box. They will be delivered to any Meſſenger with Directions ſealed up how to take them. Secrets ſo excellent in operation, and ſo friendly to Nature, that in my conſtant practice, and great experience for Twenty Years, in this City of *London*, is well known to be the moſt ſucceſsful, both for preventing, and curing, perfectly and ſpeedily the *Venereal P O X*; A Diſeaſe deſtructive to the body of Man, if not timely and carefully prevented; It proceeds from a virulent, venemous Matter ſuckt into the body by a ſtrong attractive Faculty in time of Co-pulating with an unclean Woman, which excoriates the whole paſſage of Urine, and cauſes a foul ſtinking Iſſue, or Running; this Ulceration is the cauſe of ſcalding heat of Urine, pricking, and painful ſtanding of the Yard, and if neglected, and not carefully cured cauſes ſwellings in the Cod, Buboes, or ſwellings in the Groin, and infects the body in general with the *P O X*, as by an Ulcer upon the outſide of the Yard, called a Shanker, ragged Warts in the privy Parts, pains and Scabs in the Face, Head, or Neck, and ſometimes over the whole body; Inflamma-tions and Ulcers in the Mouth and Throat. To prevent theſe dangerous Evils, be ſo kind to your ſelves, to be conſtantly provided with my Anti-Venerial Medicines, that Infalibly eradicate all poyſonous Matter and Steems that are contracted in the body, in as ſhort a time as can be

FIG. 25. *Front side of handbill from one of Groenevelt's neighbors on "Frogmorton Street," advertising a purging drink and antivenereal pills. By permission of the British Library.*

gentleman" Millington first thanked Yonge for defending the college from
William Salmon some years earlier and then "entertained [Yonge] with a
very particular account of a stone cut from him by the Dutch lithotomist
Cyprian after he [Millington] was 70 years old."[35] At the end of his life,
Cyprianus was buried in the Church of Austin Friars near the consistory: a
spot reserved for important or well-to-do people.[36]

Without a good medical practice, with a damaged reputation among the
public, and with vigorous rivals among the London lithotomists, Groenevelt
fell on hard times. He was reduced to asking his acquaintances to encourage
people to undergo the operation at his hands. In 1704 he begged Hans Sloane
to have his neighbor, who had a son afflicted with bladder stones, come and
witness Groenevelt operate on a boy of about the same size, so as to convince
him of Groenevelt's abilities.[37] Two years later, James Yonge had to tell
Groenevelt that "neither those many Instances off your success in ye like
Case with all the Arguments [Yonge] could use" could prevail upon an aged
patient of his to be cut by Groenevelt.[38]

Groenevelt's age could not have helped. Surgery was a young man's
profession, for when surgeons got old, people began to suspect their eyesight
and manual abilities. Groenevelt's sixtieth birthday came in 1708. In his
own opinion he remained vigorous, but his practice apparently continued to
decline. By early 1710, he could no longer pay his dues to the College of
Physicians.[39] "I thank God, I yet enjoy a perfect Health," he wrote in that
same year, "notwithstanding the Malice and notorious Falsities of my restless
Adversaries, who have industriously spread amongst the People that Age has
made me incapable of Practice, that my Sight is bad, my Hand-shakes, my
Strength fails, nay, that I was Dead."[40] Around Christmas, the College of
Physicians heard a petition from him read out to the assembly, in which he
asked for "a Charitable Gift to him in prison": apparently debtors' prison.
His wife seems to have returned to Amsterdam about the same time—probably
to live with relatives—where she died in December 1713.[41] All his children,
who might have helped support him in his old age, had died.[42] "It was left
to every man to give [to Groenevelt] as he pleases," noted the college
registrar.[43]

Groenevelt had enough friends left to help him barely keep his head above
water. He knew the very successful Hans Sloane, for instance. Groenevelt
had given his copy of Ten Rhijne's Dutch treatise on leprosy to Sloane but
borrowed it back for more than a year. Sloane may have intended to have
it translated into English.[44] The grand doctor seems to have felt enough of
a tie with Groenevelt to help him, since a few years later Groenevelt wrote

to Sloane about the latter's "former favours."[45] Perhaps some of Groenevelt's previous allies, like Richard Blackmore, aided him too. He did get out of prison, but all appearances suggest that he remained on the fringes of the college and in financial difficulties.

Even in his church he had become marginalized. At the turn of the century, the Church of Austin Friars was torn by a disagreement over one of its ministers, the Reverend Aemilius van Cuilemborg, who had defended Groenevelt to the consistory during the malpractice proceedings. The consistory and Van Cuilemborg had a series of disagreements, culminating in 1702, when the consistory accused him of dishonest conduct, keeping intimate company with bad people, and slander, asking for his resignation. Van Cuilemborg replied with a stiff letter; the consistory immediately fired him. Van Cuilemborg and his supporters appealed to the bishop of London. When the bishop took no action, Van Cuilemborg mounted the pulpit one Sunday without notifying the consistory beforehand, causing a stir that led to shoving and almost a generalized brawl. The consistory then asked the bishop to intervene as well, and he decided against Van Cuilemborg. The reverend wrote letters trying to explain that he was an old and confused man but innocent; finally, in October 1703, he sent his resignation, together with a claim for his pension, and died heartbroken a year and a half later.[46]

In the dispute over Van Cuilemborg, Groenevelt took what became the losing side against the consistory. In the eyes of his supporters, including Groenevelt, Van Cuilemborg was a learned and pious man who had the backing of the general congregation but who had antagonized the wealthy oligarchy in the consistory (all "honest Merchants, and esteemed on the Exchange," as they described themselves):[47] as in Groenevelt's malpractice case, a small group of elite men seemed to be trying to suppress the general good. Van Cuilemborg had previously defended Groenevelt in the consistory from the college's charges of malpractice, as well as from charges of being a "Socinian." (The latter accusation generally meant "atheist" in the contemporary language of abuse, but it may have been meant more precisely, prompted by Groenevelt's continuing association with the Polish Socinian Christopher Crell.)[48] Groenevelt firmly took Van Cuilemborg's side: he led the list of signatories of one of the two February 1703 petitions to the bishop of London asking him to restore Van Cuilemborg, and he signed the other as well; he supported Van Cuilemborg in letters to others of the congregation; he was one of three people who physically prevented the church sextons from getting near the pulpit on Sunday, 22 August 1703, when Van Cuilemborg preached without permission; he led the list of the fomenters of tumult (*oproermakers*) whom Van Cuilemborg assembled when the bishop of London came to the church to settle the dispute on 3 September; and he was the person Van Cuilemborg selected to argue his case to the bishop.[49] In the words of the consistory, Groenevelt led the group of "common people" who had been "imposed upon" by Van Cuilemborg, a group among whom were "very few of our [i.e., consistory] members, or contributors to the maintenance of our Church."[50] All this may help to explain why Groenevelt was no longer listed among the members of the church at the beginning of the eighteenth century.[51]

Groenevelt's attempts to turn his fortunes around now centered once again on publishing a book. It was another English work on stones, in which he resorted to all the rhetorical techniques at his disposal. Groenevelt advertised in the *Post Man* that he would be publishing a book on stones, soliciting remarkable observations.[52] He dedicated it to a great personage—Thomas Howard, the duke of Norfolk—from whom he seems to have received permission for the dedication.[53] Even more explicitly than before, he pushed for medical learning only insofar as it was useful to practice. "The finest Speculations, and the most Sublime Thoughts are worth little to Mankind, if they don't put something in action, so as to be made usefull to Humane Life: For *Virtus* in *Actione* consistit. I am altogether of the Opinion of a certain Author, who says; Anatomy, Chymy and Botany, and their whole circle of Sciences, that refer to Physic, are only servicable, when they conspire to improve a regular and safe Practice."[54] He mentioned Sylvius as a fine example of someone who oriented all his theory to practice, and he noted that he had himself studied under Sylvius. He included a favorable mention of his surgical student and assistant Mr. Benjamin Marten—who may have been the one to help with his English. (Marten went on to a successful practice in the treatment of consumption, even announcing that "wonderfully minute living creatures" were its cause, which was seen two centuries later as an anticipation of the germ theory.)[55] Groenevelt also assured the reader that he had the support of his "very good Friends of the College," with whom he was "in great Amity," and of whose society he had "the Honour of being a member." Finally, he lambasted empirics but noted that people needed to know where to find good surgeons and physicians. Thus, his book was not to be seen as quackish for advertising his expertise: "No Man is a Quack for Using fair means to be known," but only for engaging in an occupation he knows little about. In Amsterdam, he noted, all physicians had to have their names and profession written on the outside of their houses.[56] He urged strong measures against pretenders to medical knowledge. As for his own knowledge, derived from many years of study and practice, there could be no imputation of quackery.

The text itself presented material familiar from his earlier works, together with many illustrations taken from Tolet. He gave many case histories of people whom he had successfully cut. He also printed a letter from James Sturgeon, a surgeon from Bury St. Edmunds, concerning the case of a boy named James Seaden who had suffered from a stone in the glans, apparently sent as the result of Groenevelt's advertisement. After going on to discuss the signs and causes of stones, and the operation to remove them, Groenevelt concluded by declaring against lithontriptics.[57] Too many people, like Walter Charleton, believed that lithontriptics were possible, not because they had direct experience of them, but because they believed the claims of others. "For my part, I declare, tho' I have been as conversant with this Distemper, as any body, I never knew one freed from the Stone in the Bladder, if it was too big to pass the Urethra, but by Cutting."[58] The final few pages of the book recounted his successful operation on the twenty-two-month-old son of Captain Rogers.[59] He had begun and ended his book by trying to assure the public of his surgical abilities.

Thus, in his currently narrowing straits, Groenevelt took ever more refuge in the Grub Street trade: that poor neighborhood north of the London walls infamous for the number of hack writers who lived there hand to mouth. The educated person without means who tried to make a living by his wits, impressing (or not) coffeehouse clatches with satirical political observations or allusive poetry, seeking patronage and in the meantime hoping for a few coals and a bit of meat and ale from scribbling for the newsheets and printers: these were the denizens of Grub Street.[60] Many of the new medical men, trying to sell their skills in an increasingly competitive market and well attuned to the growing power of popular print, moved on the fringes of the Grub Street trade; indeed, some, like the surgeon John Martyn, helped to organize it, at the same time propagandizing against empirics and quacks while putting themselves forward as medical experts.[61]

For instance, one of Groenevelt's younger London Dutch medical acquaintances, Bernard de Mandeville, learned how to play the Grub Street game very well. He had written his first published words in a poem introducing the second edition of Groenevelt's book on the use of cantharides in 1703, lambasting the College of Physicians and praising Groenevelt and his new remedy: he may even have been seeking the poor Groenevelt's help in advancing his medical career in London.[62] Mandeville's first published work was *The Pamphleteers: A Satyr* (1703), which defended William III against his detractors, after which he published a series of satires for the press.[63] His medical views sounded much like Groenevelt's, albeit better tuned to his audience and pitched in excellent English. For instance, in *The Female Tatler*—aiming his attacks at Steele's *Tatler*—Mandeville declares, "Those who study Latin and Greek for their use in theology, law and medicine are despised as drudges by the true '*Litterati*,' [while in medicine] university learning is irrelevant to curing patients."[64] His first major medical work, on hysteria, made similar points. In this tale, written in the form of an entertaining but instructive dialogue, the hero, Philipirio, weans his patients from excessive somatic concerns, speaks wittily but honestly to the protagonists, and mixes his own drugs when necessary, insuring their purity and saving his patients the money an apothecary would have charged (as well as adding to his own fees). He proclaims his learning to be based upon experience, and made for use, even admitting to being an empiric who is opposed to all a priori reasoning. And of course, Mandeville himself lets the reader know that he can be reached through the bookseller, although he vigorously denies that this publicity constitutes quackery.[65]

But while the young Dutch doctor found ways to climb the greasy pole of fame using the latest Grub Street means, his elder was not nearly as fortunate. Groenevelt's book of 1710 was successful enough to have a second edition two years later.[66] But circumstances did not favor it making a large splash in his London practice. It did not speak wittily enough to a potential audience or anticipate as well as it might have the desires of patients. In fact, his views were becoming just a bit old-fashioned. Although Cyprianus had become the lithotomist of the moment, it was the French surgeon Tolet's book that people eventually took to recommending as the best work on the operation.[67] The irony was that Groenevelt's plea for medical knowledge put to use—radical enough in the 1680s and 1690s—had become the watchword of the day, making his opinions seem commonplace or even dated. Learned physicians might still admire those items that marked his medical handling of the condition, such as the lengthy preventative advice centered on dietetics, and the long and erudite discussions of various opinions about what the cause of stones might be. But these items appealed less to a vernacular audience interested in how the stones could best be treated. If no lithontriptics were possible, as Groenevelt claimed, then surgery seemed the only recourse; in that case, a learned medical-surgical treatise like Groenevelt's could hardly compete with a well-illustrated and detailed straightforward description of the operation, like Tolet's. An entirely modest success, Groenevelt's new book seems not to have changed his fortunes.

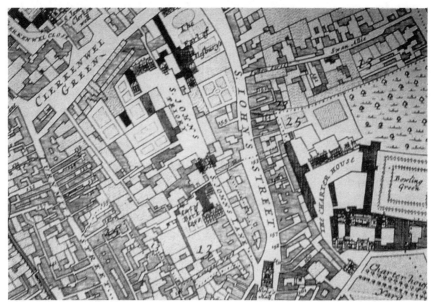

FIG. 26. *The London suburbs northeast of the city walls (point "3" in fig. 19). St. John's Court, where Groenevelt lived at the end of his life, stood in St. John's Priory, which led onto St. John's Lane and Clerkenwell Green. From William Morgan's "London etc. Actually Survey'd."*

At the age of sixty-six, then, in 1714, he himself moved to new lodgings, being "forced to come out" of London "by ye Act," he wrote Sloane.[68] Apparently he had in mind a 1712 act of London's Common Council. This declared in part "that no person whatsoever, not being free of the city," could "use, exercise, or occupy, any art, trade, mystery, manual operation, or handicraft whatsoever" upon a penalty of £5.[69] Groenevelt had never bothered to become a freeman of the city, which he could have done by joining the surgeons' company. Physicians had no need of doing so. But if, as seems likely, he resorted more and more to living as a surgeon, while being marginalized in the college, he might have been subject to this act. Whatever the reason, Groenevelt moved to a suburb just north of the city proper, near Grub Street itself, taking up rooms in St. John's Court, between Clerkenwell Green and St. John's Lane. He now lived in the parish of St. James, a parish sympathetic to Calvinism: the famous latitudinarian Gilbert Burnet was buried there in 1715. A well in Clerkenwell had been rediscovered in the late seventeenth century, which was found to contain medicinal water not unlike that of Tunbridge Wells. This well "became greatly frequented by Citizens,

and used as Chalybiate Waters for correcting Hypochondriacal Distempers,"
one contemporary wrote.[70] With plenty of traffic from people seeking medical
help, and being situated not far from St. Bartholomew's Hospital adjoining
the Smithfield market, the neighborhood may have had good possibilities for
setting up a medical practice.

He therefore put a brave public face on his fortunes. "I have taken a little
house . . . part of which i have lett [to roomers at a good rate]," he wrote
Sloane. This income "being joined with my small practice" encouraged him
to hope he would get ahead. All he needed was "a small sum of money to
pay ye charges" of moving. "I beg pardon for this liberty, butt hope it will
be ye last time that i shall have occasion that i am forced to make such a
request."[71] His slide into a penurious old age was continuing.

The poor and elderly Groenevelt came more and more to depend on Grub
Street enterprises to generate an income. He authored another Latin book in
1714, to which his name was not attached, perhaps because he did it on
commission. The publishers' preface noted that the recent publication of
Richard Mead's work on the medical influence of the sun and moon had
made clear the necessity of a work on medical theory.[72] There were few such
works available in England. The bookseller therefore seems to have stepped
in and commissioned such a work, paying Groenevelt to undertake it but
publishing it anonymously. To make this money, Groenevelt plagiarized the
excellent general textbook written by a former medical professor of the
University of Louvain, Frans vanden Zype, or Zypaeus. Zypaeus had managed to pack many new medical ideas into an old-fashioned summary of the
medical institutes: he was a fine chemist (and follower of Sylvius), an excellent
anatomist (being especially interested in the lacteal vessels and thoracic duct),
and the recipient of the secret of Louis de Bils about how to embalm bodies
for preservation.[73] His text remained a standard introduction to medicine
for twenty years and went through several editions.[74] Groenevelt simply
transformed Zypaeus's descriptive and analytical discourse into a series of
questions and answers.[75] But he also added a valuable appendix on diseases
and their recommended remedies.[76]

The new text was successful. A year later, a second edition appeared,
identical to the first except that it mentioned the names of both Zypaeus and
Groenevelt on the title page.[77] An English translation appeared in the same
year, following the 1715 Latin edition exactly.[78] The publisher included a
preface, remarking, "Whereas the following Sheets came into my Hands
without any Preface, as never intended to be made Publick, so I think it
needful to advertise the Reader, that the Reason of their appearing in this

manner, is: because I have not met with so much useful Learning, within so small a Compass, in any thing yet Extant." Groenevelt himself probably sold the translation to the publishers, which they in turn edited, although it might have been done by another medical Grub Street scribbler. Perhaps he received some money from the 1715 Latin edition to help keep him going for a time. A second English edition of his *Treatise Of the Safe, Internal Use of Cantharides in the Practice of Physick* also appeared in 1715, virtually identical to the first.[79]

But the aging Groenevelt was growing increasingly desperate. The public no longer often came to him for surgical help, a matter the doctor ascribed to unnamed enemies. Hans Sloane received yet another letter from Groenevelt asking him to help stop the rumors. Various people continued to spread abroad a false report "that [he was in]capable through age and badness of sight of per[form]ing that Operation" of lithotomy. He hoped that Sloane could help "to remove the prejudice that many people have taken against me, on that really groundless Account."[80] But such rumors all but finished his surgical career.

With a public reputation for being too old to operate well, and without a good medical practice in which he could have charged for advice, Groenevelt's career, even his life, was coming to a close. His last year saw the second edition of his plagiarized Latin textbook and its English translation, which may have paid him a few pounds. But even hopes of putting food on the table regularly had been dashed by rumor. In the middle of the next winter, at the age of sixty-eight, he died. The local minister buried him cheaply outside the parish church on 15 January 1716.[81] The ambitious and anxious soul from Lebuinus's town of Deventer, baptized in a spring of heavy rain, had passed away in poverty in a foreign metropolis.

In medicine, the internal use of cantharides which Groenevelt did so much to promote became an ordinary treatment in certain conditions; but its originator came to be largely forgotten. In surgery, the lithotomy technique he first brought to England found new advocates who worked to advance their own reputations at the expense of his. Soon enough, in the third decade of the eighteenth century, the English surgeons James Douglas and William Cheselden became the heroes of their own nation, effectively eclipsing all those who came before. As one English medical historian put it succinctly, it was Cheselden "who perfected the operation" of lithotomy.[82] Few remembered earlier experts, much less Dutch ones. The Dutch surgeon Abraham Titsingh lauded the learned Doctor Groenevelt: this gentleman of medicine had written an account of lithotomy more fully and correctly than anyone else, from whom others plucked feathers for their own renown.[83] But he was among the last to mention anything substantial about Groenevelt's contribution to the field. In medicine more generally, Groenevelt's Latin textbook had an entirely new translation into English long after his death, in 1753. The new publisher remarked, "Dr. Groenvelt by a most happy Genius, has contracted the whole Substance of Physick into so small a Compendium, that he hath rendered the Study of it both easy and pleasant."[84] But almost no one now remembered anything about the author. Even his books had become faint shadows from an earlier age, his name mentioned only in Latin medical encyclopedias. By the twentieth century, the rare historian who noticed his existence thought him to have been only an ignorant quack.

Because many of the books he wrote were considered to be of medical use after his death, a faint memory of him persisted in the pages of several reference works. The medical encyclopedists of the eighteenth century gave attention to his most important works.[85] They intended to record medical knowledge in the same way as knowledge about any other subject: according to the natural historical genre, presenting a wealth of discoveries and facts plainly so that they could be known to others and accumulated over time. One of the first of the medical encyclopedists, Johannis Mangeti, physician to the king of Prussia, thought Groenevelt's two major investigations—on bladder stones and on the internal use of cantharides—worthy of preservation and dissemination.[86] Four decades later, the famous Albrect von Haller gave positive evaluations of the same works of Groenevelt in his *Bibliotheca Chirurgica* and in his *Bibliotheca Medicinae Practicae*.[87] The second of Haller's entries became the source for most other reports of Groenevelt, including those of Vigilius von Creutzenfeld[88] and Eloy.[89] The model entries of Haller in Latin, and Eloy in French, continued to serve medical encyclopedists through the middle of the nineteenth century,[90] and Groenevelt has even been mentioned in passing by two recent books on the history of surgery for bladder stones.[91]

But by the nineteenth century, as narrative histories linked to romantic literary forms began to reshape historical writing, and as medical practice changed so as to leave Groenevelt's compositions behind, people like him dropped out of sight. Authors preferred to present medicine—like all other aspects of human life—as developing along certain grand lines rather than from a host of small, often discarded developments. As this slimmer, speculative, and more heroic history replaced the massive tomes recording when various facts became known, those like Groenevelt, whose work was never quite famous and was later superseded, simply disappeared.[92] There was little point in noticing someone who had not entered the halls of greatness.[93]

When his name reentered the printed historical annals at the end of the nineteenth century, it was not for his medical ideas but for his membership in a group. It is because of his having become a licentiate of the London College of Physicians that somewhat fanciful reports of Groenevelt's life can be found in more recent works of reference. As a licentiate of the London College of Physicians, Groenevelt earned a very short notice in William Munk's Victorian register of the college. Reading some of the college's contemporary eminence back to the seventeenth century, Munk assumed any member to have been a good physician, so he mentioned Groenevelt's medical qualifications and added a list of a few of his books.[94] Typically, Munk discreetly avoided a discussion of Groenevelt's trial by simply noting that "the circumstances are fully detailed in the Annals, but are too lengthy for insertion [in the register]."[95] Having been identified by Munk as a medical author living in England, Groenevelt went on to receive an entry in the English *Dictionary of National Biography*, published a few years later. Gordon Goodwin's entry in the *DNB* corrected Munk on one point and added another detail,[96] and the Goodwin entry also gave a brief summary of his malpractice case.[97] For the sake of literary completeness, Goodwin also added guesses as to his birth and death dates.[98]

Then, because he was a Dutchman mentioned in the English national biography, Groenevelt also received the attention of the compilers of the Dutch national biography. A. Geyl added together the entry in the English *DNB* and a German encyclopedia entry based upon Eloy[99] and further speculated about Groenevelt's patrons and the reasons for his trial.[100] Most recently, an attempt to make information about the medical history of the Netherlands available in English caused G. A. Lindeboom to collect together biographical materials on Dutch physicians. Lindeboom's short entry on Groenevelt even further digested the sketchy information and speculation in his secondary sources, correcting some misprints concerning the dates of Groenevelt's publications but otherwise leaving out important qualifying words like "probably" and "nearly" to make the whole sound more authoritative. Unfortunately, this means that Lindeboom repeated previous authors' fancies as certain truths: to give a simple example, he gave Groenevelt's (incorrect) birth and death dates—first introduced in the English *DNB*—as definite rather than probable.[101] A recent work on eighteenth-century British doctors, compiling information on thousands of people mentioned in English references, confuses matters even further: mixing together information on two people, it lengthens

Groenevelt's life by twenty years and grants him a set of English university degrees.[102] In short, over the last century, information about a seventeenth-century doctor has seemingly become more certain when in fact it has become more corrupt.

Growing up among unregenerate humankind, Joannes Groenevelt probably expected little else. He fought his fights as best he knew how, with the stubbornness of the righteous. He lived through an age like all ages, of intellectual and political turmoil, doing what he could to push people in the direction he believed best, probably without hope of transforming the world. His ideas emerged from circumstance and talk with others as much as time spent in study, his practices from opportunity as much as a disinterested desire to help relieve the suffering. But one wonders whether the predestinarian Calvinism of his youth returned to him at the end, causing him to examine his conscience in the hope that he would be counted among the elect. Would he understand that despite his own failures and the decline of human memory, his ordinary life of hard-won achievements as well as disappointment—ghostly as it now is—could enter ours, three centuries on?

The English and the Dutch had long been locked in a mutually exasperating relationship. The people of the low and marshy lands on the east side of the North Sea benefited at times from English military support and raw products for their cloth industry; the people of the large offshore island learned from the Dutch much about trade, industry, and new notions of nature. But these mutual "influences" arose from countless human contacts among people who did not always understand one another's language, much less one another's values. Mutual encounters often led to personal successes, when each side benefited from the other. But living among strangers could easily cause misunderstandings and personal tragedy as well. At the end of the Dutch Golden Age, the Netherlands had an abundance of doctors and surgeons, certainly as compared with England; the opportunities for making a comfortable living in England therefore seemed quite good to the young Groenevelt. He moved for the same reason as many others: to achieve greater success than was possible at home. But he brought with him not only his knowledge and skill but his values as well. In the end, the way he put his learning to work in concert with a utilitarian and commercial outlook, coupled with his lack of sufficient respect for gentlemanly authority and habits of medical tradition, brought him into conflict with the English medical establishment, which crushed him. Groenevelt and his dissenting friends would help to effect changes in English medicine; but such long-term developments often came at terrible personal cost.

Dr. Mandeville was therefore not the only Dutch physician who angered the native English establishment after moving to London. He may have outraged a greater variety of Englishmen than his older acquaintance, Joannes Groenevelt, and he may deservedly have acquired a greater renown, but both helped to overturn the established order. They did so in part because of the intellectual views they brought with them from the Continent. Mandeville's *Fable of the Bees*, with its famous phrase about "private vices, public benefits," argued for a clear-eyed, empirical, and utilitarian study of how self-interested human desires lead to the general good. Mandeville's constant mockery of contemporary English moral seriousness—in the form of the societies to improve manners, for instance—was no accident. As bad as Machiavelli, Hobbes, or Spinoza, according to many of his critics, he brought with him at least two important traditions: the academic analysis of natural jurisprudence that stemmed from people like the great Dutch political philosopher Hugo Grotius and his French colleagues, which based an understanding of human nature, the supreme good, and social and political relationships on the study of natural law; and a deep religious sense that true virtue is impossible to a corrupt and unregenerate humankind, a view in keeping with his Calvinist upbringing. Both views offended landed Anglican gentlemen and their pen-wielding dependents, who saw Mandeville's skeptical and academic distance as undermining all hope of improving personal and public morality and as mocking religion and virtue. He had attacked their aristocratic values and moderate theology directly. It would be Scots like Adam Smith, who had long had a connection to Continental scholarship, especially to that of the Dutch, who would make Mandeville's formula more acceptable to an increasingly commercialized England at the end of the eighteenth century.[103]

Groenevelt never tried to upset local English sentiments so thoroughly. He had a greater sense of moral earnestness in his own life. But he shared much with his younger Dutch colleague. His academic training brought him to believe that learning must be rooted in empirical studies and directed toward use; his religious upbringing made him suspicious of those who claimed to have virtue on their side; his middling background made him no automatic upholder of oligarchy, whether aristocratic or mercantile. Since his energies were directed toward finding new and better methods to heal the sick, which brought pecuniary rewards as much as renown and self-satisfaction, he was quite comfortable in a world of medical commercialism. The sick had to be able to find the best practitioners, and the best practitioners could be known not by their character but by the their works. Their works, in turn, could best be improved by practicing all of medicine rather than keeping physic, surgery, and pharmacy separate. Many of his English brethren believed in taking similar medical roads. But the medical establishment did not. Brought up in a tradition that preferred good manners to commercial enterprise and Anglican "right reason" to neo-Thomist or Cartesian rationality, those raised in the English tradition remained somewhat skeptical that works could be divorced from character. Medical practice had a pastoral aspect, they believed, in which counsel played an equal or more important part than treatment. Good counsel could only come from those whose judgments had been formed properly.[104] Inventing dangerous new remedies on the basis of some theory and trying them out on patients not only had the potential to cause great bodily harm, it showed grave lack of judgment. In their view, Groenevelt had demonstrated time and again that he ought not to stand among them as a physician; the case of Mrs. Withall affirmed their opinion and made it clear that something had to be done to stop him.

Groenevelt's efforts to find new and effective treatments for chronic diseases therefore elicited a response far from what he expected. He had scoured all the sources, written and oral, ancient and modern, and put them together with the best theories of his teachers and his own clinical experiences, developing a remedy to relieve sufferers of their ills. Yet this work of years resulted not in success but in public controversy that ripped his life apart. The world had failed to respond as he wanted it to: it refused him his modicum of fame and fortune, instead slapping him down, hard. Not lauded but vilified, he found himself subjected to a series of personal attacks, to the point of being bodily thrown in jail. Perhaps his classical education told him that this fateful turn resulted from hubris. It is certainly hard to imagine that he could any longer believe that he stood among the elect, since one sign of their chosen state was worldly success. He had traveled from a proud but increasingly provincial town to the heart of the Dutch empire and then to the English metropolis, surviving wars and plagues, learning new languages and customs, making his way on his knowledge and skill, all the time helping patients. Throughout his life up to Mrs. Withall's case, sustained by his moral education and his faith, Joannes Groenevelt might well have counted himself among those whose lives fulfilled the divine plan. But now? Had he become another Job, tested by the Devil with the permission of God? Or was he merely an ordinary person, with the failings of all Adam's descendants whom the Lord had not elected to save? If so, did he still believe in Hell?

Perhaps because it forced such questions on him, the English medical establishment encountered a stubborn person, intent on saving not just his reputation but himself. The criticism of his practice by the college censors left Groenevelt puzzled, smarting, and soon seething with the anger of the just. He believed that he was in the right as much as they believed that he was in the wrong—how could he believe otherwise? His anger soured to spite, aimed at those he considered to be personal enemies. With the stubborn pride of his ancestors, he would not bow his head to what he thought of as malicious and overbearing personal attack. With the mature skill of a survivor, he managed to fight the censors to a standstill in the courts, drawing on the support of English allies who believed in pushing medical practice forward in the way he did. His stand therefore helped to weaken the moral authority of the College of Physicians and to encourage in England the kind of practical medicine which had already come to dominate the Netherlands. But in the process, he was dragged through the muck of public scandal, in which his character and his skill were called into question. Although the kind of medicine he advocated—innovative and aggressive rather than conservative and cautious—grew ever more important, his personal practice would never recover from the blows he had received in the late 1690s. Nor would his life. Joannes Groenevelt, born a Calvinist child of the Dutch Golden Age, died alone in virtual poverty in an Anglican parish, his hopes for evidence of election snuffed out long before the end.

Appendix

Groenevelt's Library in 1682

THE FOLLOWING letter—from the British Library, Sloane Manuscripts 2729, folios 112–113—contains a list of the books left behind by Groenevelt in Delft when he left for England. It does not list any that he took with him, or the smallest (12mo) of them. But it does suggest much about his education and reading. Sibelius apparently made the "0" marks next to the books that he shipped to Groenevelt; the others were missing. As was common in the period, Groenevelt had arranged his list according to the size of the books, from large to small. I have supplied a literal translation of the letter and have tried to identify the works from the sometimes cryptic titles used by Groenevelt; when possible, I have identified likely editions (from among those printed before 1674, when Groenevelt left his library in Delft). The remarks in square brackets "[ ]" are descriptions of unidentified books rather than actual titles. It shows that a young Dutch physician of the mid-seventeenth century had access to books printed throughout western Europe.

Mÿn Heer en seer goede Vrient

Mÿn versoeck is dat UE dese moeite voor mÿ gelieve an te nemen en gaan op de Deftsche bierkaÿ bÿ de Oude Kerck tot een bierbeschoyer sÿn naam is Dirck Woutersen, dese man sal UE brengen tot seker persoon dicht bÿ sÿn huÿs, alivaar ick een groot gedeelete van mÿn Bibliotheeck gelaten hebbe, UE gelieve te vragen, wat gelt hÿ veen mij pretendeert

My dear sir and very good friend

My request is that you please take some trouble on my behalf and go to the Delft beer quay by the Old Church to a beer inspector by the name of Dirck Woutersen; this man will bring you to a certain person very near his house. Sadly, I had to leave a large part of my library there. Would you please ask how much money he claims from me? I will send you the amount

ick sal an UE per Wissel soo veel
oversenden als hem toe komt, soo
vas als ick van UE antwoort ont-
fange, 't welck ick met den Eersten
van UE verwachte, ondertusschen
versoecke van mijn natesien of UW
dese boeken daer mochte vinden,
e[rubbed out] mÿ te laten weten
wat onkosten UE sal moeten uÿtleg-
gen om dese Boeken wel opte
packen of in een ben of oude kist
ick sal UE daer vorder over schrÿven per naesten en an welcke schip-
per UE die sal doen leveren, indien
mÿn Heer de tÿt niet mochte hebben, gelieft een ander te krÿgen en
hem voor sÿne moeite te betalen
ick sal UE met danckbaarheÿt UE
gelt te rugge stuuren. De boeken
syn dese volgende.
    in Folio. miscellanen
    1. Biblia Septaagint interp.
Duÿts—
    2. Bocchii Historica descriptio
Belgiis Principum—O

    3. Via Gerh. AEmilii van
Hoogeven—O
    4. Ambrosius Colepinus unde-
cim ling.—O
    5. Donati Antonii Abaltomau
Opera Med O
    6. Ioann. Manardi Itali Epistola
Med.—O

    7. Amati Lusitani Curationum
Medicinalium Centuriae Quatuor O

    8. De Veltboune ofte Lantwin-
ninge &c.
    9. Francoylike Chirurgie door
Jaques Guilleme an Duÿts—O

that is owed him by bill of exchange, just as soon as I receive an
answer from you, which I will expect from you by the first post.
Meanwhile I ask that you look after
them for me if you find these
books there, and let me know what
it costs [for] you will have to pay
something in order to have these
books packed up or put in a box or
an old chest. I will write you there
further about sending them and
which skipper you would prefer to
do it. In case, Sir, you might not
have time, please get someone else
to do it and pay him for his trouble. I will with gratitude send the
money on to you. The books are
the following:

    In Folio, miscellaneous
    1. [Dutch translation of the Sep-
tugint]
    2. [A historical description of
the Kingdom of the Belgae, by
Bocchus]
    3. [Possibly a work of Gerard
van Hoogeveen]
    4. [Unidentified]

    5. [An unidentified author's
medical works]
    6. Joannes Mandardus, *Episto-
lorum Medicinalium libri duodevi-
ginti.* (several fol. editions, from
Basel, 1535, to Hainaut, 1611)
    7. Amatus Lusitanus, [i.e.,
Joao Rodrigues, de Castelo
Branco], . . . *Curationum medicinalium centuriae quatuor.* (many
editions, only one in folio: Basel,
1556)
    8. [Possibly a work on agri-
culture]
    9. Jacques Guillemeau, *Fran-
coylike Chirurgie* [version of M.

[no. 10. listed]
11. Thresoor van Italiaens Boeckhouden door Ioannes Buigha—O

LIBRI in Quarto
1. Felis Plateri Medica Practica O

2. Lexicon scapulae Graeco Latinium O
3. Alphonsi ACARANSA Fcti tractatus de partu—O
4. Ioann. Rodolph. Fabri. corpus Loy. peripatetic—O
5. Tho. Dempsteri Antiq. Rom.—O

6. Hieron. Cardani Commentaria in Aph. Hipp.—00

7. Sennerti Opera omnia Vol. 5—0

8. Francisc. Saches opera medica O

9. Ioann. Fernelii Medicina Universa O

10. Ioannis Veslingii Syntagma Anatomicus O

11. Henrici Regii Medicina Practica O

12. Ioann. Ant. Vander Linden Medicina Physiologica—O

Bouman] by A.M. (Dordrecht, 1597)
[no. 10. listed]
11. [Work on Italian books]

Books in Quarto
1. Felix Plater, the Elder, . . . *Praxeos medicae opus . . . in tres tomos distinctum . . .* (Basel, 1656)
2. [A Greek-Latin lexicon]

3. [Unidentified]

4. [Possibly a work on peripatetic, i.e., Aristotelian, philosophy]
5. Thomas Dempsterus, *Antiquitatum Romanarum corpus absolutissimum* (several 4to editions, from Geneva, 1620, to Leiden, 1663)
6. [Probably] Girolamo Cardano, *In Aphorismos Hippocratis commentaria luculentissima cum Graeco textu* (Pavia, 1653)
7. [Probably] Daniel Sennert, *Operum in quinque tomos divisorum,* Vol. 5. (Lyons, 1666)
8. Franciscus Sanchez, *Opera medica: His juncti sunt tractatus quidam philosophici non insubtiles* (Toulouse, 1636)
9. Joannes Fernel, *Universa medicinâ . . .* [many editions: probably that of Utrecht, 1656]
10. Joannes Veslingius, *Syntagma anatomicum, iconibus exorn.* [many editions, probably that of Amsterdam, 1666]
11. Henricus Regius, *Medicina et Praxis medica, medicationum exemplis demonstrata* [several editions, probably that of Frankfurt on Rhine, 1668]
12. Joannes Antonius van der Linden, *Medicina physiologica, nova curataque methodo ex optimis*

13. Epitheta Textoris—

14. Antonides Y Stroom

15. Zuylichems Zee-straat van Graven Hage op Schevening O

16. Daniel Voetii Physiologia O

17. Dictionaire & Ffcly Fr. flams 0

18. Avinament [Hrinament?]. med. chym. Minsich. O
19. Christophorus Heyll de constitution. Arist Med. &c. O

20. 2de deel der spaense Ty[?, cropped] 0
21. Rechten der Stadt Deventer O
22. Nymannus de vitâ foetus in utero materno

23. Harvejus de motu cordis O

24. Opera Cartesii: Vol. 2

in Octavo O
1. Anatom. Bartholini O

2. Zwelferi Pharmacopoea Aug. 0

auctoribus contracta (Amsterdam, 1653)
13. [Possibly a work on Latin epithets]
14. Antonides Y Stroom [a poem of 1671]
15. Constantijn Huygens, *De Zee-straet van 's Graven-Hage op Schevening* (The Hague, 1667)
16. Daniel Voet, *Physiologia; adjectis aliquot ejusdam argumenti disputationibus . . .* (Amsterdam, 1661)
17. *Le Grand Dictionaire François Flamen* [by E. E. L. Mellema; several editions]
18. [A work on medical chemistry]
19. Christophorus Heyl, . . . *Artificialis medicatio, constans Paraphrasi in Galeni librum de Artis Medicae Constitutione.* 2 pt. (Mainz, 1534)
20. [Perhaps the 2d volume of] *Spiegel der Jeugd*
21. [Work on the laws of the city of Deventer]
22. Gregorius Nymannus, *Dissertatio de vita foetus in utero qua . . . demonstratur, infantum in utero non matris, sed sua ipsius vita vivere, etc.* (Wittenberg, 1628)
23. William Harvey, *Exercitatio anatomica de motu cordis et sanguinis in animalibus* [three possible 4to editions]
24. René Descartes, *Opera philosophica: Editio secunda ab auctore recognita.* 3 vols. (Amsterdam, 1650)
Books in Octavo
1. Thomas Bartholinus, . . . *Anatomia* [8vo editions]
2. Joannes Zwelfer, *Pharmacopoeia Augustana [Augsburg] reformata, . . . cum animadversioni-*

3. Opera Hipp. Vol. 2. O

4. Instruction de trois langues.
franc. Aug. flam. O
5. Dictionar. Biglottori O

6. L. A. Florus in notis Salmas-
ius O

7. Parnassus Poeticus &c. O

8. Posselii Calligraphia Oratia

[torn page: 9.] Prarium Poët-
icum Weinrichi—O

10. Epistolae Bandii—O
11. Terentius in notis Schreve-
lii—O

12. Anatomia Riolani—O

13. Plateri Observ. Medicinales
O

14. Iacobus pons de discendae
& exercendae medicinae ratione O

bus J. Zwelferi [several editions,
probably Dordrecht, 1672]
3. Hippocrates, *Magni Hippocrates Coi opera omnia, graece et
latine edita.* 2 vols. (Leiden, 1665)
4. [Language text for learning
French, German, and Dutch]
5. [Perhaps] Luigi Bigi [called
Pittorio], *Pictorii Hippolyta epi-
grammaton per dialogos opus libri
sex*
6. Publius Annius Florus, *L. A.
Floris [Rerum a Romanis ges-
tarum], cum notis integris C. Sal-
masii [Claude de Saumaise]* (Amsterdam, 1660)
7. [Probably] *Parnassus, dat is,
Den blijdenbergh, der gheestelij-
cker vreught, etc.* [religious poems]
(Antwerp, 1619)
8. Joannes Posselius, the elder,
*Calligraphia Oratia linguae Grae-
cae* [several 8vo editions, from
Leiden, 1607, to Geneva, 1620]
9. Melchior Weinrich, . . .
*Prarium poeticum, hoc est phrases
et nomina poëtica* . . . (Frankfurt,
1647)
10. [Letters to imitate?]
11. Publius Terentius, . . .
*Comoediae sex post optimas edi-
tiones emendatae.* [there were two
editions of this very common work
with Schrevelio's notes: Leiden,
1662, and Leiden and Rotterdam,
1669]
12. Jean Riolan, the younger,
*Encheiridium Anatomicum et Patho-
logicum . . . figuris . . . exornatum*
(Leiden, 1649)
13. Felix Plater, the elder, *Ob-
servationem, in hominis affectibus
plerisque, corpori et animo* (Basel,
1641)
14. Jacobus Pons, *Medicus; seu
ratio ac via aptissima, ad recte tum*

15. Prosodia Smetii—O

16. Timpleri Philosophia Pract.
0

17. Julius Caesar—O

18. Iustinus en notis
Berneccari—O

19. Gutberlethi chronologia—O

20. Ursini Comp. cathecheti-
cum—O

21. N. A. Frambesarii canones
& consultationes medicinal—O

22. Nov. Test. Graeceo Lat-
inum—O

23. Apophthegmata Ly-
coetenis—O

24. M. A. Mureti Orationes—
O

discendam tum exercendam medi-
cinam . . . (Leiden, 1600)
15. Henricus Smetius, *Prosodia*
Henrici Smetii . . . *promptissima*
[many editions, from London,
1615, to Amsterdam, 1674]
16. [Probably] Clemens Tim-
pler, *Physiae seu Philosophiae Na-*
turalis systema methodicum in tres
partes digestum . . . *Pars prima*
(Hanover, 1605)
17. Caius Julius Caesar, many
editions of his whole works published in 8vo in the Netherlands
18. [Trogus Pompeius,] *Justi-*
nus cum notis selectissimus vario-
rum, Berneggeri, Bongarsy, Vossy,
Thysy, etc. (Amsterdam, 1669)
19. Henricus Gutberleth,
M. H. G. chronologia . . . *Editio*
secunda (Amsterdam, 1656)
20. Zacharias Ursinus, *Cateche-*
sis religionis Christianae, quae tra-
ditur in Ecclesiis et Scholis Palati-
natus [many editions of the
Heidelberg catechism]
21. Nicolas Abraham de La
Framboisière, *Canones et consultati-*
ones medicinales (Paris, 1619)
22. [Probably the *textus recep-*
tus, the New Testament in Greek
published by Elzevier in 1633]
23. Lycosthenes, *Apophthegma-*
tum ex optimis utriusque linguae
scriptoribus per C. Lycosthenem
(several editions, from Lyons,
1574, to Cologne, 1618)
24. [Possibly] Marc Antoine
Muret, . . . *Orationes xxiii* . . .
Eiusdem interpretatio quincti libri
Ethicorum Aristotelis ad Nicoma-
chum: Eiusdem hymni sacri et alia
quaedam poematia [many editions
of his works, and individual orations published]

25. Hafenrefferus de morbis Cutaneis O

26. Homeri Opera Volum. duo—O

27. Ionstoni Med. Practica—O

28. P. de Witte syn Catechisatie O

29. Beverwycks Heelkonst—O

30. Orationes Ciceronis Vol. duo—O

31. Nicholai Tulpii Orationes med.

32. Sollingii Orationes—O

33. Burgersdycks institutiones log O

34. Theophil. Gotri. Gramm. graeca O

35. Valerius Maximus—O

36. Henrici Bullingeri compendi religionis Christianis

25. Samuel Hafenreffer, Πανδοκειον αιολοβερμον *in quo cutis eique adhaerentium partium, affectus omnes, singulari methodo, et cognoscendi et curandi . . . traduntur* (Tübingen, 1630)

26. Two volumes of Homer's *Works,* published in many editions.

27. Joannes Jonstonus, *Idea universae medicinae practicae libris VIII absoluta* (several editions of this compendium of practical medicine)

28. Petrus de Witte, *Catechisatie over den Heidelbergschen Catechismus* (1652, with many subsequent editions)

29. Johan van Beverwyck, *Heel-Konst, ofte derde deel van de Genees-Konste, om de uytwendige gebreken te heelen* (Dordrecht, 1645)

30. Two volumes of Cicero's *Orations,* published in many editions

31. [Probably] Nicholaus Tulpius, *Observationum Medicarum libri tres: Cum aeneis figuris* (several Amsterdam editions)

32. [Probably] Cornelius Sollingen, *Embryulcia; ofte Afhandinge eenes dooden Vruchts door de handt van den Hell-Meester* (The Hague, 1673)

33. Franco Burgersdyck, *Institutionum logicarum libri duo . . . ex Aristotelis praeceptis novâ methodo ac modo formati* (several editions)

34. [A Greek grammar]

35. [The works of the Roman historian and philosopher Valerius Maximus]

36. Heinrich Bullinger, *Compendium Christianae religionis decem*

37. Nodigh Pestboeck van Docter Hearnius—O

38. Jacobi Cruci Epistolae

NOTA. Om op Mÿn Heer niet al te groot moeite te versoecken soo weet datt er om trent noch 70. Boeken meer sÿn als ick hier genaamt hebbe en gelieft die maer bÿ het getal antenemen daer syn omtrent 60. boecken in duodecimo, misschien sullen de luyden niet willen toe laten om die overte sien mÿn Heer gelieve te tenteren wat UE doen kan en mÿ te laten weten, voort soo ist dat UE uÿt mÿn naam gelieve te versoeken dat sÿ doen niet mogen openbaren tot anderen, nadien die boecken maten beslagen worden in 't schip of in haer huÿs, als sÿ haer gelt ontfangen hadden, nadien ick nog in Amsterdam een hondert pontten achter ben, 't welcks ick in tÿt sal betalen, ondertussen wilde ick mÿn Bibliotheeck gaven hebben, ick ben in 't recht van mÿn Vrouws Vader hoope daer in 't kort een einde van te hebben, sal dan contante munt geven, mÿn Heer gelieve dog selfs een tot Desen Dirk Wouters te gaan en discovreert me hem s en syn E. Vrouw, groetse vrintelÿck uÿt mÿn naam sÿ syn altÿt mÿn goede vrienden geweest en heb haer eerlÿck bedientjen en sal oock eerlÿck met haer als met ÿdereen hadelen, dat ick weg ging, quam dat ick wiert bedroge doch ick danck God, ick ben hier seer well. Laet mÿ oock dogh weten of Ue de manuscripta van Dr. Ten Rhÿnen in Hollant heeft

libris comprehensum . . . (several editions)

37. Johanes Heurnius, *Het noodigh pest-boeck* (Leiden, 1600)

38. [Probably an edition of the surgical works of Giovanni Andrea della Croce, known as Joannes Andreas Cruci]

NOTA. In order, dear sir, not to ask too much of you, you should know that there are about 70 books more than I have listed here and asked for, but by the number collected there are about 60 books in duodecimo. Perhaps the sound of all this will not make you want to do all this. Dear Sir, please examine what you can do and let me know. Furthermore, there is this: that you would please in my name request that they do not make what they do be public to others. Afterward the books must be closed up in the ship or in her house, as they had received her money, because I am still behind a hundred pounds in Amsterdam, the which I will pay back in time. In the meantime I would like to have my library. I have the rights of my wife's father, and hope to have an end of it there shortly. I shall then pay cash. Dear Sir, please go once yourself to this Dirk Wouters and tell him and his wife of me. Greet them kindly in my name. They were always my good friends and I have served them well and also will do well by them as with everyone I deal with. Tell them that I went away because I was deceived, yet I thank God I am here quite well. Let me also but know if you have had the manuscripts of Dr. Ten Rhijne printed in Holland, or what resolution you have taken in regard to them. If I laten drucken, of wat resolutie UE genoomen heeft omtrent die selve. Soo UE dienen kan ick sal sÿn UWe eygen hant over senden tot UE satisfatie als oock tot vergenoeging van d'Heer Dr. & Professor Ruysch. welck en ick wilde dat mÿn Heer uÿt myn naame gelieve to groeten. Hier mede afbrekende en verwachtende met den Eersten antwoort Verblyve

Mÿn Heer sÿn Eden Onderdamge Vrient en Dienaer.

Ioannes Groeneveld Med.

Doctor

Myn groeteniss an de Heer Joann Daems

Gelieve doch pertinent te schrÿven hoe veel gelt ick moet over maken, de Vracht van de boeken sal ick hier tot London betalen, alleen daer is 100 guld. geleent gelt en 6. of 7. jaar interest moet ick senden, tegen 4 en een half per cento dat wil ick doen en dan wat het op packen en 't scheep brengen mag koeten UE kan dat oprekenen, en sett mÿ eene summa ick sal 't overschicken, en respect an UE persoon alle tÿt betalen. Vale.

can serve you in any way I shall do so, sending over with my own hands to your satisfaction, as also to the contentment of the Heer Doctor and Professor Ruysch, whom I would like you, Dear Sir, to please greet in my name. Here I have to break off and awaiting an answer by the first post I remain

Dear Sir, your very obedient friend and servant

Joannes Groenevelt, Med.

Doctor

My greetings to Master Ioann Daems

Please just write to the point about how much money I should make over. I will pay the freight for the books here in London. There is only 100 gilders of borrowed money and 6 or 7 years' interest at 4 and one-half percent which I have to send. I will do that and then what the packing and the shipping here may cost you can add up and give me a total, which I will send to you, and will always pay respect to your person. Farewell.

Notes

INTRODUCTION
The Importance of an Ordinary Doctor

1. *Dictionnaire de médecine,* 6:345.
2. Bracken, *Midwife's Companion,* 24. I owe this reference to Cathy Crawford.
3. Lovejoy, *Great Chain of Being,* 19–20.
4. Palmer, *English Works of George Herbert,* 1:xii.
5. See Porter, "Patient's View"; Porter, *Patients and Practitioners;* Porter and Porter, *Patient's Progress;* Ulrich, *Midwife's Tale.*
6. Ginzburg, *Cheese and the Worms;* Davis, *Return of Martin Guerre;* Seaver, *Wallington's World;* Spence, *Question of Hu;* Darnton, *Great Cat Massacre.* For a discussion of microhistory, see Muir and Ruggiero, *Microhistory and the Lost Peoples of Europe.* Many American historians have been inspired by the method of "thick description," an idea of the philosopher Gilbert Ryle advocated by anthropologist Clifford Geertz: see Geertz's "Thick Description: Toward an Interpretive Theory of Culture," in his *Interpretation of Cultures,* 3–30.
7. The phrase is from Latour, *Science in Action.*

CHAPTER 1
Medical Malpractice in the Seventeenth Century

1. On the censors' committee of the college, see Cook, *Decline of the Old Medical Regime,* 77–93; for statistical information on the number of prosecutions undertaken by the censors in the seventeenth century, see 276–80, and Cook, "Policing the Health of London."
2. Annals 5:109–13 (9 Mar. 1693/4); Annals 5:115–18 (23 Mar. 1693/4).
3. Dunk, *Copy of a Letter written by E.D.,* 20: "The name of an Empirike is derived from the Greek word which signifieth experience: and by an Empirike is, as you know, understood a Practitioner in Physicke, that hath no knowledge in Philosophy, Logicke, or Grammar: but fetcheth all his skill from bare and naked experience." The English translator of Steven Blankaart's *Physical Dictionary* equated mere experience with quackery: "*Empirica Medicina,* quacking, is Curing the Sick by guess, without reason. *Acron*

Agrigentinus was the first Author of it, who neglecting the reasons of things, contented himself with bare Experience. *Quacks* first flourished among the *Ægyptians;* from this Trade came *Mountebanks*" (113).

4. Annals 5:95–99b, 97–101, 101–4. Rivett later continued to defy the censors.

5. Annals 6:77, 79 (4 and 18 Aug. 1693).

6. Ibid., 6:154; 7:100 (9 Apr. 1697). Although Hamilton was a licentiate of the college, the record does not show what he might have said about Withall's condition prior to Groenevelt's treatment. Hamilton, who had studied at Leiden and then Paris, became a fellow of the college after Queen Anne made him one of her physicians-in-ordinary. He also later obtained a knighthood. Munk, *Roll*, 2:12–13.

7. The commonly used index of wage rates comes from Phelps Brown and Hopkins, "Seven Centuries of Building Wages," and idem, "Seven Centuries of the Prices of Consumables," both in Carus-Wilson, *Essays in Economic History*. For a recent discussion of real wages in England based on the Phelps Brown and Hopkins series, see Wrigley and Schofield, *Population History of England*, 638–41.

8. Annals 7, Eels: 146; Hobbs: 140, 141, 142–43, 144.

9. Annals 7:140, 141, 142–43 (Jan. and Feb. 1698/9). Saufay explained to the college censors that he practiced as a surgeon, although he did not belong to the London Company of Barber-Surgeons, and that he had a license to practice from the archbishop; the censors decided not to pursue charges of illicit practice against him on the condition that he dropped his suit against Baddingbroek.

10. Annals 6:154.

11. Ibid., 7:170, 171.

12. Ibid., 5:82.

13. Willcock, *Laws Relating to the Medical Profession*, 111–12.

14. Annals 6:154.

15. Nicolas Lémery, *Traité universel des drogues simples* (Paris, 1698), cited in Van Gils, "Spaansche vlieg," 378.

16. *Dictionnaire de médecine*, 6:336.

17. Groenevelt, *De Tuto Cantharidum*, 10.

18. Geyer, *Tractatus physico-medicus de cantharidibus*. For a modern study, see Pinto and Selander, *Bionomics of Blister Beetles*, 9–10.

19. "Cantharidum sucos dante parente bibas." Ovid, *Ibis*, line 306.

20. Anonymous letter to Sir Hans Sloane, 27 Nov. 1731, British Library, Sloane MS. 4034 (hereafter, Sloane 4034), fol. 77.

21. Annals 6:155.

22. Faye Getz and I have searched without success the parish records of St. Saviours Southwark, whence Mrs. Withall came according to the Annals 6:155, looking for christenings from Jan. 1691/2 to 1695, marriages from Jan. 1674 to 1695, and burials from 1695 to 1710 (Greater London Records Office, X39/2b and X39/3b).

23. For a description of contemporary Southwark, see Boulton, *Neighbourhood and Society*.

24. Spufford, *Great Reclothing of Rural England*.

25. These identifications come from the depositions they later swore, as recorded in Annals 7:100–103 (9 Apr. 1697).

26. Annals 6:175–76 (7 Nov. 1694).

27. Ibid., 6:155; 5:62b, 63a, 65a (28 Sept. 1687).

28. Ibid., 6:155.

29. Ibid.

30. Annals 6:156.

31. Ibid., 6:158 (3 Aug. 1694); 6:174 (2 Nov. 1694).

32. Ibid., 6:175.

33. He mentions this explicitly in his *De Tuto Cantharidum,* 97–98.

34. Groenevelt later changed his testimony to having made pills with two grains of cantharides per pill, for a total dose of thirty-six grains: Annals 7:104–5.

35. Annals: 6:175–76.

36. Somewhat confused by who was who, Registrar Gill now called Prunella Beckett "Susanna."

37. Annals 6:176.

38. Ibid., 6:176–77.

39. Born in 1650, Tyson earned his M.D. from Corpus Christi College, Cambridge, in 1680. In 1679 he became a fellow of the Royal Society; he joined the College of Physicians as a candidate on 30 Sept. 1680 and became a fellow on 2 Apr. 1683. He also obtained appointments as physician to Bridewell and Bethlehem hospitals: Foster, *Alumni Oxonienses,* 1528; Venn, *Alumni Cantabrigienses,* 4:287; Ashley Montague, *Edward Tyson.*

40. Tyson, *Phocaena; Carigueya; Orang-outang.*

41. Annals 5:96b (19 Mar. 1688/9); "Proposed Act of 1689," *House of Lords Journals,* 14:241. For more on this affair, see Cook, *Decline of the Old Medical Regime,* 215–20.

42. Annals 6:186.

43. Torlesse received permission to make copies from the Annals on 5 June 1695; the argument between Tyson and Gill occurred on 5 July, 12 Aug., and 6 Sept.: Annals 6:210, 218–20, 223, 231.

44. Annals 6:198–99, 200–201, 201–6, 209, 212, 222 (5 Apr. to 2 Aug.).

45. Ibid., 6:230 (6 Sept. 1695).

46. The other censor was William Dawes: Annals 7:1–3; Annals 7:4.

47. Annals 7:5 (1 Nov. 1695).

48. Ibid., 7:105.

49. Ibid., 7:9–10.

50. Van Gils, "Spaansche vlieg," 378. Van Gils also writes that using the hard parts of the beetle internally would certainly not be poisonous. William Salmon agreed, in his *Pharmacopoeia Londinensis,* 259. About the Hippocratics and cantharides, Lloyd, in his *Science, Folklore and Ideology,* notes: "To the usual list of potent and possibly dangerous drugs (such as hellebore) commonly prescribed by the Hippocratic writers, the gynaecological treatises add some for which they show their own particular predilection, notably cantharides" (82).

51. Groenevelt, *De Tuto Cantharidum.*

52. Quoted in Van Gils, "Spaansche vlieg," 378.

53. Groenevelt, *Arthritology,* 2–16.

54. Sylvius, *Idea praxeos medicae,* bk. 1, cap. iv, para. 8, p. 589; cap. lvi, para. 1–5, p. 593.

55. Groenevelt to Casparus Sibelius, 31 Mar. 1682, Sloane 2729, fols. 116–17.

56. Groenevelt, *Arthritology*, 11–16, 20–22.

57. Thijssen-Schoute, *Nederlands Cartesianisme*, 258–60; Hall, "Acid and Alkali"; Metzger, *Doctrines chimiques en France*, 199–219.

58. Ruestow, "Rise of the Doctrine of Vascular Secretion."

59. Boyle, *Experiments, Notes, &c.*; Baumann, *François Dele Boe Sylvius*, 206.

60. Boyle, *Works*, 4:291.

61. Colbatch, *Physico-Medical Essay Concerning Alkaly and Acid*, preface.

62. François André, *Entretiens sur l'acid et l'alcali, où sont examinées les objections de M. Boyle contre ces principes* (Paris, 1672; reprinted 1677, 1681); transl. by "J.W." as *Chemical Disceptations*. Also see Hall, "Acid and Alkali," 17; Metzger, *Doctrines chimiques en France*, 207–8, 217–18. André was a royal physician to Louis XIV and professor of medicine at Caen: *Nouvelle Biographie Générale*, 2:556.

63. For instance, the physician Walter Harris, friend of Thomas Sydenham, warned readers not that alkalies were of no use but that too many people had a great enthusiasm for fixed alkali salts and needed reminding of the useful natural alkalies like pearl, oriental bezoar, crabs' eyes, chalk, coral, "etc.": Harris, *Pharmacologia Anti-Empirica*, 85; Harris also believed that children's diseases were caused by the moistness of children degenerating into acids, and hence that they were best treated with alkalies: Harris, *Exact Enquiry*, 5.

64. Bontekoe, *Fragmenta, dienende tot een Ondewys van de beweginge, en Vyandschap . . . van het Acidum met het Alcali* (The Hague, 1683), transl. into Latin by Cornelis Blankaart as *Fundamenta Medica, sive de Alcali et Acidi effectibus per modum fermentionis et effervescentiae* (Amsterdam, 1688). I have used the text found in Bontekoe, *Alle de philosophische, medicinale, en chymische werken*, vol. 2, pt. 2, pp. 186–267 (hereafter, *Werken*).

65. Bontekoe, *Werken*, 224.

66. Bontekoe, *Werken*, 262–63.

67. Salmon, *Pharmacopoeia Londinensis*, 259.

68. Blankaart, *Lexicon Medicum Renovatum*, 167–68.

69. *Dictionnaire de médecine*, 6:242.

70. Blankaart, *Lexicon Medicum Renovatum*, 167–68.

71. For instance, it was recommended as an ingredient for an eye ointment and a plaster in the *Pharmacopoea Ultrajectina*, 76, 78.

72. According to the early nineteenth-century *Dictionnaire de médecine*, camphor was a well-known anaphrodisiac, calming erections in cases of gonorrhea and even causing the organs of generation to disappear in people who breathed the scent of camphor too much. It may even have been known to the medievals for such an effect (6:244, 255–57). The anaphrodisiac properties of camphor caused it to be used in the nineteenth century as a treatment for priapism, gonorrhea, satyriasis, and nymphomania: Sigerist, "Alexandre Ricord's Dissertation," 472. Schroeder, *Pharmacopoeia Medico-Chymica*, 717: "Illis vis venerrem ac libidinem compescendi, inflammationesque extinguendi." I have been informed that it is rumored that until fairly recently, the Dutch army mixed a bit of camphor in the bread served to soldiers while they were in camp to help keep their sexual appetites low during periods away from home.

73. Groenevelt, *De Tuto Cantharidum*, 98–101, the case of one Mrs. Anthony.

74. Clark, *History of the Royal College of Physicians*, 455.

CHAPTER 2
A Place in the World

1. B. H. Slicher van Bath, "Welvaart op Wankele Basis: De Sociaal-Economische Omstandigheden Gedurende de Middeleeuwen," in Slicher van Bath et al., *Geschiedenis van Overijssel,* 97; Dumbar, *Kerkelyk en Wereltlyk Deventer,* 2:177–83.

2. For a translation of the earliest life of Lebuinus, see Talbot, *Anglo-Saxon Missionaries in Germany,* 229–34. Also see Dumbar, *Kerkelyk en Wereltlyk Deventer,* 2:183; R. R. Post, "De Kerk in het Midden: De Middeleeuwse Kerk," in Slicher van Bath et al., *Geschiedenis van Overijssel,* 106–16.

3. Keuning, *Kaleidoscoop der Nederlandse landschappen,* 30–66.

4. Verhulst, "Origins of Towns in the Low Countries"; W. Jappe Alberts, "De Middeleeuwen, Staatkundig Beschowd," in Slicher van Bath et al., *Geschiedenis van Overijssel,* 61–69; Van Houtte, *Economic History of the Low Countries,* 22–23.

5. Reitsma, *Centrifugal and Centripetal Forces;* Dollinger, *German Hansa,* 122–23, 251–52, 298–302; Jappe Alberts, *Nederlandse Hanzesteden.*

6. Huizinga, *Erasmus and the Age of Reformation,* 7; Oberman, *Devotio Moderna;* Post, *Modern Devotion.*

7. Geyl, *Revolt of the Netherlands,* 62.

8. The exact causes of the development of the late medieval economy of Holland are hotly debated: the above follows the argument of Van Zanden, "Op zoek naar de 'missing link.'" But see De Vries, "Modernity of the Dutch Republic"; idem, *Dutch Rural Economy;* TeBrake, *Medieval Frontier;* and Van der Wee, "Antwoord op een industriël uitaging."

9. For recent views on the early formation of a "state" in the low countries, see Blockmans, "Corruptie, patronage, makelaardij, en venaliteit"; Tracy, *Financial Revolution in the Habsburg Netherlands;* idem, *Holland under Habsburg Rule,* 64–89; and Rodríguez-Salgado, *Changing Face of Empire;* on the sixteenth century in Overijssel, see Reitsma, *Centrifugal and Centripetal Forces.*

10. For two standard accounts of the revolt in English, see Geyl, *Revolt of the Netherlands;* and Parker, *Dutch Revolt.* On the importance of the dispute over new bishoprics, see Postma, "Nieuw licht op een oude zaak."

11. Reitsma, *Centrifugal and Centripetal Forces,* 72–116.

12. Frijhoff, "Deventer en zijn gemiste universiteit."

13. Koch, "Reformation in Deventer." Also see Hofman, "Deventer in de tweede helft der 16e eeuw en daarna"; De Hullu, "Bijdrage tot de kerkelijke geschiedenis van Deventer"; Reitsma, *Centrifugal and Centripetal Forces,* 204–95.

14. Reitsma, *Centrifugal and Centripetal Forces,* 204–95.

15. There would continue to be occasional religious troubles in Deventer, as when a Catholic named Hendrick Achtervelt assassinated the Protestant minister Franciscus Schorickmen in 1599 (Van Deursen, *Plain Lives,* 226); but the dominance of the Reformed faith could no longer be doubted.

16. Timekeeping has often been associated with modernity and sometimes also with Protestantism. See Toulmin and Goodfield, *Discovery of Time;* Landes, *Revolution in Time;* Mayr, *Authority, Liberty, and Automatic Machinery.*

17. Schenkeveld, *Dutch Literature,* 106.

18. Gemeentelijke Archief Deventer (hereafter, GA Deventer), "Klapper Hervormde Dopen Deventer: 1647–1656."

19. Christopher and Gelmer, twins, had been baptized on 9 July 1643, the first Jan on 26 Dec. 1645: GA Deventer, "Klapper Hervormde Dopen Deventer: 1638–1646." On the customs of naming children, see the interesting remarks of Imhof, "Old Mortality Pattern to the New."

20. GA Deventer, "Klapper Hervormde Dopen Deventer 1591 juli 2–1616 mei 28." Although baptized as Judith, and occasionally mentioned in the archives by that name, she is more commonly named as "Goedeken," "Guede," or "Gude" and tended to sign her own name "Guedeken"; later in life, as when her son Joannes got married, she went by "Odilia" or "Odielia."

21. GA Deventer, "Ondertrouw Klapper, 1624–1650"; Gemeentelijke Archief Zutphen (hereafter, GA Zutphen): "Trouwvermeldingen." It is in this last document that she is mentioned as a recent widow.

22. See McLaren, *History of Contraception.*

23. See Van Dorsten, *Poets, Patrons, and Professors;* Frijhoff et al., *Geschiedenis van Zutphen.*

24. There is a one-page account of the family in the "Genealogie" folders in GA Zutphen.

25. GA Deventer, "Attestaties, Belijdenissen Herv. Kerk 1632–1816 (hereafter, "Attestaties")," June 1641.

26. Van Deursen, *Plain Lives,* 8–10; Dutch women not only worked publicly but held great domestic authority: ibid., 82–84. Also see Schama, *Embarrassment of Riches,* 375–480.

27. GA Deventer, RA 141a/513–28: "Boedelinventaris, 1518–1811," (18 Mar. 1664).

28. The financial transactions are given in GA Deventer, RA 134f/395: "Renuntiatien van 17 May 1636 tot 1 December 1643" (28 Oct. 1640); RA 134g/304: "Testamenten en Renuntiatien van 28 Nov. 1643 tot 6 Mart 1655" (no. 1; 28 May 1648), 134g/467 (no. 2; 14 Apr. 1651), and 134g/501–2 (16 Oct. 1651); RA 104c/230: "Bekende Schulden van 27 Jan. 1637 tot 16 July 1649" (1 Oct. 1644); RA 104d/130: "Bekende Schulden van 27 Jan. 1637 tot 16 July 1649" (no. 2, 17 Oct. 1651).

29. GA Deventer, RA 141a/513–28: "Boedelinventaris, 1518–1811" (18 Mar. 1664). About 200 gilders at Amsterdam in 1670 could have bought a last of wheat (2 tuns—large barrels—or about 2 metric dead-weight tons), 100 gilders a last of rye, or 15 gilders a tun of herring. In Leiden in 1620, a twelve-pound loaf of rye bread cost 6.4 stuivers (at 20 stuivers per gilder). A captain in the Dutch navy earned 30 gilders per month, a common sailor about 10. Posthumus, *History of Prices in Holland,* 2:770, 783; Van Deursen, *Plain Lives,* 6; Boxer, *Dutch Seaborne Empire,* 337, 342.

30. For a description of Dutch children and child rearing, see Schama, *Embarrassment of Riches,* 481–561.

31. Schenkeveld, *Dutch Literature,* 86, poem transl. by August F. Harms.

32. First published in 1630, expanded in 1634; for a modern edition, see Smit, *Jacobus Revius.*

33. Ten Harmsel, *Jacobus Revius,* 143.

34. For a somewhat different discussion of *deftig, deugdzaam,* and *gezellig,* see Regin, *Traders, Artists, Burghers,* 129–31, 144.

35. GA Deventer, "Attestaties."
36. There is no mention of the Groenevelts in *Rijksarchief in Overijssel*.
37. See esp. Van der Wall, *De mystieke chiliast Petrus Serrarius;* Fix, *Prophecy and Reason;* and Israel, *European Jewry.*
38. Israel, *European Jewry,* 155.
39. On the Dutch Reformed faith before the Remonstrant/Contra-Remonstrant argument, see Nijenhuis, "Variants within Dutch Calvinism."
40. See esp. Groenhuis, *Predikanten.*
41. Schöffer, *Lage landen,* 233.
42. Bussemaker, *Geschiedenis van Overijssel,* 5–7.
43. Posthumus Meijes, *Jacobus Revius,* 26–33.
44. Verbeek, *Descartes and the Dutch,* 5.
45. The most widely translated English author in Dutch was the English Puritan minister William Perkins; the translation of Lewis Bayley's *Practice of Piety* was the single most frequently printed piece of religious prose (with thirty-two editions between 1620 and 1688): Schenkeveld, *Dutch Literature,* 145.
46. Posthumus Meijes, *Jacobus Revius,* 33–35.
47. On the raising of Dutch children generally, see Van Deursen, *Plain Lives,* 115–33.
48. For what follows, see De Booy, *Weldaet der scholen.*
49. They were among the books he had left in Delft: see appendix.
50. See appendix. A modern English edition is *The Heidelberg Catechism with Scripture Texts.*
51. GA Deventer, RA 141a/513–28: "Boedelinventaris, 1518–1811."
52. Postma, *Nederland in vroeger tijd,* 84–85, cites a contemporary source as saying that more than 4,533 people died of the epidemic in Deventer in 1656, although this figure may be somewhat exaggerated. The population of Deventer in 1579 had been about 10,500 to 11,000 (Koch, "Reformation in Deventer," 29), but it shrank by about one-third during the religious troubles and sieges of the late 1580s and 1590s, never to regain its number. Another estimate of Deventer's population (after the plague) puts it at around 7,000: Van Houtte, *Economic History of the Low Countries,* 136. It had grown back only to about 8,500 in 1795: TeBrake, *Regents and Rebels,* 12. Van der Woude, "Demografische ontwikkeling," estimates that the plagues of 1617, 1625, and 1635 killed perhaps 10 percent of the people of large cities (5:144–45).
53. Postma, *Nederland in vroeger tijd,* 84–85. Although Deventer is not specifically mentioned, see Van Andel, "Plague Regulations in the Netherlands," and Dijkstra, *Epidemiologische beschowing,* 50–60.
54. GA Deventer, RA 108a/121: "Testamenten 16e eeuw tot c. 1656" (6 Aug. 1656).
55. Postma, *Nederland in vroeger tijd,* 84.
56. De Booy, *Weldaet der scholen,* 37.
57. See appendix (quarto, no. 20).
58. De Booy, *Weldaet der scholen,* 278: *Spiegel der Jeught, ofte een kort verhael der voornaemste Tyrannye ende Barbarische Wreetheden Welcke de Spangiaerden hier in Nederlandt bedreven hebben aen menigh duysent menschen.* On history teaching, see 60–64.
59. Schama, *Embarrassment of Riches,* 51–125.

60. The classic statement of this point remains Weber, *The Protestant Ethic and the Spirit of Capitalism*. Many have raised objections and caveats to the Weber thesis: for a Dutch example, see Van Stuijvenberg, " 'The' Weber Thesis."

61. Petrus de Witte, *Catechisatie over den Heidelbergschen Catechismus* (Hoorn, 1652, with many subsequent editions).

CHAPTER 3
The Education of a Dutch Physician

1. Frijhoff, " 'Non satis dignitatis . . .' "; idem, "Wetenschap, beroep en status"; and generally, idem, *Société Néerlandaise et ses gradués*.

2. Van Slee, *Illustre School te Deventer*, 41.

3. Huizinga, *Erasmus and the Age of Reformation*, 7; Cameron, "Humanism in the Low Countries," 139, 143.

4. Frijhoff, "Deventer en zijn gemiste universiteit," 46, 47; Van Slee, *Illustre School te Deventer*, 7–11.

5. For a description of the rich educational resources before the Reformation in two cities, see De Booy, *Kweekhoven der wijshied*, 67, 122; Brugmans, *Gedenkboek van het Athenaeum*, 13–20.

6. Van Slee, *Illustre School te Deventer*, 24, 19–20.

7. Fortgens, *Schola Latina*, 11, 15.

8. Van Slee, *Illustre School te Deventer*, 30; the last professor of the Illustrious School to sign the document was Groenevelt's theology professor, Antonio Perizonius, in 1661.

9. Zeeland issued school regulations in 1583, Friesland 1588, Gelderland in 1611, and Holland and West Friesland in 1625: Fortgens, *Schola Latina*, 54. On the school regulations of 1654, see De Booy, *Weldaet der scholen*, 30–34; and De Booy, *Kweekhoven der Wijshied*, 70.

10. Van Slee, *Illustre School te Deventer*, 69, 66.

11. De Booy, *Kweekhoven der wijshied*, 121–25; Fortgens, *Schola Latina*, 31–42.

12. De Booy, *Kweekhoven der wijshied*, 121; Fortgens, *Schola Latina*, 63.

13. See appendix (octavo, nos. 11, 30). In Utrecht, Latin lessons began with the "Distichs" of (pseudo-) Cato and then followed with Cicero and Terence: De Booy, *Kweekhoven der wijshied*, 121. Groenevelt may also have used Cato, but in his letter he mentions only his books larger than 8vo, and there were many 12mo editions of Cato.

14. See appendix (octavo, nos. 7, 9).

15. See appendix (octavo, no. 17).

16. See appendix (octavo, nos. 26, 34).

17. Since the surviving registers of burials for the Deventer Reformed church begin in 1674, it is impossible to be certain of the date of Frans Groenevelt's death. But officials reported an inventory of his widow's property on 18 Mar. 1664: GA Deventer, RA 141a/513, vol. 1: "Boedelinventaris, 1518–1811."

18. GA Deventer, RA 108a/121: "Testamenten 16e eeuw tot c. 1656" (6 Aug. 1656).

19. GA Deventer, RA 141a/513–28: "Boedelinventaris, 1518–1811."

20. Schama, *Embarrassment of Riches*, 405.

21. GA Deventer, RA 141a/513–28: "Boedelinventaris, 1518–1811."

22. Rowen, *Princes of Orange.*

23. Bussemaker, *Geschiedenis van Overijssel,* 22–25; Formsma, "Nieuwe geschiedenis," in Slicher van Bath et al., *Geschiedenis van Overijssel,* 127.

24. On the second Anglo-Dutch war, see Wilson, *Profit and Power,* 111–42; Geyl, *Orange and Stuart,* 163–300; Rowen, *John de Witt,* 448–64.

25. Postma, *Nederland in vroeger tijd,* 84–85; Formsma, "Nieuwe geschiedenis," 128; Bussemaker, *Geschiedenis van Overijssel,* 110–27.

26. Van Slee, *Illustre School te Deventer,* 221.

27. Frijhoff, "Deventer en zijn gemiste universiteit," 76.

28. Van Slee, *Illustre School te Deventer,* 27; on the importance of Alsted for Protestant millenarianism, esp. in England, see Webster, *Great Instauration,* 12–15.

29. Van Slee, *Illustre School te Deventer,* 108–9, 120–21, 40; Frijhoff, "Deventer en zijn gemiste universiteit," 52; Lindeboom, *Descartes and Medicine,* 10.

30. Van Slee, *Illustre School te Deventer,* 68–69, 63.

31. Ibid., 64: the professor, Gutberleth, was reprimanded. On the philosophy of Pierre de la Ramée, or Ramus, see Ong, *Ramus and Talon Inventory;* idem, *Ramus: Method, and the Decay of Dialogue;* Howell, *Logic and Rhetoric in England;* Van Berkel, *Isaac Beeckman,* 279–90; Grafton and Jardine, *Humanism to the Humanities.*

32. Van Slee, *Illustre School te Deventer,* 69.

33. Ibid., 96.

34. See appendix (quarto, nos. 5, 21; folio, no. 8, may also have pertained to how the Dutch legal system worked).

35. Van Slee, *Illustre School te Deventer,* 136–37.

36. Ibid., 30, 118; on Descartes's followers making philosophy independent of theology, see Verbeek, *Descartes and the Dutch,* esp. 76–77.

37. Van Slee, *Illustre School te Deventer,* 110–11.

38. See appendix (octavo, no. 16). On philosophy being studied in the last two years of the Deventer Triviale School, see Van Slee, *Illustre School te Deventer,* 69.

39. GA Deventer, RA 141a/515: "Boedelinventaris, 1518–1811."

40. See appendix (octavo, no. 24).

41. See appendix (octavo, nos. 18, 19, 35).

42. Van Slee, *Illustre School te Deventer,* 126–27.

43. Ibid., 77–78, 91.

44. Thijssen-Schoute, *Nederlands Cartesianisme,* 30–34; Verbeek, *Descartes and the Dutch,* 87; on Perizonius as a moderate Cartesian, Thijssen-Schoute, "Cartésianisme aux pays-bas," 244.

45. See Ottley, *Introduction to the Old Testament in Greek;* idem, *Handbook to the Septuagint;* Jellicoe, *Septuagint and Modern Study;* and J. C. H. Lebram, "Ein Streit um die Hebräische Bibel und die Septuagunta," in Lunsingh Scheurleer and Posthumus Meyjes, *Leiden University in the Seventeenth Century,* 21–63.

46. See appendix (folio, no. 1).

47. De Jong, "Study of the New Testament."

48. See appendix (octavo, no. 22).

49. He also possessed the work of the Zurich Reformer Heinrich Bullinger, a more liberal statement of the Reformed faith than Witte's: see appendix (octavo, no. 36).

50. Van Slee, *Illustre School te Deventer*, 70.

51. He was baptized in November as Casparus Sibelius à Goor Lubbarti, the son of Joannes Lubbarti van Goor (minister in Bloemendaal) and Elisabeta Sibelia (the only surviving daughter of Caspar Sibelius, minister), on 15 Nov. 1646: GA Deventer, "Klapper Hervormde Dopen Deventer: 1638–1646." On the grandfather Casparus Sibelius or Sibel, see Van der Aa, *Biographisch Woordenboek der Nederlanden*, 10:199–200; Posthumus Meijes, *Jacobus Revius*, 1:xlvi–xlviii, 2:147ff., 156–57.

52. He matriculated in mid-Sept. 1664: Van Slee, *Illustre School te Deventer*, 220.

53. Dapper matriculated to the athenaeum in mid-Nov. 1664, being inscribed as "Oenensis," that is, from a town nearby: Van Slee, *Illustre School te Deventer*, 220. Members of his family—and later he—regularly served on the town council for Deventer from the early seventeenth century: Dumbar, *Het Kerkelyk en Wereltlyk Deventer*, 1:110–53; GA Deventer, Jhr. H. H. Röell, coll., "Deventer Vroedschap," vol. 2.

54. The two entries for Ten Rhijne (6:1213; 9:861) in the *Nieuw Nederlandsch Biographisch Woordenboek* differ as to whether he was baptized in Jan. 1649 or 1647: the latter date was an error of his earlier biographers. He matriculated to the Illustrious School in Aug. 1665: Van Slee, *Illustre School te Deventer*, 220.

55. GA Deventer, Jhr. H. H. Röell, coll., "Deventer Vroedschap," vol. 2; GA Deventer, "Klapper Hervormde Dopen Deventer: 1647–1656," (Jan. 1649); he also matriculated to the Illustrious School in mid-Jan. 1665: Van Slee, *Illustre School te Deventer*, 220.

56. GA Deventer, "Attestaties."

57. On the costs of travel, see De Vries, *Barges and Capitalism*, 76–77.

58. *Album Studiosorum Academiae Lugduno Batavae.*

59. Frijhoff, *Société Néerlandaise et ses gradués*, 62.

60. On town-gown relations, see Grafton, "Civic Humanism," esp. 64–67.

61. University of Leiden, "Archieven van Senaat en Faculteiten der Leidsche Universiteit, Recensielijsten," no. 38 (1668). In addition to Groenevelt, the widow housed Hermannus Ruys (no place given), Joannes Weerden from "Aquisgranensis," Fredericus Cristoffel from Veltdorp, Fredericus Gimtor from Harlingen, Theodorus Huete from Hasselt in Overijssel (just outside Zwolle), and four students from Zwolle: Petrus Crans and three brothers, Henricus Holt, Hermannus Johannes Holt (both of whom had been to the Deventer school), and Hermannus Henricus Holt. In 1669, the *recensielijst* naturally shows some turnover in her house; one of the new lodgers was one Henry Pratt from England.

62. See the map in Frijhoff, *Société Néerlandaise et ses gradués*, 111. The four other Dutch universities included Franeker, Utrecht, Groningen, and Harderwijk.

63. For a narrative, see Fruin, *Siege and Relief of Leyden*.

64. See Van Dorsten, *Poets, Patrons, and Professors;* Grafton, *Joseph Scaliger*.

65. For a brief overview in English of the early years of the university, see J. J. Woltjer's introduction to Lunsingh Scheurleer and Posthumus Meijes, *Leiden University in the Seventeenth Century*, 1–19; and Jurriaanse, *Founding of Leyden University*. The registers of matriculations to the university show about three hundred new students per year: while some of the students (foreigners in particular) spent only a few months or even days at the university, others spent two years or more; additionally, young men and

tutors who did not register at the university spent time in Leiden getting acquainted with the place and its teachings.

66. Verbeek, *Descartes and the Dutch,* 34–70, 79–81.

67. Ruestow, *Physics,* 43–46. Also see Dibon, *Philosophie néerlandaise,* 80–119.

68. Frijhoff, *Société Néerlandaise et ses gradués,* 139: Deventer also had the highest percentage of law graduates of the thirty-eight cities. It was about in the middle of thirty six cities according to the annual number of citizens who took university degrees: ibid., 143.

69. Frijhoff, "Deventer en zijn gemiste universiteit," table on 69, shows that medicine was a very infrequently chosen career path (5.2 percent) for students from Overijssel. Sibelius, Ten Rhijne, and Dapper also graduated in medicine (Sibelius and Dapper switching from theology); Van Duren graduated in law. Two other students in medicine at Leiden were from Deventer during the 1660s, although neither had matriculated in the Illustrious School: Clemens Nenlo (17 Feb. 1661) and Theodorus Muller (18 Apr. 1669) (*Album Studiosorum Academiae Lugduno Batavae*).

70. Cook, "Good Advice and Little Medicine."

71. GA Deventer, RA 141a/527: "Boedelinventaris, 1518–1811": 800 gilders to the first, 1,200 to the second.

72. Van Dorssen, "Willem ten Rhijne," 139–41.

73. Lindeboom, "Medical Education," 203.

74. Th. H. Lunsingh Scheurleer, "Un amphithéâtre d'anatomie moralisée," in Lunsingh Scheurleer and Posthumus Meyjes, *Leiden University in the Seventeenth Century,* 217–77.

75. De Beer, *Diary of John Evelyn,* 2:53. The knife and a picture of the man in question are now on display at the Museum Boerhaave in Leiden.

76. Ibid., 2:52.

77. Karstens and Kleibrink, *Leidse Hortus;* Veendorp and Baas Becking, *Hortus Academicus Lugduno Batavus;* Prest, *Garden of Eden.*

78. Beukers, "Clinical Teaching."

79. Hett, *Memoirs of Sir Robert Sibbald,* 56–57.

80. Dewhurst, *John Locke,* 261, commas added.

81. The best single treatment of Sylvius remains Bauman, *François dele Boe Sylvius* (hereafter, *Sylvius*). For a rather unsympathetic summary in English of his major ideas, see King, *Road to Medical Enlightenment,* 93–112.

82. On the reception of Harvey's theory in the Netherlands, see Van Lieburg, "Zacharias Sylvius," and idem, "Isaac Beeckman."

83. Beukers, "Mechanistiche principes bij Franciscus dele Boë, Sylvius," emphasizes that the terms *iatrochemical* and *iatromechanical* philosophies were coined after the seventeenth century, so that trying to sort out the medical ideas of those like Sylvius into one camp or the other is a false dichotomy.

84. Beukers, "Clinical teaching"; idem, "Het laboratorium van Sylvius."

85. See appendix (folio, nos. 6, 7; quarto, nos. 1, 19; octavo, nos. 2, 13, 25, 29, 31, 37).

86. See appendix (quarto, nos. 7, 18; octavo, no. 27). Perhaps Groenevelt also followed the lectures of Marggraff, who was still teaching chemistry in Leiden privately.

Marggraff's lectures were later published by one of his English students: Christopher
Love Morley, *Collectanea Chymica Leidensia* (Leiden, 1684).
87. Lindeboom, *Ontmoeting met Jan Swammerdam,* 12; Swammerdam, *Miraculum
naturae.*
88. Groenevelt, *Dissertatio Lithologica,* 10–11.
89. See appendix (quarto, nos. 10, 12, 22; octavo, nos. 1, 12, 32).
90. He possessed no herbals but several pieces on *materia medica;* as for works of
medical theory and general physiology, he also possessed several: see appendix (quarto,
nos. 6, 8, 9, 16, 23; octavo, nos. 14, 21).
91. On Drélincourt, see Lindeboom, "Dog and Frog," 289–90.
92. Lonie, "The 'Paris Hippocrates' "; Nutton, "Hippocrates in the Renaissance."
93. See Smith, *Hippocratic Tradition.*
94. See appendix (octavo, no. 3).
95. Lindeboom, "Medical Education," 203.
96. Cunningham, "Sir Robert Sibbald."
97. Lindeboom, *Florentius Schuyl,* 94–95.
98. In Schuyl, *Pro veteri medicina* (Amsterdam, 1670).
99. See Van Berkel, *Isaac Beeckman.*
100. Verbeek, *Descartes and the Dutch.*
101. Ibid., 13–33.
102. Bauman, *Sylvius,* 36; Lindeboom, *Florentius Schuyl.*
103. See Carter, *Descartes' Medical Philosophy;* Dankmeijer, "Biologische studies
van René Descartes."
104. See appendix (quarto, no. 24).
105. Sloane 2729, fols. 116–17, 118, 157v.
106. Fockema Andreae and Meijer, *Album Studiosorum Academiae Franekerensis,*
no. 6918.
107. Jensma et al., *Universiteit te Franeker;* Napjus, *Hoogleeraren in de geneeskunde.*
108. GA Deventer, "Attestaties."
109. 3 Mar. 1668: *Album Studiosorum Academiae Lugduno Batavae.*
110. Dapper is mentioned in the "Recensielijsten" (University of Leiden) in 1669,
1670, 1671, and 1672, although he returned to Deventer from Leiden as "doctor in de
medicijnen" on 24 June 1671: GA Deventer, "Attestaties."
111. Willem ten Rhijne, *Disputatio . . . de dolore intestinorum a flatu; Praes. F.
de la Boe Sylvio* (Leiden, 1668); D. Schoute, intro. to *Opuscula,* 19:xlii–xliii.
112. I owe this thought to Harm Beukers, who observed that many of the Leiden
students went elsewhere during the epidemic.
113. Van Thiel, *Anopheles en malaria,* 3.
114. Lindeboom, *Florentius Schuyl,* 64; Bauman, *Sylvius,* 39–40; it reopened at the
end of November.
115. *Album Studiosorum Academiae Rheno-Traiectinae,* 63.
116. On the Cartesian controversies, see Thijssen-Schoute, "Cartésianisme aux pays-
bas"; idem, *Nederlands Cartesianisme;* De Hoog, "Currents of Thought"; McGahagan,
"Cartesianism in the Netherlands"; Van Berkel, "Descartes in debat met Voetius"; Ver-

beek, *Querelle d'Utrecht;* French, "Harvey in Holland"; and Verbeek, *Descartes and the Dutch.*

117. See appendix (quarto, no. 11).

118. Ysbrand van Diemerbroek, *De peste libri IV* (Arnhem, 1646).

119. Beukers, "Clinical teaching," 140–41; I owe several further bits of information about Diemerbroek's teaching to Harm Beukers.

120. Sibelius left for Utrecht on 25 Feb. 1667, matriculating there only in 1668; on 9 Aug. 1669 he received a certificate in Deventer stating that he was leaving for Geneva: GA Deventer, "Attestaties"; *Album Studiosorum Academiae Rheno-Traiectinae,* 63. It is possible that Groenevelt joined Sibelius in Utrecht before the latter left. On the two belonging to the student society, see Schutte, *Wapenboeken,* 190.

121. Van Duren left Deventer for Utrecht on 13 Sept. 1669 and eventually matriculated in law at Leiden on 1 Oct. 1670: GA Deventer, "Attestaties"; *Album Studiosorum Academiae Lugduno Batavae.* He did not matriculate at the University of Utrecht, but this formality was also ignored by Sibelius, who apparently spent some time in Utrecht before matriculating.

122. Groenevelt to Sibelius, Sloane 2729, fol. 160.

123. Ketner, *Album Promotorum Academiae Rheno-Trajectinae,* 26.

124. Cavlier, *De Calculo Renum, & Vesicae;* Spechtius, *De Celebri;* Hulleman, *De Calculo renum & vesicae;* Straselius, *De Calculo renum & vesicae;* Curtius, *De calculo renum et vesicae:* this thesis has been printed with an introduction on the life of the author, an English translation, and a facing-page Latin and Lithuanian edition as Budrys, Paprockas, and Tamosaitis, *Alex[ander] Carolus Curtius, Inaugural Medical Dissertation;* Van der Heyden, *De Calculo vesicae;* Van Campen, *De calculo renum;* Hutchinson, *De calculo;* Middegaels, *De calculo vesicae.* According to Molhuysen, *Bronnen tot de geschiedenis der Leidsche Universiteit,* 3:296* Thomas Nierop also completed a medical thesis on stones at Leiden on 1 Oct. 1658, but I have not been able to locate an extant copy of it.

125. This is especially true for the theses of Cavlier, Middegaels, Van Campen, Hutchinson, Hulleman, and Spechtius.

126. See esp. Spechtius, Hulleman, and Cavlier, the last two of which recommend the use of saxifrage as a lithontriptic, a venerable remedy for the problem.

127. Van der Heyden, *De Calculo vesicae,* sig. B.

128. Van der Heyden also mentions "in collegio chirurgico" with regard to Van Horne.

129. Groenevelt, *De calculo vesicae.* In the dedication, "Patriae" may very well refer to Deventer rather than the United Provinces.

130. Of Sylvius, Groenevelt writes the following laudatory parenthesis: "ab Excellentissimo, multaeque experientiae Viro, D. Francisco De le Boe Sylvio, M.D. & Practicae in almâ Lugduno-Batavâ Academiâ Professore ordinario, de meis studiie totâque Medicinâ plurimum merito" (*De calculo vesicae,* sig. Bv).

131. Smalzius is mentioned briefly on p. B2.

132. His teacher Sylvius believed that spirit of niter might have some efficacy as a lithontriptic when injected into the bladder: François dele Boë Sylvius, *Opera medica,* 117, 136.

234 *Notes to Pages 74–81*

133. His teacher Sylvius, for instance, only wrote of trying to free a urethra blocked by a stone through squirting a liquid up into the bladder if the stone was large, or trying to make it pass by giving large quantities of diuretics if it was small, not mentioning surgery at all: Sylvius, *Idea praxeos medicae,* chap. 57, para. 23.

CHAPTER 4
Learning to Cut for the Stone

1. GA Deventer, RA 134i: "Renunciatien, 9 Oct. 1668–23 March 1688," (31 Mar. 1670).
2. Formsma, "Nieuwe geschiedenis," 128–29; Bussemaker, *Geschiedenis van Overijssel,* 127–98; Houck and Dixon, *Deventer onder de Stadhouders.*
3. Van der Hoeven, "Het Chirurgijn-gilde te Deventer"; also see Van Gelder, Grendel, and Wittop Koning, "Deventer en de Farmacie."
4. The number of physicians per person in Overijssel generally was one to about twenty-five hundred (about 35 percent fewer than in the province of Holland), although there would have been more physicians per person in the towns, like Deventer: Frijhoff, *Société Néerlandaise et ses gradués,* 231.
5. Caspar Sibelius to John Locke, 5 Apr. 1692, in De Beer, *Correspondence of John Locke,* 4:441.
6. Van Lieburg, "Pieter van Foreest"; Russell, *Town and State Physician.*
7. GA Deventer, Jhr. H. H. Röell, coll., "Deventer Vroedschap," vol. 2; Dumbar, *Kerkelyk en Wereltlyk Deventer,* 1:78–110.
8. Groenevelt, *Rudiments of Physick,* iv. For more on these works, see chapter 8.
9. Schillings, *Matricule de L'Université de Louvain,* 255, no. 342: one Joannes Groenvelt is mentioned as a matriculant in 1661, but as someone from Amsterdam, at a time when our Groenevelt was just entering adolescence in Deventer; Zypaeus is entered on 30 Jan. 1670 (303, no. 453).
10. On the Louvain medical faculty, see Sondervorst, *Geschiedenis van de Geneeskunde in België;* also publ. as *Histoire de la médicine belge.*
11. See appendix (quarto, no. 17); Van Dorssen, "Willem ten Rhijne," 142.
12. Gemeentelijke Archief Amsterdam (hereafter, GA Amsterdam), 497/417: "Kerk ondertrouw."
13. GA Amsterdam, 142/282: "Dopen."
14. As many as two-thirds of the people married in Amsterdam had not been born there: De Vries, *European Urbanization,* 185; Hart, *Geschrift en getal,* 115–81.
15. GA Amsterdam, PA 27/20: "Nomina Medicorum, 1641–1753."
16. Quoted in Regin, *Traders, Artists, Burghers,* 80.
17. Lindeboom, "Jan Swammerdam als microscopist," 98; for more on Hudde, see Van Berkel, *In het voetspoor van Stevin,* 53.
18. Frijhoff, *Société Néerlandaise et ses gradués,* 237; on the physicians of Amsterdam more generally, see 236–40.
19. GA Amsterdam, PA 27/20: "Nomina Medicorum, 1641–1753."
20. Wittop Koning, "Voorgeschiedenis."

21. Haver Droeze, *Het Collegium Medicum Amstelaedamense;* Wittop Koning, "Oorsprong"; also see the intro. of Wittop Koning, *Facsimile.*

22. De Moulin, "Paul Barbette, M.D."; Baumann, "Job van Meekren."

23. Aveling, *Chamberlens and the Midwifery Forceps,* 179; Geyl, *Geschiedenis van het Roonhuysiaansch geheim.*

24. Erasmus's Latin letters detailing his condition are printed with facing English translation in *Opuscula,* 17:2–9; the reference to Linacre is on 2–3.

25. See Frame, *Complete Works of Montaigne,* 861–1039; he also commented on stones at length in his often republished essay "De l'expérience." Also see Brockliss, "Development of the Spa."

26. Winn, *John Dryden.*

27. *Philosophical Transactions* 17, no. 202 (July, Aug. 1693): 817–24: "Dr. Mullineux [Molyneux] his Account of a Stone of an extraordinary bigness, spontaneously voided through the Urethra of a woman in Dublin" (the published report of T. Molyneux's "Of a Calculus from a female," read at RS, 8 Nov. 1683 [*sic* for 1693]: Royal Society, "Classified Papers," vol. 14, no. 35); *Diary of Samuel Pepys,* 1:283, 310, 320–21.

28. Batty Shaw, "East Anglian Bladder Stone," 222. The author publishes a picture of the stone and notes that it was kept for many years after in the library of Trinity College, Cambridge; in 1956, it was in the Department of Urology at Addenbrooke's Hospital.

29. *Opuscula,* 17:6–7.

30. Blankaart, *Physical Dictionary,* 269.

31. Hildanus, *Lithotomia Vesicae,* 4.

32. Keynes, *Works of Sir Thomas Browne,* 4:399 (no. 240).

33. Translation of "De l'expérience," Frame, *Complete Works of Montaigne,* 836–37.

34. *Diary of Robert Hooke,* 13 (Nov. 1672).

35. Report of William Stukeley, quoted in Westfall, *Never at Rest,* 869.

36. *Diary of Samuel Pepys,* 6:51–52; also see 5:165, 241.

37. Pagel, *Paracelsus;* Yates, *Rosicrucian Enlightenment;* Webster, *Great Instauration;* Trevor-Roper, "Paracelsian Movement"; Moran, *Alchemical World of the German Court.*

38. Crosse, *Formation, Constituents, and Extraction of the Urinary Calculus,* 166–231.

39. Van Helmont, *Opuscula medica inaudita. I. De lithiasi.*

40. Beverwijck's *Steen-stuck* of 1652; there is an edition with facing-page English translation in *Opuscula,* 17:11–129.

41. Sherley, *Philosophical Essay,* 24, unpaginated intro.

42. Ibid., 1. Boyle, *Some Considerations,* 31–35, considers the production of stones in the body in a heavily Helmontian manner.

43. *Philosophical Transactions* 14, no. 157 (20 Mar. 1683/4): 523–33; vol. 16, no. 182 (26 June 1686): 140–45.

44. *Philosophical Transactions,* 18 (Jan. 1693/4): 30–32: "Observatio Anatomica rara de Calculo in Rene invento à Cl. Viro D^{re} Wittie, R.S. haud ita pridem Communicata"; in the same issue is "Of a Stone found in the Gall-Bladder of a Woman [during dissection]. By Mr. J.T." 111–22.

45. *Philosophical Transactions* 18, no. 209 (Mar., Apr. 1694): 103–4: "An Account of a stone of a Prodigious size extracted by Section out of a Woman's Bladder, now living, on the Eighth day of November, 1693. by Mr. Basil Wood, Surgeon"; vol. 19, no. 220 (Mar., Apr., May 1696): 250–53: "A Letter of Mr. Charles Bernard, giving an Account of Two Large Stones, were for twenty Years past Lodg'd in the Meatus Urinarius, and thence cut out by him the 28th of September last"; vol. 19, no. 222 (Sept., Oct. 1696): 310–11: "An Account of a Stone of the Bladder, which weighed 51 Ounces, or Three Pounds Three Ounces, and a Stone out of the Bladder successfully, which adhered to it. By Dr. Charles Preston" (report from studies in Paris and Ghent). Volume 12 of the manuscript "Classified Papers" of the Royal Society (on anatomy and surgery) also contains many unpublished reports on stones submitted by members.

46. Blankaart, *Collectanea medico-physica . . . MDCLXXX*, 43–44, 49–50, 70–71.

47. Wangensteen and Wangensteen, *Rise of Surgery*, stress dehydration as a cause of bladder stones, 65–66.

48. Wilhelm Fabricius von Hilden, whose original German treatise appeared in Latin as *Lithotomia Vesicae* (Basil, 1628); it was translated into English as Hildanus, *Lithotomia Vesicae;* it was reprinted by William Cheselden in 1723. This is according to the English edition of 1640, p. 6.

49. Rather, "The 'Six Things Non-Natural' "; Bylebyl, "Galen"; Niebyl, "Non-Naturals."

50. See Jones, "Life and Works."

51. Hildanus, *Lithotomia Vesicae*, 10–12.

52. Paré, *Oeuvres*, pt. 17, chap. 37.

53. For a discussion of how heat bakes the earthy material into stones, see Beverwijck, *Steen-stuck*, in *Opuscula*, 17:39–41.

54. Groenevelt, Λιθολογια, 9–12.

55. Hildanus, *Lithotomia Vesicae*, 8–9.

56. Groenevelt, Λιθολογια, 12–14; also in his *De calculo vesicae*, thesis 8.

57. Groenevelt, Λιθολογια, 14–19; *De calculo vesicae*, theses 10 and 12.

58. Groenevelt, Λιθολογια, 21–29; *De calculo vesicae*, thesis 13.

59. Thoren, *Lord of Uraniborg*, 468–69.

60. Hildanus, *Lithotomia Vesicae*, 16–29; Paré, *Oeuvres*, pt. 17, chap. 35.

61. Groenevelt, Λιθολογια, 36–39; *De calculo vesicae*, theses 15 and 16. The physician Beverwijck, however, still believed that physical diagnosis in this case was less reliable than ascertaining the symptoms: *Steen-stuck*, in *Opuscula*, 97.

62. *Diary of Robert Hooke*, 13 (Nov. 1672).

63. Viseltear, "Joanna Stephens"; Viseltear noted, however, that calcined shells contained a high proportion of lime, "an agent which indeed was capable of dissolving certain varieties of stone *in vitro*" (200).

64. Royal College of Physicians, SR 173: Anon. copybook, fol. 56.

65. Van de Ven, "Een steensnijding in 1653." Also Van Andel, "Geneesmiddelen tegen den steen."

66. *Diary of Robert Hooke*, 13 (Nov. 1672).

67. See Porter, *Medical History of Waters and Spas*.

68. Groenevelt, Λιθολογια, 46–54; *De calculo vesicae*, theses 19, 21, and 23; on remedies to lessen pain and cause urination, Λιθολογια, 56–69.

69. Copy of letter of Matthew Bacon to Sir Henry Walgrave, 4 Jan. 1653, Sloane 1833, fols. 15–15v.

70. Justin-Godart, "L'Opération de la taille"; Raymond, "Lithotomie musciale." The 1969 recording I have heard includes a voice announcing the title of each section: "Das Alte Werk," Telefunken, SAWT-9549-B.

71. According to James Douglas, quoted in Cope, *William Cheselden,* 29.

72. Luyendijk-Elshout, "Death Enlightened."

73. Parsons, *History of St. Thomas's Hospital,* 2:64; McInnes, *St. Thomas' Hospital,* 57.

74. *Diary of Samuel Pepys,* 1:97–98, 8:129, 5:247, 8:191, 198.

75. Van de Ven, "Een steensnijding in 1653," 3306.

76. On what follows, see Avalon, "Une auto-opération"; De Lint, "Comment Jan De Doot"; Boerma, "Wondergeval van Jan de Dood."

77. I have only seen a later edition: Tulp, *Observationes Medicae,* bk. 4, observ. 31.

78. For accounts of the history of lithotomy, see Ellis, *History of Bladder Stone;* Wangensteen and Wangensteen, *Rise of Surgery,* 65–92; Nöske, *Lithotomia Vesicae.*

79. Titsingh, *Heelkundige verhandeling,* 94–95; Banga, *Geschiedenis van de genees- kunde,* 798.

80. Celsus, *De medicina,* bk. 7, sec. 26 (3:425–47 in the Loeb Classical Library edition); he describes the use of a scoop.

81. Hildanus, *Lithotomia Vesicae,* 96–97; also see Paré, *Oeuvres,* pt. 17, chap. 43.

82. Wangensteen and Wangensteen, *Rise of Surgery,* 68.

83. Van de Ven, "Een steensnijding in 1653"; Hildanus, *Lithotomia Vesicae,* 97– 99. Also see Beverwijck, *Steen-stuck,* in *Opuscula,* 123–25.

84. Hildanus, *Lithotomia Vesicae,* 99–100; also see Beverwijck, *Steen-stuck,* in *Opuscula,* 125–27, and Paré, *Oeuvres,* pt. 17, chap. 44.

85. The account of what follows is mainly from Dirk Cloes, an apprentice of Cypri- naus's, quoted in Titsingh, *Heelkunde verhandeling,* 94–95. The information that Cypri- anus was sued is from Banga, *Geschiedenis van de geneeskunde,* 798, but it should be noted that Banga seems to be relying on Titsingh, who mentions Cyprianus's surgical misfortunes but not a suit.

86. The Colot family practiced lithotomy for more than 150 years, beginning with Laurent Colot, lithotomist to Henri II of France in 1556: Wangensteen and Wangensteen, *Rise of Surgery,* 601. Philippe offered to teach students his technique for 13,000 or 14,000 livres per annum salary from the government, plus a pension: *Collection de documents pour servir a l'histoire des hôpitaux de Paris,* 201. His son, François, was in Ghent in 1680 after having been in England: Blankaart, *Collectanea medico-physica . . . MCDCLXXXI en LXXXII,* 174–75.

87. Groenevelt, Λιθολογια, 65–66.

88. Keynes, *Works of Sir Thomas Browne,* 4:27.

89. GA Amsterdam, PA 366, no. 231: *Privilegien, Willekeuren en Ordonnantien,* 24–25 (sec. 21); 66 (the fee amounted to 4 Flemish pounds per year); 85.

90. Titsingh, *Heelkunde verhandeling,* 95.

91. Lindeboom, *Dutch Medical Biography,* col. 1824; Bitter, "Stadsoperateurs en steensnijders."

92. Van der Heyden, *Calculo vesicae,* sig. B; Groenevelt, *De calculo vesicae,* sigs. C2–C3.

93. I owe this fact to Harm Beukers, who has noticed this phenomenon in several theses done under Sylvius.

94. Gemeentelijke Archief Leiden (hereafter, GA Leiden), Gilden Archieven, No. 350: " 't Boeck van de Mr. Chirurgijns," fol. 5.

95. Groenevelt, *De calculo vesicae,* sigs. C2–C3.

96. The opinion of Cornelis van de Voorde, in Banga, *Geschiedenis van de geneeskunde,* 509.

97. Groenevelt, *Dissertatio Lithologica,* "ad lectores."

98. GA Amsterdam, "Begraven" Klappers, buried on 18 May 1674.

99. *Privilegien, Willekeuren en Ordonnantien,* 85–86, which says that Velthuis first practiced in 1673; but see the next paragraph.

100. Groenevelt, *Dissertatio Lithologica,* "ad lectores": ". . . me advocari curavit, suaque, mihi dono dedit instrumenta Lithotomica, enixe rogans, ut illa in illius memoriam et miserorum commodum susciperem."

101. Ibid.: "non solum inclinante, sed et urgente natura, hanc operationem aggressus fui."

102. Groenevelt, Λιθολογια, 66: "With this manner, and with such Instruments the Famous Monsieur *Collot* has cured very many by a sedulous and frequent inspection, of whose Operation the Author of this Treatise has successfully practiced, and does practice this manner of Cure."

103. While very few physicians practiced surgery, a few Dutch surgeons were beginning to earn M.D.'s in the late seventeenth century, like Johannes Rau of Amsterdam. These Dutch surgeon-physicians are noticed by Temkin as in the forefront of a medical revolution, in his "Role of Surgery."

104. The Hippocratic "Oath" is often printed in translation: for one version, see *Hippocratic Writings,* 67.

105. Groenevelt, *Dissertatio Lithologica,* "ad lectores."

106. From 16 to 21 June: Formsma, "Nieuwe geschiedenis," 129–30.

107. See Geyl, *The Netherlands,* 96–147; Rowen, *John de Witt,* 815–84; Haley, *English Diplomat;* Sonnino, *Louis XIV.*

108. Ekberg, *Failure of Louis XIV's Dutch War.*

109. Formsma, "Nieuwe geschiedenis," 130.

110. Laguette, "Beleg en herovering van Grave"; Patist, *Het beleg van de Stad Grave;* De Luine, *Relation de tout ce qui s'est passé pendant le siége de Grave.*

111. Groenevelt [Greenfield], *Treatise of the Safe, Internal Use of Cantharides.* The book is a translation from Groenevelt's *De Tuto Cantharidum,* and so even though the dedication to Portland was printed in 1706 for the first time, the period of twenty five years makes sense when calculated from the date of the original Latin treatise.

112. Kerkhoff, *Over de geneeskundige vergorging in het Staatse Leger;* Gemeentelijke Archief Grave (hereafter, GA Grave), RANB I.400: "Resolutieboeken, 1656–1681"; RANB II.400: "Ingekomen stukken, 1670–72, 1673–76"; RANB I.300: "Rekeningen, 1671–1674."

113. They were also later burned, and the remains can now be consulted only on microfilm; the future may turn up something yet.

114. A silver coin weighing 0.25 grams.
115. Sloane 2729, f.5; fols. 112–13.

CHAPTER 5
An Immigrant Doctor in London

1. Among the many works discussing the Dutch influence on England, see Colie, *Light and Enlightenment;* Geyl, *Orange and Stuart;* Haley, *British and the Dutch;* Israel, *Anglo-Dutch Moment;* Murray, *Flanders and England;* Van Dorsten, *Anglo-Dutch Renaissance;* Wilson, *Holland and Britain.*
2. For example, Cotta, *Short Discoveries of the Unobserved Dangers,* 111–12.
3. Annals 3:172a (10 July 1637).
4. Keevil, *Hamey the Stranger;* idem, *Stranger's Son;* Birken, "Dr. John King (1614–1681) and Dr. Assuerus Regimorter (1615–1650)"; Cook, "Living in Revolutionary Times," 129–32. Like Baldwin Hamey, Sr., Gerard Boet, a native of Gorcum and an M.D. of Leiden (1628), moved to London and became a licentiate of the London college in 1646, but none of his offspring became fellows in later years; Munk, *Roll,* 225.
5. "Advertisements, medical," British Library, C.112.f.9 (hereafter, "C.112.f.9"), no. 61: 4to, 2 sides.
6. "Advertisements, medical," British Library, 551.a.32 (hereafter, "551.a.32"), no. 201. They could be seen at the Hand and Urinal, St. Martins-Le-Grand, from 8 to 12 o'clock, and 1 to 8.
7. C.112.f.9, no. 36: 4to, printed on both sides. This person claimed to have "his Majesties License, and Speciall Approbation, and could be seen from 8 to 12 and 2 to 7."
8. 551.a.32, no. 186; C.112.f.9, no. 40; 551.a.32, no. 156; C.112.f.9, no. 128. For other variants on the latter handbill, see C.112.f.9, nos. 51 and 63.
9. For an account of the trial of witches at Bury St. Edmunds in 1665 in which Browne was involved, see Thomas, *State Trials,* 2:52–73; more generally, MacFarlane, *Witchcraft in Tudor and Stuart England;* Gijswijt-Hofstra and Frijhoff, *Witchcraft in the Netherlands.*
10. Bloch, *Royal Touch;* Barlow, "King's Evil."
11. Wrigley, "Simple Model of London's Importance"; Fisher, *London and the English Economy.*
12. This is an estimate of the number around 1670; by 1693, the broadside *Catalogue of the several Members of the Society of Apothecaries . . . 1693* listed 410 members.
13. The Barber-Surgeons' Company had 289 members in 1641, about 32 percent surgeons and 34 percent barbers: Dale, "Members of the City Companies."
14. On the number of members of the College of Physicians, see Cook, *Decline of the Old Medical Regime,* 275.
15. Haley, *English Diplomat in the Low Countries,* 287.
16. Knuttel, *Catalogus,* no. 9996.
17. Ibid.: three slightly different versions are listed as nos. 10129, 10130, 10131.
18. Public Record Office, Chancery Lane, S.P. 29/311/210 (also see fols. 86–93).

19. Annals 4:127b (1 Feb. 1677/8): Groenevelt's M.D. is given as 18 Mar. 1672 instead of 1670.

20. Shaw, *Letters of Denization*, 114: "John Groenwaldt, alien born."

21. Pettegree, *Foreign Protestant Communities*, 14–16, 283; Grell, *Dutch Calvinists*, 18. Naturalization, granted by the Parliament, had greater value than denization, since it effectively made a foreigner English.

22. London Guildhall, Dutch Church at Austin Friars: 7382, "Register of Baptisms 1602–1874, Marriages 1602–1874, and Burials 1671–1853" (unfoliated; hereafter, Guildhall MS. 7382). Also see Moens, *Marriage, Baptismal, and Burial Registers*, 29.

23. See Lindeboom, *Austin Friars;* Pettegree, *Foreign Protestant Communities;* Grell, *Dutch Calvinists*.

24. In his first extant letter to a Dutch friend he gives his return address as "in Frogmorthen street against Drapers Hall London" (Sloane 2729, fols. 85–85A, 16 Oct. 1681); he later said he could be addressed at "against ye lower end of drapers hall in Frogmorthon street" (Sloane 2729, fols. 151–151A, 18 Dec. 1683); in the preface to *The Oracle for the Sick* of 1687 (on which, see chapter 6), he gave his address as "in Throgmorton Street, next door but one to Broad-street."

25. London Guildhall, Dutch Church at Austin Friars: 7406, "Register of Members of the London-Dutch Church 1681–1690," fol. 54, also has Groenevelt located in the Minories next to the Drapers.

26. Hessels, *Register of the Attestations*, 106: Thurs., 15 Oct. 1676.

27. Guildhall MS. 7382; and Moens, *Marriage, Baptismal, and Burial Registers*, 29. Elias was baptized on 4 Nov. 1677; Christina on 2 Apr. 1679.

28. London Guildhall, Dutch Church at Austin Friars: 7401, v.2, "Register of Members of the Consistory 1666 to 1685"; 7389, v.1, "Kerek Rek[ening] Boek van 1658 tot 1705"; 7408, "Gen'l memoranda book 1594–1714"; 7410, "Deacons Memoranda 1615–1741."

29. Mandeville, *Hypochondriack and Hysterick Passions*, xiii.

30. Henry "Cruttenden" set up as a printer in Oxford from 1681 to 1694, where he got into trouble with the licenser for printing an edition of the classical author Cornelius Nepos and where he helped to set up a Catholic press: Plomer, *Dictionary of the Printers and Booksellers*, 91.

31. *Transcription of the Registers of the Worshipful Company of Stationers*.

32. Arber, *Term Catalogues:* the price is listed on 12 Feb. 1677. This compares with other popular works like Sermon's *Friend to the Sick*, an 8vo of 275 pages priced at 2s. 6d. by Clavel in his *General catalogue of books;* or Pechey's *Plain and Short Treatise of an Apoplexy*, a 12mo, priced 6d. according to *Term Catalogues* for Nov. 1708 and Feb. 1709.

33. According to Mangeti, *Bibliotheca Scriptorum Medicorum*, 1:527, Richard Browne later helped Groenevelt with the English of his *Arthritology*.

34. Groenevelt, Λιθολογια, 8.

35. Ibid., 65, 66–67.

36. The order of English noble rank is prince, duke, marquess, earl, viscount, and count. In Dorchester's case, he was granted his title by Charles I, whom he served loyally during the civil war. He gave his very large library to the London College of Physicians,

and because of his learning he was made a member of Gray's Inn as well, making him a barrister.

37. In the disputes over chemical medicine of the 1660s, both sides tried to claim Dorchester as one of their own: both Nedham, *Medela Medicinae,* and Johnson, 'Αγυρτο-Μαστοξ, dedicated their books to Dorchester.

38. Van de Velde, "Werken van Stephanus Blankaart"; Van de Velde, "Werken van den geneeskundige Cornelis Bontekoe."

39. Van Meek'ren, *Heel- en Genees-Konstige Aanmerkkingen,* forward.

40. Sloane 2729, fols. 85–85A: Letter to Casparus Sibelius, 16 Oct. 1681: "voorspost & voort 't gene wÿ alle na suchten."

41. Sloane 2729, fols. 120–120A (9 May 1682); fol. 160 (20 May 1684).

42. Allen, "Medical Education"; Lewis, "Faculty of Medicine"; O' Malley, *History of Medical Education;* Poynter, *Evolution of Medical Education;* Robb-Smith, "Cambridge Medicine"; Rook, "Medical Education at Cambridge."

43. This requirement was enacted in the Laudian statutes of 1636, which governed Oxford for about two hundred years: Ward, *Oxford University Statutes,* 1:53–54.

44. Cook, "New Philosophy and Medicine"; idem, "Physicians and the New Philosophy."

45. Jones, "Thomas Lorkyn's Dissections"; Frank, "Image of Harvey."

46. Nedham, preface to Sylvius, *New Idea of the Practice of Medicine,* sig. b6.

47. Ibid., sig. c2.

48. For more, see Cook, "The Troubles of Adriaan Huyberts in London" (forthcoming).

49. Cook, *Decline of the Old Medical Regime,* 58.

50. McAdoo, *Structure of Caroline Moral Theology,* 27; Wood, *English Casuistical Divinity,* 5.

51. Securis, *Detection and Querimonie,* sig. Biiiiv. This is consonant with Aristotle's notions of virtue as derived from practical reason, and with contemporary Anglican notions of conscience as habits of mind: McAdoo, *Structure of Caroline Moral Theology;* Wood, *English Casuistical Divinity;* Sherman, *Fabric of Character;* Gottlieb, "Aristotle and Protagoras."

52. Cook, "Good Advice and Little Medicine."

53. Cook, "Troubles of Adriaan Huyberts."

54. Perhaps he is the Gerrit van der Meulen who married Elizabeth Niellius on 26 Jan. 1674 in Amsterdam: GA Amsterdam, 497/417: "Kerk ondertrouw."

55. Annals 4:127b.

56. For more, see the forthcoming work on Starkey by William Newman.

57. Groenevelt to Sibelius, 16 Oct. 1681, Sloane 2729, fols. 85–85A. Perhaps Culpeper's book was meant for Sibelius's friend Frederick Ruysch, supervisor of the midwives in Amsterdam.

58. Sloane 2729, fol. 143 (13 July 1683), referring to Wiseman's *Severall Chirurgicall Treatises* (London, 1676; reprinted 1686).

59. Huyberts, *Corner-Stone Laid,* 32; Cook, "Troubles of Adriaan Huyberts."

60. Sloane 2729, fol. 169 (30 Oct. 1684), referring to John Jones, *Noverum dissertationem de morbis abstrusioribus tractatus primus: De febribus intermittentibus* (London,

1683). As far as I know, this work has gotten no notice from medical historians, Jones being an "unknown." For what little there is on him, see Munk, *Roll.*

61. Stubbe, *Campanella Revived,* 22, lumps "the Merretts and Sydenhams" together; also see idem, *Lord Bacons Relation of the Sweating-Sickness;* Cook, "Physicians and the New Philosophy," 246–71.

62. Sydenham's MS essay on anatomy is reprinted in Dewhurst, *Thomas Sydenham,* 85–93; Bates, "Thomas Sydenham," 357–61, also believes that the MS is Sydenham's even though it is in Locke's hand.

63. On Sydenham, see Dewhurst, *Thomas Sydenham;* Bates, "Thomas Sydenham"; Meynell, *Materials for a Biography;* and Cunningham, "Thomas Sydenham."

64. Sloane 4376, f. 75. Dr. Richard Mead also possessed a copy of this letter: Sloane 4292, f. 143.

65. Groenevelt to Sibelius, 27 June 1682, Sloane 2729, fols. 122–23; fol. 169 (30 Oct. 1684); Thomas Sydenham, *Opuscula* (Amsterdam, 1683).

66. Sloane 2729, fols. 181–82 (7 Apr. 1685), mentioning *[Methodus curandi febres.] Observationes medicae circa morborum acutorum historiam et curationem . . . Edito quarta ab authore adhuc vivo emendatior et auctior reddita* (London, 1685); and Sloane 2729, fol. 202 (Mar. 1687), mentioning *Schedula monitoria de novae febris ingressu* (London, 1686).

67. Sloane 2729, fols. 122–23 (27 June 1682): "Zidnum De Febribus geloove ick hebt gliy in Hollant, het is oock een braven man ick ben speciaal met hem bekent." The fact that Groenevelt spelled Sydenham's name as it sounded rather than as it appeared on paper suggests that he had only just met him. He referred to Sydenham's *Methodus curandi febres* (London, 1666, with second edition in 1668).

68. Sloane 2729, fol. 202 (Mar. 1687).

69. Crell Spinowski, *Calculo renum et vesicae.* This is an average-size (fourteen-page) production, with thirty-one theses, but it does not mention lithotomy (nor Groenevelt), nor does Crell give citations to specific books or page numbers or prescriptions for lithontriptics (which he thinks have some efficacy).

70. After mentioning his father and mother in the dedication, he continues "nec non D.D. Jacobo Nutley, D.D. Henrio Hedworth, D.D. Thomae Firmin, amicis Fautoribusque honoratissimis." Firmin took special interest in helping Polish Socinians and Calvinists.

71. Matthews, "Philip Guide"; his papers are in Sloane 2655; his probated will of June 1716 is in the Public Record Office, Chancery Lane, Wills 1714-30, no. 86, 116.

72. Guide, *Observations Anatomiques,* a forty-five-page 12mo together with a two-page "expliquation de la Machine" and diagram, dedicated to Monseigner de Lamoignon, premier president of the Parlement of Paris; idem, *Traité de la Nature du Mal Venerien,* a thirty-eight-page 8vo in the form of a letter to M. Bourdelot, first physician to the queen of Sweden.

73. Guide, *De la Vertu Singulière du Vin Rouge,* a forty-six-page 16mo; Royal Society, "Classified Papers," vol. 14 (1), "Physick."

74. Sloane 1394, an anonymous list of birthdates for horoscopes, fol. 171; British Library, Add. MS. 29,551, fols. 146–47, a letter of Richard Browne to Christopher Hatton, from Oxford (Pembroke College?), 1 Dec. 1665; Longfield-Jones, "Buccaneering Doctors"; Munk, *Roll,* 1:390; *Dictionary of National Biography* (hereafter, *DNB*).

75. Browne's works up to 1687 include: Περι ’αρχων *Liber in quo recepta veteribus*

rerum principia funditus evertuntur et nova, ut in natura vere sunt, stabiliuntur (London, 1678); Browne, transl., *The Cure of Old Age, and Preservation of Youth. By Roger Bacon . . . Also a Physical Account of the tree of life by Edw. Madeira Arrais, translated* (London, 1683); Plutarch, *Of Natural Affection towards one's Offspring,* transl. Richard Browne (London, 1684); [Olaus Borrichius], *Prosodia Pharmacopaeorum: or the Apothecary's prosody* [transl. and ed.] by Richard Browne (London, 1685).

76. Browne may have been the person to have printed an English translation of Groenevelt's *Dissertatio* in *Chirurgorum comes: Or the Whole Practice of Chirurgery* (London, 1687). Browne helped Groenevelt with the English of his *Arthritology* according to Mangeti, *Bibliotheca Scriptorum Medicorum,* 1:527.

77. See Peachey, "Two John Peacheys."

78. Pechey, *Store-house of Physical Practice,* sigs. A2–A2v; this work is a rearranged, expanded, and translated version of his *Promptuarium Praxeos Medicae* (1693), which had a second edition in 1694.

79. Pechey, *London Dispensatory,* preface. This is a translation and expansion of the London *Pharmacopoeia* published by the College of Physicians, with the addition of the uses and doses of the medicines (a matter omitted from the official *Pharmacopoeia*).

80. Pechey, *Collections of Acute Diseases,* the first part of which was published in 1686. Pechey's later *Whole Works of the Excellent Practical Physician, Dr. Thomas Sydenham,* is a slightly edited version of the *Collections.* Although it has been doubted that Sydenham knew anything about Pechey's translation on the assumption that if he had he would have approved of it and so have been mentioned by Pechey, another translator of Sydenham, James Drake, says that Sydenham neither encouraged nor discouraged him in his project: *Treatise concerning the Gout lately published in Latine by Dr. Sydenham,* translator's preface.

81. Pechey, *Collections of Acute Diseases,* dedication to first part.

82. Pechey, *Collections of Acute Diseases,* dedication to fifth and final part.

83. [Browne?] *Chirurgorum comes,* sig. A2v.

84. London Guildhall, Society of Apothecaries: 8290, "Papers relating to disputes and suits between the Society and the Barber-Surgeon's Company, 1690–1708," includes "A Committee for the Surgeons Bill," of 24 Oct. 1690, to which Groenevelt subscribed.

85. Sloane 3915, "Minites of Ye Comm. of Ye Coll. of Phys: 1681–1697": the letters signed by the king were drawn up by Sir Thomas Millington and Drs. Goodall and Bateman and passed on to the king via Sir John Holt (fols. 26v–27v); also see Cook, *Decline of the Old Medical Regime,* 196–209.

86. Sloane 2729, fol. 126, 29 Aug. 1682: "Ioannes Groenevelt & Coll. Med. Lond. Socius," or: "Joannes Groenevelt, Fellow of the College of Physicians of London."

87. Among the large literature on the Royal Society, see Hunter, *Establishing the New Science;* Purver, *Royal Society.*

88. Cook, "New Philosophy and Medicine"; idem, "Physicians and the New Philosophy."

89. From his stopover at the newly established Dutch colony at the Cape of Good Hope would come a later book on the natural history of the cape and the local people, the "Hottentots." Ten Rhijne, *Schediasma de Promontorio Bonae Spei;* it was later translated as *An account of the Cape of Good Hope and the Hottentotes,* 4:768–82.

90. Royal Society LB.C.8, fols. 240–42; since Oldenburg had recently died, the

letter is summarized but not printed in Hall and Hall, *Correspondence of Henry Oldenburg*, 13:368; the letter was brought to a meeting on 18 January 1682: Birch, *History of the Royal Society*, 4:119–20.

91. Wrop, *Briefwisseling*, vol. 6, letters nos. 6995, 7001, and 7011.
92. Busschof and Roonhuis, *Two Treatises*, 73–76.
93. Busschof and Roonhuis, *Two Treatises;* [Temple], *Miscellanea*, 189–238; Temple's story is summarized in Rosen, "Sir William Temple" (although Rosen was unaware that "Zulichem" was Huygens).
94. Royal Society, LB.C.8, fols. 276–78; Birch, *History of the Royal Society*, 4:122.
95. Groenevelt to Sibelius, 24 Jan. 1682, Sloane 2729, fol. 109.
96. *Album Studiosorum Academiae Lugduno Batavae*.
97. Sloane 2729.
98. Groenevelt to Sibelius, Mar., Apr., and June 1682, Sloane 2729, fols. 112–13, 116–17, 118, 119, 122–23; Birch, *History of the Royal Society*, 4:140, 143 (Apr. 5 and 19, 1682).
99. Ten Rhijne, *Dissertatio de arthritide*. The portion of the work on acupuncture has been translated: Carrubba and Bowers, "Treatise on Acupuncture."
100. Sloane 2729, fol. 140 (30 May 1683). Groenevelt explained that he was out of pocket much more than the cost of the two books in helping to produce them. Aston also wrote Sibelius: Sloane 2729, fol. 137 (10 May 1683). The Royal Society ordered on 9 May 1683 that a copy of the book be placed in its library (Birch, *History of the Royal Society*, 4:204).
101. *Philosophical Transactions* 13, no. 148 (10 June 1683): 221 [*sic* for 222]–35. Further reports about the use of moxa in the East Indies from Busschoff appeared in Blankaart, *Collectanea medico-physica . . . MCDCLXXXI en LXXXII*, 14–20; Ten Rhijne, *Verhandelinge van het Podagra en Vliegende Jicht*.
102. Sydenham, *Tractatus de Podagra et Hydrope;* transl. into English in 1684 by James Drake, and several times thereafter. The passage occurs at the third paragraph from the end.
103. Letter of Dr. Johannes Jacob Wepfer to Casparus Sibelius, 20 Aug. 1684, quoted in a letter of Sibelius to Locke, De Beer, *Correspondence of John Locke*, 2:635.
104. Hunter, *Royal Society and Its Fellows*, 41, 61, 64.
105. An English extract of a Dutch letter of Ten Rhijne to Groenevelt containing his offer is in the Royal Society, LB.C.8, fols. 446–48, dated as received on 21 Mar. 1682/3; a Latin letter from Ten Rhijne to Aston about the same subject is in LB.C.9 fols. 373–76. On Ten Rhijne's rivalry with Cleyer, see Van Dorssen, "Willem ten Rhijne," 134–228; also on Cleyer, Van der Pas, "Earliest European Descriptions of Japan's Flora." In Ten Rhijne's letter, he notes that while he would like to receive any works of interest from the Royal Society, he could not read English. Also see Aston to Ten Rhijne on behalf of one Mr. Watts on 2 Dec. 1682 (Royal Society, LB.C.8, fols. 359–60); Ten Rhijne also sent a specimen of a camphor tree to the Apothecaries' Garden in Chelsea: Birch, *History of the Royal Society*, 4:169 (6 Dec. 1682).
106. Rogers, *Oratorio Anniversaria*.
107. Annals 5:9b (9 Feb. 1682/3: "Doctori Sylvae Hebraei perlecta"); Groenevelt wrote to Sibelius: "[D]e Heer Dr Sylvius hier sÿnde heb het geluk voor een dagh of 2. gehad van sÿn Ede Compagnie en sÿn Ede beswaart" ("The Heer Dr. Sylvius is here; I

have had the good fortune to have shared for a couple of days his great company and his great burden"): Sloane 2729, fol. 143 (13 July 1683). Sylvius moved on to Dublin, where he incorporated his degree at Trinity College, and became one of the three most active members in the Dublin Philosophical Society: Hoppen, *Common Scientist,* 42, 44; he was also made a member of the Royal Society of London, although he never returned to London to be inducted: Hunter, *Royal Society and Its Fellows,* 234–35; Birch, *History of the Royal Society,* 4:106, 127, 128, 416, 528.

108. Letter of 16 June 1682 to the college, entered into Annals 5:1b. Conway had supported Greatrakes, on whom see Duffy, "Valentine Greatrakes"; Steneck, "Greatrakes the Stroker."

109. Letter transcribed into Annals 5:2a.

110. Annals 5:12a.

111. Ibid., 5:7a, 8b, 10a, 11b.

112. "[V]iro nempe eruditione & experientiâ notissimo . . ." The letter to Groenevelt was surely in English, but it is known only in Latin, since it—and Groenevelt's reply— were published by Mangeti as an example of the frauds of empirics who offered lithontriptics. While it is addressed only from "J. G. Eques Auratus", the date and circumstances point to Godwin as the author. The letter had arrived in Mangeti's hands shortly before he published Barbette, *Opera Omnia,* pt. 2, pp. 162–63; presumably Groenevelt made the translation into Latin, since it is unlikely that Mangeti knew English well. Groenevelt cut the younger Godwin in May: Sloane 2729, fol. 160 (20 May 1684).

113. Sloane 2729, fols. 151–151A (18 Dec. 1683). Also fol. 155 (25 Jan. 1684); fol. 160 (20 May 1684).

114. Nöske, *Lithotomia vesicae,* 39.

115. Tolet, *Traité de la Lithotomie.*

116. Idem, *Treatise of Lithotomy.* The dedication to Hobbs is dated 23 Sept. 1682.

117. James Mullins, Jr., was the senior lithotomist at St. Bartholomew's; Thomas Hobbs joined him as his junior in 1680 but quickly became the better-known operator: Moore, *History of St. Bartholomew's Hospital,* 737. Hobbs became a licentiate of the London College of Physicians in Dec. 1684, about a year and a half after Groenevelt: Munk, *Roll.*

118. Groenevelt, *Dissertatio Lithologica.* There is a passing reference to Tolet as a lithotomist on 10–11. The *Term Catalogue* of June 1684 lists Groenevelt's *Dissertatio* as being a 12mo published by T. Malthus, which may be a second impression (mistaking an 8vo for a 12mo), but is more likely to be a mix-up, since Malthus published a Lianardo Di Capoa, *Uncertainty of the art of physick,* transl. J[ohn] L[ancaster] (London, 1684), a 12mo registered with the Stationers' Company on 13 Nov. 1683: *Registers of the Company of Stationers.* On the other hand, Groenevelt was by now acquainted with Thomas Sydenham (see next chapter), who used Peruvian bark supplied by Mr. Malthus in 1687 (it was not uncommon for booksellers to sell medicines), so that Malthus might have been interested in carrying Groenevelt's book. On Malthus carrying Peruvian bark: British Library, Add. MS. 33,573, fol. 158, letter of Sydenham to Major Hale, 17 Dec. 1697.

119. "amore Christiano at languentium aegrotorum misericordia": *Dissertatio Lithologica,* "Ad lectores."

120. Groenevelt, *Dissertatio Lithologica,* 84–85; Sylvius, *Opera Medica,* 136, "De Methodo Medendi," bk. 2, chap. 14, para. 50.

121. Sloane 2729, fol. 160 (20 May 1684).

122. Groenevelt, *Dissertatio Lithologica* (1687); this edition reduced the type size, being seventy pages in length.

123. [Browne?] *Chirurgorum comes*, 626–43. Krivatsy's *Catalogue of Seventeenth Century Printed Books in the National Library of Medicine*, no. 9426, mistakenly describes a portion of the work as translating Groenevelt's Λιθολογια. The editor may have been one of Groenevelt's closest medical associates in London, R. Browne, who is listed as the author of the work in 1685 in the *Registers of the Company of Stationers*.

124. [Browne?] *Chirurgorum comes*, 626.

125. Barbette, *Opera Omnia*, pt. 2, pp. 155, 161–65.

126. Sloane 2729, fol. 169 (30 Oct. 1684); fols. 181–82 (7 Apr. 1685); fol. 202 (Mar. 1687).

127. They included Drs. Heidegger, March, and Sylvius (Sloane 2729, fol. 143, 13 July 1683); and the Amsterdam publisher Van den Velde (Sloane 2729, fol. 160, 20 May 1684).

128. Sloane 2729, fol. 109 (24 Jan. 1682); fols. 124–124A (30 June 1682).

129. Sloane 2729, fol. 5 (29 Nov. 1674), which contains a note from the lender, Sibmacher, that it had been paid with interest on 28 Apr. 1682 [new style]; Groenevelt asks Sibelius to take care of the matter by an enclosed bill of exchange in fols. 116–17 (31 Mar. 1682 [old style]).

130. See appendix; also Sloane 2729, fols. 112–13 (10 Mar. 1682); 116–17 (31 Mar. 1682); 118 (2 Apr. 1682); 120–120A (9 May 1682); 124–124A (30 June 1682); and (29 Aug. 1682).

131. Sloane 2729, fols. 112–13 (3 Mar. 1682); see appendix. There was a Jan Jansz. buried in Amsterdam on 8 Mar. 1682 [new style], who may have been Cristina's father: GA Amsterdam, "Begraven" Klappers.

132. Sloane 2729, fols. 122–23 (27 June 1682); Sloane 2729, fol. 126 (29 Aug. 1682).

133. "Ick ben soo ongeluckig geweest om in 't lange van Ue niet gehoort en hebbe, indien eenige discontent an Ue bÿ mÿ door neglect of anders gegeven hebbe ick bidde excuse, of soo ick noch eenig in Ue schult moghte sÿn in 't gene Ueden an mÿ heeft overgesonden sal Ue ten Dancke voldoen." Sloane 2729, fol. 202 (Mar. 1687). Note that fifteen years after he emigrated, Groenevelt used English words ("discontent" and "neglect") in a Dutch letter.

134. Public Record Office, Chancery Proceedings, C7/137/65.

135. John Browne's *Compleat treatise of the muscles* (London, 1681) was taken from Molins' *"Muskotomia": or, the anatomical administration of all the muscles of the humane body* (London, 1648). The quotation is from James Yonge's *Medicaster medicatus, or a remedy for the itch of scribling* (London, 1685), quoted in Russell, "A Seventeenth Century Surgeon," 396; the subscription list is reproduced on 504. Browne sent "a remarqueable Account of a Glandulous Liver" to the Royal Society: Royal Society, B.2.37.

136. McInnes, *St. Thomas' Hospital*, 57, 59.

137. Groenevelt stated that they had drawn up the articles on about 30 July 1686; Browne claimed that the agreement was to take effect from 1 May 1686.

138. Annals, 6:77, 79: Hawes complained of Groenevelt before a censors' meeting

of the College of Physicians on 4 Aug. 1693; the case was heard with both parties present on 18 Aug.

139. Public Record Office, Chancery Proceedings, C7/137/65.

140. There is no record of Francis Groenevelt's death in the records of the Church of Austin Friars, although by 1710 Groenevelt wrote that God had taken all his children from him: Groenevelt, *Compleat Treatise of the Stone and Gravel,* xiii.

141. These notes are contained in Groenevelt's copy of the second edition of his *Dissertatio Lithologica* (1687) (Royal College of Physicians, SR 259), which had been bound with each page interleaved with a blank sheet: a printer's device for making corrections in the text for a further edition. The quoted admonition is on the verso of the first page, dated 18 Jan. 1692/3. Most of the notes seem to have been written in this book at about the same time as the dated manuscript preface, and are indexed, but a later note in a margin next to a prescription for his cantharides remedy (inserted shortly after the opening remarks) refers the reader to his treatise on the subject of 1697.

CHAPTER 6
The Troubles with Withall

1. A later document of October says that the last of the seven articles was to take force "from the 1st of March last past," meaning March 1687: Sloane 2655, fols. 151–53v.

2. "Advertisements, medical," British Library, 551.a.32, no. 3, from Cornelius à Tilburg.

3. Sloane 2655, fols. 154, 157v–58.

4. "Advertisements, medical," British Library, nos. 226, 26. These handbills bear no date, so the sequence is inferred on the supposition that they increased the number of hours put in at the repository.

5. Groenevelt et al., *Oracle for the Sick.* Since the title page contains no date (or publisher), The British Library tentatively dated the work from 1685; the copy at the Wellcome Institute Library has written in ink "London Printed 1687."

6. In this pamphlet, they said that one of them would be there every day of the week from 7 until 8 o'clock (in the morning?), and all would be present from 2 to 6 in the afternoon on Mondays and Thursdays.

7. On the controversies about physicians making their own medicines, see Cook, "New Philosophy and Medicine"; idem, "Physicians and the New Philosophy."

8. *Oracle for the Sick,* "To the Reader," and 8–9.

9. Annals 5:60b.

10. On the penny-post system, see Todd, *William Dockwra;* Staff, *Penny Post.*

11. Rattansi, "Paracelsus"; Webster, "English Medical Reformers"; for example, Cooke, *Unum Necessarium,* and Culpeper, *Physicall Directory.*

12. The long account is in Annals 5:68a (25 Nov. 1687), based on a record written out on 27 Sept.; the dismissal of the beadle, Mr. Foster, was noted in 5:69a (29 Nov.); Russell was fined on 14 Jan. 1687/8 (5:72a).

13. Annals 5:66a–67b (Sept. and Oct. 1687).

14. Ibid., 5:70b–71a (9 and 21 Dec. 1687): Browne pulled rank on the latter day

by claiming that he could not come to the meeting because he had been sent for by the very wealthy and influential Sir Joshua Child. He was accused by John Elliott and John Bateman.

15. Ibid., 5:72a–b (7 and 21 Jan. 1687/8); his accuser this time was Elliott.

16. Ibid., 5:91a–b (4 and 18 Jan. 1688/9). Browne brought a Mr. William Cox with him to testify to Tyson's having said this. Tyson was fined £4.

17. Ibid., 5:67a, 70b (21 Oct., 16 Dec. 1687).

18. Ibid., 5:86b (13 Aug. 1688).

19. Sloane 2655, f. 151–153v, dated 26 Oct. 1688; the document is printed in full in Peachey, "Two John Peacheys," 130–31.

20. On these royal practitioners, see Cook, "Living in Revolutionary Times"; *Collection of Ordinances and Regulations*, 407.

21. He first shows up in Annals, 6:88–89 (17 Nov. 1693).

22. 20 May 1689, *Cal. St. Papers*, Warrant Book 34, p. 340.

23. "Advertisements, medical," British Library, 551.a.32: no. 3; repeated with small variations in nos. 54, 159, 160, 117, 158; quarto illustrated advertisements of his in British Library C.122.f.9, nos. 6, 7.

24. *Post Man*, no. 539 (17–19 Nov. 1698). For more on Dutch practitioners in London, see chapter 5.

25. Locke's political radicalism has been most forcefully advanced by Ashcraft, *Revolutionary Politics*.

26. On Locke's time in the Netherlands, see Cranston, *John Locke*, 231–311; Dewhurst, *John Locke*, 224–81; Thijssen-Schoute, "Nederlandse vriendenkring van John Locke."

27. Bodleian Library, Locke MS. F.7, fols. 157, 161–62 (1/10 and 11/21 Dec. 1683). He also mentioned Sibelius and Sibelius's home on 6 Jan. and 14 Apr. 1684 [New Style]: Locke MS. F.8, fols. 1–2, 58.

28. From 7 to 19 Sept.: Locke MS. F.8, fols. 129–70; much of this part of Locke's journal is reprinted in Dewhurst, *John Locke*, 245–60, since Locke spent much time copying out medical information from Sibelius's notebooks. Sibelius followed up on their exchanges in a letter to Locke of 4/14 Oct.: De Beer, *Correspondence of John Locke*, 2:633–38; Sibelius corresponded with Locke on a medical case and some new information from Ten Rhijne in letters of 3/13 June, 4/14 Aug., and 9/19 Sept. 1686: ibid., 3:8–11, 22–25, 265–67. Locke also copied out parts of Ten Rhijne's *Schediasma de Promontorio Bonae Spei* of 1686 (Locke MS. C.31, fols. 51–62v), which he later translated for his friend the Whig publisher A. Churchill: Ten Rhijne, *Account of the Cape of Good Hope and the Hottentotes*.

29. Sibelius stopped in Amsterdam on his way to London, so that three of Locke's Dutch correspondents sent letters to him via Sibelius, the third addressed on 23 Jan./2 Feb. 1692: De Beer, *Correspondence of Locke*, 4:368–72, 374–75.

30. Sibelius to Locke, 5 Apr. 1692, with a return address "living at Doctor Greenfields house," De Beer, *Correspondence of Locke*, 4:439–42.

31. Locke to William Molyneux on 16 July 1692: Cranston, *John Locke*, 359.

32. Ashcraft, *Revolutionary Politics*, 537.

33. Sibelius had written a letter about his plans for Ireland and Sidney's train in a letter to his Deventer friend Simon Tyssot de Patot, to which Tyssot replied in an undated

letter commiserating about Sibelius's failure: Tyssot de Patot, *Lettres Choisies*, 1:364–67. Also see Rosenberg, *Tyssot de Patot*, 15. Sidney's tenure as Lord Lieutenant was also an utter failure, so that he had to be recalled early in 1693.

34. Sibelius delivered some letters from Locke to his Dutch friends in Amsterdam in early June: De Beer, *Correspondence of Locke*, 4:692–96.

35. For more on this turbulent period, see Cook, *Decline of the Old Medical Regime*, 210–40.

36. Annals 5:91a, 91b, 92a, 94a (4 and 18 Jan., 1 and 8 Feb. 1688/9).

37. This part of the prescription was also called "the *Signature* (from *Signetur*, let it be labelled). . . . [It] declares the dose, method, and time of administration; the proper vehicle, regimen, etc., as far, at least, as related to the patient and his attendants. . . . The Signature is sometimes written in the language of the country, but most often in abbreviated Latin in order to save time; thus it is left to the dispenser to make a clear and concise translation" for the patient: Bennett, *Medical and Pharmaceutical Latin*, 55.

38. When the college voted on whether to enforce this statute over Dr. Bernard's objections (he argued that the nobility and gentry would not want the directions for their treatment to be known in English), twenty-three voted to enforce it, six against: Annals 5:90a, 21 Dec. 1688.

39. On 14 Feb., Tyson, John Radcliffe, Robert Pitt, and Nehemiah Grew were questioned on the subject, but Tyson refused to answer the censors' questions. On 1 Mar. Tyson was fined another £4 for breaking the statute on English directions four times; Radcliffe and Grew were fined 40s. for breaking it twice; Pitt was fined 20s. for breaking it once. Annals 5:94a–b, 94b–95a.

40. Annals 5:99a–b (3 May and 7 June 1689).

41. Pechey had now settled into the Angel and Crown on King Street, which he advertised in a series of handbills, some of which are extant in British Library, "Advertisements, medical," 551.a.32.

42. The censors ordered Pechey sued for the fine in the law courts, confident in their ability to exact punishments for bad behavior from their own members: Annals 5:89a, 89b, 91a, 91b: 15 Nov. and 7 Dec. 1688, 4 and 18 Jan. 1688/9 .

43. Sloane 3915, fol. 73v (18 Oct. 1689).

44. Annals 5:107b, 109a (3 and 17 Jan. 1689/90).

45. Ibid., 6:14–16 (20 July and 12 Aug. 1692).

46. President Thomas Burwell, Registrar Thomas Gill, Treasurer John Lawson, *consiliarii* Samuel Collins and Thomas Witherley, and censors Humphrey Brook, John Clarke, William Briggs, and Frederick Slare: Annals 6:30 (30 Sept. 1692).

47. The exception was the period after they received the new charter from James II in 1687: see Cook, *Decline of the Old Medical Regime*, 272, 274, 277–80.

48. Annals 6:63 (5 May 1693).

49. Ibid., 6:70, 87, 105: on 20 June 1693 the college ordered its beadle to demand Pechey's dues again, but on 3 Nov. the beadle testified that because of the outcome of the previous trial, Pechey told him to "tell the President he would pay none, let him take his Course." On 2 Feb. 1693/4, the censors ordered him prosecuted again for failure to pay the dues owed since the statutes had been last dated and sealed.

50. Ibid., 6:107–8 (1, 2, and 3 Mar. 1693/4). While Dr. Ridley lectured on the brain, Pechey, Guide, Brown, and Crell were among the licentiates who refused to attend;

on the third day of the lecture, many of those who had begun to attend, like Groenevelt, failed to return.

51. Ibid., 6:68 (2 June 1693); the witnesses besides Groenevelt were Thomas Parker and his wife and John Hamersley.

52. For instance, Turquet de Mayerne, *Treatise of the Gout;* Maynwaring, *Frequent, but unsuspected progress of pains;* Sydenham, *Treatise concerning the Gout;* Atkins, *Discourse shewing the nature of the gout;* Colbatch, *Treatise of the Gout.*

53. Groenevelt, *Arthritology.*

54. Groenevelt, *Treatise Of the Safe, Internal Use of Cantharides,* 287–88.

55. Groenevelt, *Arthritology,* sigs. A2–A3.

56. For a more detailed description of the contents, see chapter 1.

57. Groenevelt, *Arthritology,* 24.

58. The *Pharmacopoea Ultrajectina,* 19, lists cantharides among the fifteen simples under "animalia, eorum partes, & excrementa" but gives no recipes containing it, even among the unguents and plasters; the *Pharmacopoeia Collegii Regalis Londini* did not mention cantharides among the "animalium partes, excrementa, aliaque aliis desumpta," 41–47.

59. For example: Schroeder, *Pharmacopoeia Medico-Chymica,* 864–65; also see the lengthy and favorable summary of previous opinion given in Bartholin, *Historiarum anatomicum,* cent. 5, hist. 82, "Cantharidum usus internus," 159–61.

60. *Dictionnaire de médecine,* 6:334–35. Millipedes instead of cantharides were recommended by Michael Ettmuller as a specific for bladder stones (*Opera Omnia,* pt. 2, pp. 203–5—although he recommended cantharides for kidney stones, pt. 2, p. 184); Bontekoe had included millipedes next after cantharides in his description of animal medicines as penetrating alkaline salts and diruetics (Bontekoe, *Fragmenta,* 224); Groenevelt also recommended millipedes as a potential lithontriptic in his *Dissertatio Lithologica,* 84–85.

61. Blankaart, *Lexicon Medicum Renovatum,* 172; Groenevelt to Sibelius, 20 May 1684, Sloane 2729, fol. 160.

62. Bodleian Library, Ashmole MS. 1432, a collection of medical recipes associated with the Oxford physician John Cokkys, p. 7. I owe this reference to Faye Getz.

63. In his *De Tuto Cantharidum,* he claimed to have cured more than one hundred women of urinary obstructions over the years using his medicine (sig. B); the earliest case he mentioned in which he used it successfully was that of Mrs. Anthony in 1679 (98–106).

64. Celer, *Late Censors Deservedly Censured,* 14–16. Little is known about Torlesse, except that he fought hard for the privileges of the college but died in poverty: see Torlesse, *Bygone Days,* 21; Munk, *Roll,* 364.

65. "Draft agreement between Fellows and members of R.C.P. to support President and Censors of College in their execution of the laws and statutes," 1695, Royal College of Physicians, 2012/9.

66. The others listed by the registrar were Pitt, Bernard, Baynard, Blackburne, How, Blackmore, Tancred Robinson, Gelsthorp, Gibbons, Gould, Chamberlen, Cole, and Cade: Annals 7:13 (23 Dec. 1695).

67. See Rosenberg, "London Dispensary for the Sick-poor"; and Cook, "Rose Case Reconsidered."

68. Annals 7:14 (23 Dec. 1695).

69. The legal question was examined in: "By what name may the College of Physicians commence any suit at law," 1695, Royal College of Physicians, 2022/1. The question turned on the interpretation of the words in the charter: "Praesidens Colleg. seu Commun.," which both lawyers agreed did not make good sense in grammatical English but could be construed as "Presidens et Collegium sive communitatis," or "President and College," on the theory that the "et" had been left out.

70. Annals 7:15 (21 Feb. 1695/6).

71. The medicines for the dispensary (presumably the list of medicines rather than the medicines themselves) were first viewed and approved on 25 June 1696: Annals 7:29.

72. This advice from counsel was reported on 6 Apr. 1696: Annals 7:20–21.

73. Meetings of 22 and 23 Sept. 1696; the controversy occurred at the 30 Sept. meeting: Annals 7:35–36, 36–80 (these pages include a full transcription of the new statutes), 82–83. Also see "Acts, Ordinances, and Bylaws relating to licentiates," 1696, Royal College of Physicians, 2013/1.

74. Annals 7:84 (6 Nov.).

75. Quoted from Registrar Gill's abbreviated list of statutes, "Collections Relating to the College of Physicians," Sloane 3914, fols. 61–61v.

76. Annals 7:85–86. In addition to Tyson and Groenevelt, the walk-out included Bernard, Baynard, How, Blackmore, Tancred Robinson, Carr, Gibbons, Gould, Chamberlen, Cole (ten of the thirty-eight fellows present); Hoy and Coward (two of the five candidates); Moor (one of the two honorary fellows); and Chauncey, Crelle, Martin, Coatsworth, Upton, Botterell, Rolfe, Oliver, Walker, Morton, and Crichton (eleven of the twenty-one licentiates).

77. This was threatened on 18 Dec.; the petition of the opponents of the new college was read in a meeting on 26 Jan. 1696/7: Annals 7:89, 93. The petitioners were Josiah Clerk, William Stokeham, Francis Bernard, Robert Pitt, George How, Richard Blackmore, and William Gibbons. The visitors (Lord Keeper Sir John Somers, Lord Chief Justice of the King's Bench Sir John Holt, Lord Chief Justice of the Common Pleas Sir George Treby, and the Lord Chief Baron of the Exchequer Sir Edward Warden) asked that the college bring copies of its charters and bylaws for their inspection, and they later asked to see a copy of the college's surrender of the charter of Charles II: Annals 7:93–96, 97. Given that the justices continued no further, and that later legal proceedings of the college were based upon the charter of Henry VIII, it would appear that the "visitors" decided that the charter of Charles II had been freely given up, and so there was no legal basis for any proceedings (including their own visitation) not authorized by the college's founding charter.

78. Clerk, Tyson, Slare, Pitt, Bernard, How, Baynard, Tancred Robinson, Gelsthorp, Blackmore, Gould, Chamberlen, Cole, Palmer, and Rose all refused to subscribe money to the scheme: Annals 7:91, 93 (22 Dec. and 26 Jan. 1696/7).

79. Annals 7:97.

80. Ibid., 7:104–5.

81. Ibid., 7:109.

82. *Post Boy,* no. 305 (17–20 Apr. 1697); *Protestant Mercury,* no. 154 (21–23 Apr. 1697).

CHAPTER 7
Becoming a Cause Célèbre

1. *Post Boy*, no. 305 (17–20 Apr. 1697); *Protestant Mercury*, no. 154 (21–23 Apr. 1697).
2. *Reply to the Remarks upon the Reasons*, a single-sheet printed folio in the Bodleian Library, Rawlinson MS. C. 419, fol. 2 (new foliation); Celer, *Late Censors Deservedly Censured*, 27.
3. Greenfield [Groenevelt], *Treatise Of the Safe, Internal Use of Cantharides*, dedication.
4. Mayhew and Binny, *Criminal Prisons of London*, 586–611.
5. Celer, *Late Censors Deservedly Censured*, 27.
6. They were Serjeants Wright and Darnall and Misters Northey and Eyres. John Darnall, the elder (d. 1706), defended several important but difficult cases, becoming a serjeant in 1692 and a king's serjeant in 1698; he was knighted on 1 June 1699 (*DNB*). Edward Northey (1652–1723) was called to the bar at Middle Temple in 1674, in 1697 became a bencher in that society, and in 1701 became attorney general; he was knighted on 1 June 1702 (*DNB*). Precisely which Mr. Eyres defended Groenevelt is unclear, since there were several distinguished lawyers and judges with that name. I also cannot be certain about the identification of Serjeant Wright.
7. The date of the hearing is given in the *Protestant Mercury*, no. 154 (21–23 Apr. 1697). It agrees with the report in the Annals about his case being heard on "the first day of this Terme" (Annals 7:110, 112), since the Easter term usually began seventeen days after Easter, which was on 4 Apr. in 1697; Cheney, *Handbook of Dates*, 67–68, 159.
8. This is according to the report in the Annals by Registrar Gill: Annals 7:110–11.
9. "An Act for the Kings most gracious general and free pardon," 6 & 7 Wm. & M. c.20, *Statutes of the Realm*, vol. 6.
10. "Warrant for Committment of J. Groenvelt to Newgate" (9 Apr. 1697), Sloane 1786, fols. 157–58.
11. Sloane 3914, fol. 54.
12. Annals 7:110–11.
13. Royal College of Physicians, envl. 237: "Brief of Counsel for Complainent." The book in question is Lister, *Octo Exercitationes Medicinales*, 221–63, where he writes of administering cantharides in one case (243) and discusses cantharides at some length in a way similar to Blankaart's on 253–54.
14. Sir Thomas Powys (1649–1719) had become the attorney general in 1687 and conducted the infamous prosecution of the seven bishops; during the reign of William III, he defended many state prisoners and pleaded many cases before Parliament (*DNB*). Sir Creswell Levinz (1627–1701) had been the attorney general before Powys (in 1679), wrote the notorious proclamation against "tumultuous petitioning" in same year, and served as one of Judge Jeffreys' colleagues in "the bloody assize." But James II removed him early in 1686, and he had then served as counsel for the seven bishops in 1688 (*DNB*). Levinz had also served as counsel to the College of Physicians during his years as attorney general. I cannot be sure of the identification of Sir Bartholomew Shore.
15. Royal College of Physicians, envl. 235, no. 1: "Case of Mala Praxis. Declaration

of William Withall and his wife Susannah concerning the treatment of Dr. John Groenveldt. Easter Term 9 William III."

16. Annals 7:111. This entry is a copy of "Objections of Defendants Counsel to the Warrant issued by the Censors Committing Dr. John Groenveldt to Newgate Prison," Royal College of Physicians, envl. 236, no. 2. The notes of the college attorney on Groenevelt's case up to this point are in "Rough notes in hand of Mr. Swift the College Attorney to the Censors return to Dr. Groenveldt's case against them on an action of trespass and false imprisonment," Royal College of Physicians, envl. 236, no. 3.

17. De Beer, "English Newspapers," 121–23; Harris, *London Newspapers,* 33–42, 47, 55–64; Walker, "Advertising in London Newspapers," 130; Elliott, *State Papers Domestic Concerning the Post Office,* 10; Habermas, *Structural Transformation;* De Krey, *Fractured Society.* According to Walker, "Advertising in London Newspapers," 117, the number of medical advertisements increased by about five times between 1696 and 1700.

18. *Post Boy,* no. 305 (17–20 Apr. 1697).

19. Hessels, *Ecclesiae Londino-Batavae Archivum,* 3:2727–28, letter of Cuilemborg to "Dr Johannes Greenfield."

20. Given the dates (21–23 Apr. 1697) on no. 154 of the *Protestant Mercury,* it would have appeared on 23 Apr., two days after Groenevelt's Wednesday hearing.

21. Narcissus Luttrell noted Groenevelt's release in his diary on Thurs., 22 Apr. 1697, and since Luttrell did so a day before the only newspaper notice of it, and since the other two major papers (the *London Gazette,* and the *Post Man*) contained no information about the matter, it would appear that he heard the information by word of mouth. Luttrell, *Brief Historical Relation,* 4:214.

22. De Beer, "English Newspapers," 122, 126.

23. *Protestant Mercury,* no. 154 (21–23 Apr. 1697).

24. Annals 7:112–13.

25. De Beer, "English Newspapers," 122–23, 125.

26. *Post Man,* no. 316 (6–8 May 1697).

27. The censors agreed to stand together in their own defense and, since the notice had been published at their direction, to order the college attorney to defend the publisher, Richard Baldwin: Royal College of Physicians, envl. 236, no. 1: "Declaration by the Censors signed Thomas Burwell, Richard Torlesse, Williams Dawes, Thomas Gill, 18 May 1697"; Royal College of Physicians, envl. 235, no. 2: "Instructions of the Censors to Mr. Richard Swift. 18 May 1697."

28. Royal College of Physicians, envl. 237: "Brief of Counsel for Complainent."

29. *Reply to the Remarks upon the Reasons.*

30. See Cook, "Sir John Colbatch."

31. Annals 7:121 (17 Sept. 1697) records the date of Garth's oration; the published version was advertised in the *Post Boy,* no. 379 (7–9 Oct. 1697). For a modern English translation and brief commentary, see Ellis, "Garth's Harveian Oration."

32. The statutes were read to the candidates and licentiates in a required meeting on 25 June 1697. On the same day, the fellows were asked to sign the document pledging support for the dispensary. Annals 7:117.

33. See the "Minites of Ye Comm. of Ye Coll. of Phys: 1681–1697," Sloane 3915.

34. London Guildhall, Society of Apothecaries: 8200, "Court of Assistants, Minute Books, Vol. 4: 1694–1716" (hereafter, Guildhall MS. 8200), fol. 14, 29 July 1695.

Goodall was also mocked in two satirical handbills distributed in London: "Advertisements, medical," British Library, C.122.f.9, nos. 28 and 29.

35. Annals 7:122.

36. Goodall to Sloane, 26 Nov. 1697, Sloane 4036, fol. 375.

37. "An Act for Preventing Dangers which may happen from Popish Recusants," 25 Car.II.c.2, *Statutes of the Realm,* vol. 5.

38. Annals 7:124.

39. Luttrell, *Brief Historical Relation,* 4:316, Thurs., 9 Dec. 1697.

40. "Brief of Counsel for Complainent," Royal College of Physicians, envl. 237 (two copies of the brief exist).

41. Lawson, Collins, Lister, and Tyson. Torlesse is the missing name from among the previous censors. He was not on Swift's list of witnesses for the trial, possibly because he had a personal grudge against Groenevelt, and would not have been as reliable a witness in cross-examination.

42. For Gibbons' practice, see Royal College of Physicians, SR 108/40, (30 July 1700); and H. Crowe to Gibbons, Sloane 4062, fol. 273; Robert Baskerville to Gibbons, Sloane 4077, fol. 284.

43. Indeed he was: Barrett, *History of the Society of Apothecaries,* 106.

44. The list of subscribers is given in Annals 7:223–27.

45. John Lawson, Samuel Collins, Martin Lister, Edward Tyson, Charles Goodall, Sir Thomas Millington, Edward Hulse, Richard Morton, Frederick Slare, Walter Harris, Walter Charleton, Edward Browne.

46. Sir Thomas Millington and Sir Edmund King.

47. First physician John Hutton and physicians-in-ordinary Millington and Christian Harrell (who is said to have been the chemical physician who helped prepare the stock for the dispensary).

48. Thomas Gibson, John Soame, Samuel Garth, Hans Sloane, John Colladon, Henry Sampson, Thomas Coxe.

49. Dr. Cyprianus, Mr. Knowles, Mr. Wiseman, Mr. Pettiver, Mr. Sheibell, and Dr. Hobbs.

50. Dewhurst, *John Locke,* 305; there is much information about Cyprianus in De Beer, *Correspondence of John Locke.*

51. Cyprianus published a paper in *Philosophical Transactions* 29, no. 221 (June, July, Aug. 1696): 291–92; his burial is recorded in London Guildhall, Church of Austin Friars: 7383, "Register of Burials in the London Dutch Church" (hereafter, Guildhall MS. 7383), 2 May 1718. For a brief summary of his life, see Lindeboom, *Dutch Medical Biography,* cols. 391–94.

52. *Catalogue of the Library of the late learned Dr. Francis Bernard,* preface; also see Lawler, *Book Auctions in England,* 185–201. Many of the medieval manuscripts now in the Sloane Collection had been in Bernard's possession. For a very brief description of his life, see Munk, *Roll,* 1:417–18.

53. Because he opposed the college dispensary, Gibbons was mocked by Garth (*Dispensary*) as an incompetent. For a brief description of his life, see Munk, *Roll,* 1:449–51.

54. On Blackmore, see Boys, *Sir Richard Blackmore and the Wits;* and Solomon, *Sir Richard Blackmore.* He was a very devout Christian, a kind of late-century Puritan,

and deeply involved in the movement to reform manners. On that subject, see Bahlman, *Moral Revolution of 1688;* and Goldsmith, *Private Vices, Public Benefits*, 21–27.

55. Celer, *Late Censors Deservedly Censured*, 14–16.

56. Luttrell, *Brief Historical Relation*, 4:316.

57. I have checked the *Post Man*, the *Gazette*, the *Post Boy*, the *Flying Post*, the *Protestant Mercury*, and the *Foreign Post* from late November to mid-December without finding any notice of the trial.

58. Groenevelt, *De Tuto Cantharidum*. This book was advertised in the *London Gazette*, no. 3358, 13–17 Jan. 1697/8, for 1s. 6d.; it was also advertised in the *Term Catalogues* (Arber) in Feb. 1697/8.

59. Groenevelt, *Tutus Cantharidum*. The book is identical to the first Latin edition, except for the addition of pages 135–57, giving further support to Groenvelt's use of cantharides from the period between his trial and 1703. It was advertised in the *Term Catalogues* in Dec. 1703, with the additions at the end sold separately.

60. Groenevelt, *Treatise Of the Safe, Internal Use of Cantharides*. The book was reissued in 1715. The English quotations given below are adopted from the 1710 edition only after having been checked against the original Latin.

61. Groenevelt, *De Tuto Cantharidum, Tutus Cantharidum,* and *Treatise Of the Safe, Internal Use of Cantharides,* reader's preface. There is no record of a hearing before the censors in this case in 1692–93, although of course Registrar Gill could simply have failed to record a hearing in which no result eventuated.

62. The mention of Torlesse occurs only in the English translation, which appeared after his death, not the original Latin exemplars. As a matter of fact, Torlesse had been dropped as censor at the college elections of Sept. 1697, although he had been on the committee during previous hearings of the case.

63. Groenevelt, *De Tuto Cantharidum, Tutus Cantharidum,* and *Treatise Of the Safe, Internal Use of Cantharides,* reader's preface.

64. Ibid.

65. Groenevelt, *Treatise of the Safe, Internal Use of Cantharides.*

66. Annals 7:124. All those present were also told by the president that they would have to obey the statutes more carefully.

67. Although often said to have been a royal physician for many years under William, Millington is mentioned for the first time as second physician to the king in the account books on the new list of expenses for the Chamber to begin at Christmas 1701, superseding all previous establishments: *Calendar of Treasury Books, 1702*, pt. 1, p. 119; he is recorded in subsequent accounts, too: ibid., pt. 1, p. 283; ibid., pt. 2, pp. 1021, 1027.

68. Quoted from the *London Gazette*, no. 3348 (9–13 Dec. 1697).

69. See Ellis, "Garth's Harveian Oration"; Garth, *Dispensary.*

70. Cook, "Living in Revolutionary Times."

71. Royal College of Physicians, 2003/27–28: "Censors petition to the King re their omission to take the oaths of Allegiance and supremacy on taking the Censorial office with Counsel's opinion."

72. Public Record Office, S.P. 44/238/171: "Petition of Dr. William Dawes," 9 Jan. 1697/8: Dawes was "well known to be very zealous for his Majesty's service." S.P. 44/238/179: "Petitions of Dr. Thomas Burwell, Dr. Richard Torless, and Dr. Thomas Gill," 21 Jan. 1697/8.

73. *Reply to the Remarks upon the Reasons.*

74. Ibid.

75. *Reasons Humbly Offered,* point 4.

76. "An Act for the giving Time to several Persons to qualify themselves for their Offices, Trusts, and Employments," 20 Apr. 1698, House of Lords Journals, 16:269.

77. "An Act for giving Time to several Commissioners of Excise therein named, and their Officers, to qualify themselves for their Employment in the Duties on Leather," 4 May 1698, *House of Lords Journals,* 16:272.

78. Annals 7:132 (28 Apr. 1698): Millington, Browne, and Morton were to wait on the Lord Chancellor, Torlesse and Gill to obtain a copy of the bill, and Torlesse, Bateman, and Gill "to attend the Lords House."

79. *House of Lords Journals,* 16:279 (10 May 1698); Annals 7:133 (18 May 1698).

80. Brewer, *Sinews of Power,* 241–42.

81. *Case of the Censors,* a one-sheet folio folded to pocket size, with the title printed on one part of the back which would appear on the outer side of the folded sheet: Bodleian Library, Rawlinson MS. C.419, fol. 1 (new foliation).

82. *Post Man,* no. 476 (14–16 June 1698).

83. "Brief of Counsel for Complainent." Perhaps Groenevelt's daughter had married Gardener, but the sense of the word *kinsman* is much more likely to mean only that the two were close.

84. *Catalogue of the several Members of the Society of Apothecaries London.*

85. London Guildhall, Society of Apothecaries: 8202, vol. 3, "Wardens' Account Book, 1692–1718" (unpaginated), 7 Jan. 1697/8.

86. The dispensary had probably opened in late February or early March of 1698: the college placed advertisements about it in the *Post Boy,* no. 452 (26–28 Mar. 1698) and no. 460 (14–16 Apr.). Also see Rosenberg, "London Dispensary for the Sick-poor"; Ellis, "Background to the London Dispensary." Clark, *History of the Royal College of Physicians,* 2:442–47, gives an incorrect date.

87. "Letter of Srgt. Tho. Adamson to Mr. Doody," undated, Sloane 4026, fol. 385.

88. *Reasons Humbly Offered.* While the British Library suggests a date of 1700 for the sheet, given the other documents surrounding the affair it was clearly printed in the spring of 1698.

89. *Oath Taken by the Censors.* Again, the British Library suggests a date of 1700 for the sheet, although it seems clear that it goes with the debate over the censors' oaths in 1698. Whether it was printed by the censors or Groenevelt's party is not certain, but given the contents I suspect that the latter group had it printed to go along with Groenevelt's *Reasons Humbly Offered.*

90. *Case of the Censors.*

91. *Reply to the Reasons Against the Censors* (Bodleian Library, Rawlinson MS. C.419, fols. 4–5).

92. *Reply to the Remarks upon the Reasons.*

93. A letter from the master of Emmanuel College suggests that he was at least a competent student: J. Balderston to anon., 4 May 1695, Bodleian Library, Rawlinson MS. C.419, fol. 28 [new foliation].

94. Given Badger's apparent poverty, the society did excuse him a £20 fine and paid him a "gift" of £10: Guildhall MS. 8200, fol. 31 (22 May 1696) and 38 (25 Aug. 1696).

Badger also marketed a medicine called his "Oblion": Porter, *Health for Sale,* 107. For more on Badger, see Cook, *Decline of the Old Medical Regime,* 227–28, 235–36.

95. *State of Physick in London.* At the end the pamphlet was signed "From the College. Th.G., & R.M. Cuss."

96. [Badger], *Doctor Badger's Vindication of Himself,* reprinted in *Short Answer to a Late Book,* 27–28. The anonymous author of this last work concludes that "this Badger and Groenvelt were two, whom the Apothecaries took particularly into their favour for their known Aversion to the College of Physicians" (30).

97. Unsigned, unaddressed, and undated copy of letter of John Badger to Society of Apothecaries, Sloane 4026, fol. 391. Other manuscript versions of Badger's account of his dealings with the society are in Sloane 4026, fols. 383, 384, 386–87v. These would all seem to be drafts of the letter Badger sent the Society of Apothecaries (Guildhall MS. 8200, fol. 143 [15 Oct. 1701]), which he later edited and published as his *Vindication.*

98. For instance, Salmon advertised his "Elixir Vitae, or, Elixir of Life," and his "Pills, Drops, and Balsam," in a collection of "Advertisements, medical," British Library, 551.a.32, nos. 126, 128, 190.

99. Annals 5:103a–b (4 and 11 Oct. 1689); Annals 6:65, 69, 70 (27 May, 16 and 20 June 1693).

100. Worshipful Company of Barbers, "Court Minute Books, 1689–1701," 4 Sept. 1694.

101. On the vicissitudes of Salmon's case, see Annals 6:171, 199, 208; 7:167; and "The President and College of Physicians vers. Salmon," 1 Ld. Raym. 680–83, *English Reports,* 91:1353–55; "The College of Physicians against Salmon," 5 Mod. 327, *English Reports,* 87:685–86. Also see "The President and College of Physicians, London, versus Salmon," 2 Salkeld 451, *English Reports,* 91:391.

102. *State of Physic in London,* 3–25 (the pamphlet begins on p. 3). The dispensary was said to save the public 15s. in the pound (18).

103. One tract of the physicians later acknowledged: "Rich and Noble Persons have been furnish'd with Medicines in their respective Cases from the Dispensaries" (*Observations upon the Case of William Rose,* 12–15), while Dr. Robert Pitt persuaded John Locke to order his medicines from the dispensary (Dewhurst, "Dr. Robert Pitt's Letters to John Locke," 262). Ellis, "Background to the London Dispensary," 210, quotes a contemporary source saying that during the first three years the physicians dispensed 13,192 prescriptions at cost—this must have severely cut into the business of apothecaries.

104. *Post Man,* no. 460 (7–10 May 1698).

105. Salmon, *Rebuke to the Authors of A Blew-Book,* 3–4. Salmon's pamphlet was advertised in the *Post Boy,* no. 507 (2–4 Aug. 1698). Since both this pamphlet and the one to which it replies were printed by Whitlock, it is just possible that the first pamphlet had indeed been issued by someone else to represent the views of the current censors— an even further level of disinformation.

106. Salmon, *Rebuke to the Authors of A Blew-Book,* 4, 7. The point about the members of the college not being any better educated than their opponents had been the centerpiece of Badger's attacks in 1695.

107. Salmon, *Rebuke to the Authors of A Blew-Book,* 17.

108. *A Short, But Full Vindication, of the Late Censors of the Colledge of Physicians, London, against the scandalous aspersions and false insinuations of Dr. Groenvelt* ap-

peared very shortly after Salmon's pamphlet had appeared, being advertised in the *Post Man,* no. 499 (6–9 Aug. 1698), the *Post Boy,* no. 500 (16–19 July 1698), and ibid., no. 513 (16–18 Aug. 1698). Unfortunately, I have been unable to find an extant copy of this tract. "Lysiponius Celer" refers to an unknown work by Thomas Burwell, perhaps meaning this *Short, But Full Vindication.*

109. Celer, *Late Censors Deservedly Censured.* The preface is signed "September 26, 1698." The British Library and Kennedy, Smith, and Johnson, *Dictionary of Anonymous and Pseudonymous English Literature,* both identify Groenevelt as the author of this tract. The best evidence seems to be the letters "M.D.L." (probably meaning M.D. and licentiate) which appear after Celer's name on the title page, the general fact that it defends Groenevelt, and several phrases: the author is "publickly opposing the Censors Violence" as Groenevelt then was (sig. A2); and "as I have endeavour'd it in my Tract," apparently referring back to *De Tuto Cantharidum* (A2v). Still, Groenevelt may once again have found someone else to author this pamphlet in his defense rather than writing it himself.

110. Celer, *Late Censors Deservedly Censured,* 1, 5, 13, 23–24.

111. Ibid., 6, 14–15, 27, 12.

112. Richard Boulton, *A treatise of the reason of muscular motion* (London, 1697); idem, *A Treatise Concerning the Heat of the Blood: And also of the Use of the Lungs* (London, 1698). This last, dedicated to Rev. Dr. Jo. Meare, principal of Brazen-Nose and vice-chancellor of Oxford, had earned the imprimatur of the college (dated 5 Mar. 1697/8) during Goodall's censorship.

113. Boulton, *Letter to Dr. Charles Goodall;* a comment by Boulton on p. 11 suggests that he had received news that Goodall might be interested, and he first approached him in a letter of 18 May 1698.

114. Ibid., 11–12; also see Goodall to Sloane, Sloane 4037, fol. 143.

115. Boulton later reprinted two signed testimonials (probably from servants of the printer) to this effect in Boulton, *Letter to Dr. Charles Goodall,* 6; on p. 10, Boulton says Goodall did not just do this with his book but also "corrected" Yonge's *Sidrophel Vapulans.*

116. Yonge, *Sidrophel Vapulans.* Yonge's book was advertised in the *Post Boy,* no. 596 (28–31 Jan. 1699).

117. Boulton, *Letter to Dr. Charles Goodall;* the letter is dated 18 January 1698/9; it was advertised for sale in the London newspaper the *Post Man,* no. 579 (21–23 Feb. 1699).

118. Goodall to Sloane, 11 Dec. 1698, Sloane 4037, fol. 140.

119. *Protestant Mercury,* no. 341 (3–8 Feb. 1698/9).

120. *Post Boy,* no. 601 (14–16 Feb. 1699).

121. For instance, the poetical broadsides "Vindiciae Pharmacapolae, Or an Answer to the Doctors Complaints against Apothecaries"; "Spite and Spleen: Or the Doctor Run Mad: To the Worthy Dr. T[y]s[o]n"; and the longer poem (by Ward?) *Hell in an Uproar.*

122. Brown, *Physick Lies a Bleeding;* John Colbatch became "Jack Comprehensive," Badger "Tom Gallypot," and Goodall "John Galen." Although this satire is published in Brown's *Works* in 1707, someone published a notice in the *Post Man* (no. 318, 11–13 May 1697) saying that Brown denied it was authored by him.

123. Garth, *Dispensary.*

124. Part 6 was given an April date on the title page and advertised as just out in the 2–4 May 1699 edition of the *Flying Post,* no. 621.

125. Meetings had to be twice canceled after Groenevelt's trial: Annals 7:127, 150 (22 Dec. 1697 and 26 June 1699).

126. The lengthiest account of the case is in "Dr. Groenvelt v. Dr. Burwell et al, Censors of the College of Physicians," 1 Ld. Raym. 454–72, *English Reports,* 91:1202–14.

127. "Dr. Groenvelt versus Dr. Burnell & al.," Carthew 492, *English Reports,* 90:883.

128. See Cook, " 'Against Common Right and Reason.' "

129. "Dr. Groenvelt versus Dr. Burnell & al.," Carthew 492–93, *English Reports,* 90:883.

130. "Dr. Groenvelt versus Dr. Burnell & al.," Carthew 494, *English Reports,* 90:884.

131. "Groenvelt versus Burnell & Al.," Holt, K. B. 537, English Reports, 90:1195–96.

132. "Groenvelt versus Burwell & Al.," 1 Salkeld 397, *English Reports,* 91:344; also see "Groenvelt versus Burwell & al.," Holt, K.B. 395, *English Reports,* 90:1117.

133. Also "Groenwelt versus Burwell," Holt, K.B. 184, *English Reports,* 90:1000; "Groenwelt versus Burwell," 1 Salkeld 144–45, *English Reports,* 91:134.

134. See Jaffe and Henderson, "Judicial Review and the Rule of Law"; and De Smith, *Judicial Review of Administrative Action,* 94–96, 513.

135. "Groenvelt versus Burnell & Al.," Holt, K.B. 537, *English Reports,* 90:1195–96.

136. See Cook, "Good Advice and Little Medicine."

137. "Dr. Groenvelt versus Dr. Burnell & al.," Carthew 493, *English Reports,* 90:884.

138. Also see "Dr. Groenvelt versus Dr. Burnell & Al.," Carthew 421, *English Reports,* 90:844; "Groenvelt versus Burwell," 1 Salkeld 263, *English Reports,* 91:231.

139. See Cook, "Practical Medicine and the British Armed Forces"; idem, "Rose Case Reconsidered."

140. See Cook, "Rose Case Reconsidered."

CHAPTER 8
One Life's Shipwreck and Its Ghosts

1. Luttrell, *Brief Historical Relation,* 4:654 (8 June 1700). I have found no mention of the trial in the *London Post,* the *Post Man,* the *Post Boy,* the *Flying Post,* the *London Gazette,* or the *Protestant Mercury.*

2. Groenevelt, *Treatise Of the Safe, Internal Use of Cantharides,* dedication.

3. Annals 7:158 (25 June 1700).

4. Ibid., 7:160, 163.

5. Ibid., 7:167, 169, 170, 171, 172, 174, 175, 176, 178, 180.

6. For example, on 22 Dec. 1702 a letter of grievance against the college (signed by Tyson, F. Slare, Dawes, Welman, How, Blackmore, T. Robinson, Gibbons, Carr,

Gelsthorpe, Chamberlen, Cole, and Cade) was read; during the debate, Blackmore accused many of the fellows of being intellectually unqualified to sit there, Pitt retorted that Blackmore was the least qualified because he had not been graduated from one of the English universities and had never been examined for entry into the fellowship, and Blackmore stalked out, followed by Tyson, Baynard, Blackburne, How, T. Robinson, Gelsthorpe, and Gibbons. Annals 7:197.

7. Robert Pitt thought that about twenty physicians were refusing to join the college: Dewhurst, "Dr. Robert Pitt's Letters to John Locke," 261.

8. "College of Physicians vers. Levett," 1 Ld. Raym. 472, *English Reports,* 91:1214; Annals 7:167, 168, 174, 179.

9. Annals 7:167; the college won its case in 1702.

10. Cook, "Rose Case Reconsidered."

11. E. Dade to Sloane, 12 Apr. 1698, Sloane 4037, fol. 57–57v.

12. William Cockburn, "A Discourse of the Operation of a Blister when it Cures a Fever," *Philosophical Transactions* 21, no. 252 (May 1699): 167–70.

13. "Part of a Letter from Mr. James Yonge to Mr. John Haughton, F.R.S. concerning the internal use of Cantharides," dated from Plymouth, 17 July 1702, *Philosophical Transactions* 23, no. 280 (July–Aug. 1702): 1210–12. Houghton had been the one to deal with Groenevelt regarding Ten Rhijne's treatise in the early 1680s and so may have been well disposed to him still.

14. Groenevelt, *Tutus Cantharidum,* 2d ed., a 12mo, listed in Arber, *Term Catalogues,* in Dec. 1703. Yonge's letter was also printed on 135–40 of this second edition.

15. Sloane 3335, "Mr James Younge Surg. of Plimouth his letter to Dr. Groenevelt concerning Cantharides," dated 27 Dec. 1706, fols. 75v–76v; a copy of most of the letter is in Sloane 2146, fols. 1v–2.

16. "A Letter from Mr. James Yonge, F.R.S. to Dr. Hans Sloane, S.R. Sec. concerning a Bunch of Hair voided by Urine," dated from Plymouth, 28 Sept. 1707, *Philosophical Transactions* 26, no. 323 (Sept.–Oct. 1709): 414–15.

17. Greenfield, *Treatise of the Safe, Internal Use of Cantharides.*

18. Spinke, *Quackery Unmask'd,* 34–35, 36, 44–46; the affidavit, dated 3 Mar. 1709, was by one "J.C.," who claimed that at the Swan Tavern on St. Bartholomew's Lane he had heard Mr. Stephens claim to be the translator of Groenevelt's treatise (46). Francis McKee first mentioned Spinke's book to me.

19. Marten, *Treatise of all the degrees and symptoms of the venereal disease.*

20. Foxon, "Libertine Literature in England," 31.

21. Greenfield, *Treatise of the Safe, Internal Use of Cantharides,* 185–86.

22. Sloane 2146, fol. 1, "Letter to Dr. Groenvelt," 7 Mar. 1706/7.

23. The original Latin letter from Smyth to Groenevelt, 4 Feb. 1706/7, is in Sloane 4034, fol. 79; copies can be found in Sloane 2146, fols. 2v–3, and (together with a rough English translation) in Sloane 3336, fols. 58–60v.

24. The original of this reply of 3 Mar. 1706/7 seems to be the one at Sloane 4064, fols. 133–133v; copies are at Sloane 2146, fols. 3–4, and 3336, fols. 58–60.

25. Mangeti, *Bibliotheca Scriptorum Medicorum,* 1:526–27; Von Haller, *Bibliotheca Chirurgica,* 1:392; idem, *Bibliotheca Medicinae Practicae,* 3:271; Vigilius von Creutzenfeld, *Bibliotheca Chirurgica,* 1:1624.

26. Boerhaave, *Prealectiones Academicae de Lue Venerea,* 225–27; a somewhat watered-down version is Boerhaave, *Traité des Maladies Vénériennes,* 140–41, 188–89.

27. Goade, *Boerhaave's Materia Medica,* 69.

28. Bracken, *Midwife's Companion,* 24; I owe the reference to Cathy Crawford.

29. Risse, *Hospital Life in Enlightenment Scotland,* app. D: "Drug usage at the infirmary: The example of Dr. Andrew Duncan, Sr.," by J. Worth Estes, 370.

30. Bracken, *Midwife's Companion,* 24.

31. "Advertisements, medical," British Library, 551.a.32, no. 139.

32. Thomas Molyneux, "Some Additional Remarks on the Extracting the Stone of the Bladder out of those of the Female Sex," *Philosophical Transactions* 20, no. 236 (Jan. 1698): 14, where Molyneux refers to "Greonevelt" among others for support of the view that the largest stones occur in men rather than women.

33. Parsons, *History of St. Thomas's Hospital,* 2:141.

34. Cyprianus published *Epistola historiam exhibens . . . ad Th. Millington Medicum regium Londinensem* in London in 1700, which received a French translation in Amsterdam in 1707: Lindeboom, *Dutch Medical Biography,* col. 392.

35. Poynter, *Journal of James Yonge,* 215.

36. Guildhall MS. 7382, 2 May 1718; also listed for the same date in Guildhall MS. 7383.

37. Groenevelt to Sloane, 27 Oct. 1704, Sloane 4039, fols. 409–409v.

38. "Mr. James Younge Surg. of Plimouth his letter to Dr. Groenevelt concerning Cantharides," 27 Dec. 1706, Sloane 3335, fol. 75v.

39. Annals 6:296 (5 May 1710), when he was dunned for back dues and referred to Dr. Clark.

40. Groenevelt, *Compleat Treatise of the Stone and Gravel,* xiv.

41. Her name is unusual for the time; a Christina de Ruÿter was buried on 13 Dec. 1713 in Amsterdam: GA Amsterdam, "Begraven" Klappers, 1103/25. I can find no reference to her burial in London.

42. Groenevelt, *Compleat Treatise of the Stone and Gravel,* xiii.

43. Annals 6:305 (22 Dec. 1710).

44. Groenevelt to Sloane, 27 June 1707, Sloane 4040, fol. 376; Groenevelt to Sloane, 14 Dec. 1708, fol. 105.

45. Groenevelt to Sloane, 29 Sept. 1714, Sloane 4043, fols. 299–300.

46. Lindeboom, *Austin Friars,* 156–58; Hessels, *Ecclesiae Londino-Batavae Archivum,* 3:2729–36, 2763–64.

47. Hessels, *Ecclesiae Londino-Batavae Archivum,* 3:2761.

48. Ibid., 3:2727–28, letter of Van Cuilemborg to Groenevelt, 8 Oct. 1702; Bloom and James, *Medical Practitioners in the Diocese of London,* 51, prints a certificate signed by Crell, Groenevelt, John Crickton, and Sam. Munford, 31 Mar. 1698.

49. Hessels, *Ecclesiae Londino-Batavae Archivum,* 3:2734–35, 2746–49, 2753, 2760 (the two petitions of February contain the names of many women congregants).

50. Ibid., 3:2761; indeed, Groenevelt does not seem to have given any noted sums of money to the church: Guildhall MS. 7389, v. 1; Guildhall MS. 7408; Guildhall MS. 7410.

51. London Guildhall, Dutch Church at Austin Friars: 7405, "Lidmaten Boek."

52. Groenevelt, *A Compleat Treatise of the Stone and Gravel,* 107–11.
53. Ibid., sig. A3: "when such as I, are admitted to make their Addresses to Persons of the Duke of Norfolk's distinguish'd Quality . . ."
54. Ibid., vii–viii. The author he refers to may be Pechey: see his *Store-house of Physical Practice,* sig. A2.
55. Singer, "Benjamen Marten"; Cummins, "Some Early British Phthisiologists"; Williamson, "Germ Theory of Disease."
56. Groenevelt, *A Compleat Treatise of the Stone and Gravel,* viii–xiv, xvi, xviii–xx, xxii–xxiii.
57. Ibid., 230–80.
58. Ibid., 277.
59. Ibid., 281–86.
60. Troyer, *Ned Ward of Grubstreet;* Rogers, *Grub Street.*
61. Williamson, "John Martyn and the *Grub-Street Journal*"; Hillhouse, *Grub-Street Journal.* Groenevelt's translator John Marten and the surgeon John Martyn of the *Grub-Street Journal* were different people.
62. Ward, "Unnoted Poem by Mandeville," reprints the Latin text of Mandeville's poem and Marten's translation of it in 1706. I owe this reference to Francis McKee.
63. Goldsmith, *Private Vices, Public Benefits,* 28–33.
64. Ibid., 42, 44.
65. Mandeville, *Hypochondriack and Hysterick Passions;* for a discussion of this work, see Cook, *Bernard Mandeville,* 60–76; Monro, *Ambivalence of Bernard Mandeville,* 48–74.
66. Groenevelt, *Compleat treatise of the stone,* 2d ed.
67. The English translator of *Boerhaave's Aphorisms* recommended Tolet as "the best Treatise, about the Stone, and the Operations for the same" (432), despite the fact that his publisher had earlier brought out Groenevelt's book. The section on the stone in this book (427–32) contains almost no theory about how the stone might form, only a description of the symptoms attending its doing so. He also mentions Cyprianus (430).
68. Groenevelt to Sloane, 29 Sept. 1714, Sloane 4043, fols. 299–300.
69. Noorthouck, *New History of London.*
70. Stow, *Survey,* bk. 4, p. 69; for a physical and historical description of the neighborhood, see 61–69.
71. Groenevelt to Sloane, 29 Sept. 1714, Sloane 4043, fols. 299–300.
72. Groenevelt, *Fundamenta Medicinae,* sigs. A4–A4v.
73. Mangeti, *Bibliotheca Scriptorum Medicorum,* 2:699; Eloy, *Dictionarie historique,* 4:625–26; Sondervorst, *Histoire de la médecine belge,* 114–15. Although a famous professor of Louvain/Leuven, little is known about him. I am indebted to Mark Derez and Geert Vanpaemel for their assistance in tracing Zypaeus.
74. Zypaeus, *Fundamenta medicinae reformatae physico-anatomica* (1683); I have seen the 1687 and the 1692 editions. There was another Brussells edition in 1693.
75. For example: Zypaeus, *Fundamenta* (1687), 39: "1. Humores, de quibus hic, naturales sunt, de praeter naturalibus agetur postmodum itaque sic sumptus, *humor est substantia liquida palpabilis in corpore nostro ex cibo potuque secundum naturam progenita.* / 2. Dicitur *liquida,* ut excludantur faeces et partes solidae." Groenevelt, *Fundamenta,*

19–20: "Quid est Humor? / Humor est *substantia liquida, palpabilis,* in *Corpore nostro,* ex cibo et potu *secundum Naturam progenita.* / Quare dicitur liquida? / Ut excludantur faeces, et partes solidae" (italics in the originals).

76. For a further discussion of this text, see Cook, "Physick and Natural History."

77. Zypaeus, *Fundamenta medicinae,* 2d ed.; the British Library catalogue mistakenly gives the publication date as 1725.

78. [Groenevelt], *Grounds of Physick;* the full title mentions Groenevelt as the author.

79. The only differences were the publisher and the fact that the second edition did not include a final advertisement at the back for Martin's book on gonorrhea. It sold for 4s.

80. Groenevelt to Sloane, 4 Mar. 1714/15, Sloane 4044, fol. 20; the interpolations are due to a tear in the paper, perhaps made to remove the names of Groenevelt's enemies.

81. Greater London Records Office, P76/JS1/8, "Marriages, Baptisms, and Burials, 1711–26, St. James Clerkenwell"; Stow, *Survey,* 64: the minister earned £2 10s. for burials in the churchyard, £5 for burials within the church.

82. Power, *Short History of Surgery,* 41.

83. Titsingh, *Heelkundige Verhandeling,* 236–37.

84. Groenevelt, *Rudiments of Physick.*

85. The two books that received the most learned interest were his *Dissertatio Lithologica* of 1684 and 1687, transl. into English in 1687 and 1710 with a second edition of the latter in 1712; and his *De Tuto Cantharidum* of 1698 and 1703, translated into English in 1706; he also received some recognition for his *Fundamenta Medicinae Scriptoribus* of 1714, 1715, and 1743, translated into English on two separate occasions in 1715 and 1753.

86. Barbette, *Opera Omnia,* 155, 161–62; Mangeti, *Bibliotheca Scriptorum Medicorum,* 1:526–27.

87. Von Haller, *Bibliotheca Chirurgica,* "308. Johannes Groenevelt," 1:392; idem, *Bibliotheca Medicinae Practicae,* 3:270–71. The latter volume is organized according to medical "schools," Groenevelt being included among the Sydenhamians. Von Haller also briefly mentions Groenevelt's work on calculi and his textbook of medicine in his *Bibliotheca Anatomia,* 1:726, 2:489.

88. Vigilius von Creutzenfeld, *Bibliotheca Chirurgica,* 1:455–56, 1624.

89. Eloy organized his material according to person rather than subject: see "Groenevelt (Jean)," in Eloy, *Dictionarie historique,* 2:389–90. The moral of Eloy's story was the backwardness of London physicians: Groenevelt "soutient son opinion sur l'usage interne des Cantharides contre la censure de quelques Médecins de Londres, qui l'avoient déséré au College Royal, comme un homme qui introduisoit des pratiques abusives & dangereuses."

90. Virtually word-for-word copies of the Von Haller and Eloy entries on Groenevelt can be found in Ploucquet, *Literatura Medica Digesta,* 1:169, 178, 182, 184, 187, 188, 189, 194, 205; *Dictionaire des sciences médicales,* 4:525–26; Dezeimeris, *Dictionnarie historique,* 2:632–33; Bayle and Thillaye, *Biographie médicale,* 2:92–93.

91. Ellis, *History of Bladder Stone,* 27; Nöske, *Lithotomia Vesicae,* 42–44.

92. For instance, Groenevelt was no longer thought worthy of mention by Callisen, *Medicinisches Schriftsteller-Lexicon.*

93. Because medical ideas are today often distinguished from scientific ones, and only the most important ideas are ordinarily thought worthy of historical study, Groenevelt and his like have received no notice in Gillispie, *Dictionary of Scientific Biography*.

94. Munk gave the incorrect date of Groenevelt's M.D. from Utrecht recorded in the college Annals (18 Mar., 1672: in fact it was 1670) and took the trouble to find his matriculation at Leiden, but he made no use of the earlier favorable references to Groenevelt and his work in the medical encyclopedists.

95. Munk, *Roll*, 1:401–2. Or was this an implicit refutation of the Frenchman Eloy?

96. Goodwin corrected Munk's mistaken date of Groenevelt's graduation from Utrecht—presumably by checking the catalogue of the British Library, which contains a copy of Groenevelt's Utrecht dissertation—and mentioned his being a physician to the garrison at Grave in 1673, a fact given in the preface to Groenevelt's *Treatise of the Safe, Internal Use of Cantharides*.

97. For an account of Groenevelt's case, Goodwin made use of Luttrell's *Brief Historical Relation*.

98. Gordon Goodwin's entry "Groenveldt," in *DNB*, 8:712. The guess at a birthdate of 1647 undoubtedly derived from the fact that when Groenevelt matriculated at Leiden in Sept. 1667, he gave his age as twenty years old (it is now recognized that such entries were often inaccurate); why Goodwin suggested a death date of 1710 cannot be guessed, since he mentions one of Groenevelt's books being published in 1714.

99. Hirsch, *Biographisches Lexicon*, 2:862.

100. *Nieuw Nederlandsch Biographisch Woordenboek*, 1:978–79.

101. Lindeboom, *Dutch Medical Biography*, cols. 730–31.

102. Wallis and Wallis, *Eighteenth-Century Medics*, "John Greenfield," 244, confuse our doctor with the Leiden physician and jurist Joannes Groenvelt who helped Boerhaave with editing and publishing ancient Greek medical authors. On the latter Groenevelt, see Lindeboom, *Herman Boerhaave*, 150.

103. Mandeville, *Fable of the Bees;* Monro, *Ambivalence of Mandeville;* Goldsmith, *Private Vices, Public Benefits;* idem, "Regulating Anew."

104. Cook, "Good Advice and Little Medicine."

Bibliography

MANUSCRIPTS

Bodleian Library

Ashmole MS. 1432: Collection of medical receipts.
Locke MS. F.7: Diary.
Locke MS. F.8: Diary.
Locke MS. F.9: Diary
Locke MS. C.11: Correspondence.
Locke MS. C.18: Correspondence.
Locke MS. C.31: Manuscript translation from Ten Rhijne.
Rawlinson MS. C.419: Broadsides, handbills, and correspondence re: medical quarrels of the 1690s.

British Library

Add. MS. 29,551: Correspondence.
Add. MS. 33,573: Correspondence.

Birch MS. 4460, pt. 7: "Extracts from the learned and Ingenious dr. Hen. Sampsons MS Daybook, 1698."

Sloane MS. 1394: Assorted Correspondence.
Sloane MS. 1786: Assorted Papers re: Medical Affairs.
Sloane MS. 1795: Album Amicorum of Casparus Sibelius.
Sloane MS. 1833: "Dr. E. Browne, Anatomical Notes and Collections."
Sloane MS. 2146: Assorted Papers re: Medicine.
Sloane MS. 2655: "MS of and Relating to Dr. Philip Guide."
Sloane MS. 2729: Correspondence of Casparus Sibelius.
Sloane MS. 3335: Book of Letters and Receipts of Interest to James Petiver.
Sloane MS. 3336: Assorted Papers re: Medicine.
Sloane MS. 3914: Collections Relating to the College of Physicians.

Sloane MS. 3915: "Minites of Ye Comm. of Ye Coll. of Phys: 1681–1697."
Sloane MS. 4026: Medical Correspondence.
Sloane MS. 4034: Assorted Papers re: Medicine.
Sloane MS. 4036: Medical Correspondence.
Sloane MS. 4037: Medical Correspondence.
Sloane MS. 4039: Medical Correspondence.
Sloane MS. 4040: Medical Correspondence.
Sloane MS. 4043: Medical Correspondence.
Sloane MS. 4044: Medical Correspondence.
Sloane MS. 4056: Correspondence.
Sloane MS. 4062: Medical Correspondence.
Sloane MS. 4064: Assorted Papers re: Medicine.
Sloane MS. 4292: Medical Correspondence.

Corporation of London Records Office

MC1: "Mayor's Court Original Bills."
MC6/514: "Mayor's Court Interrogation."

Gemeentelijke Archief Amsterdam

"Begraven" Klappers
142/282: "Dopen."
497/417: "Kerk ondertrouw."
PA 27/20: "Nomina Medicorum, 1641–1753."
PA 366, no. 231: *Privilegien, Willekeuren en Ordonnantien, Beteffende het Collegium Chirurgicum Amstelaedamense* (Amsterdam: Pieter vanden Berge, 1736).

Gemeentelijke Archief Deventer

"Klapper Hervormde Dopen Deventer 1591 juli 2–1616 mei 28."
"Klapper Hervormde Dopen Deventer: 1616–1637."
"Klapper Hervormde Dopen Deventer: 1638–1646."
"Klapper Hervormde Dopen Deventer: 1647–1656."
"Ondertrouw Klapper, 1624–1650."
"Attestaties, Belijdenissen Herv. Kerk 1632–1816."
Jhr. H. H. Röell, coll., "Deventer Vroedschap," vol. 2.
RA 104: "Bekende Schulden van 27 Jan 1637 tot 16 July 1649."
RA 108a: "Testamenten 16e eeuw tot c. 1656."
RA 134f: "Renuntiatien van 17 May 1636 tot 1 December 1643."
RA 134g: "Testamenten en Renuntiatien van 28 Nov. 1643 tot 6 Mart 1655."
RA 134i: "Renunciatien, 9 Oct. 1668–23 March 1688."
RA 141a: "Boedelinventaris, 1518–1811."

Gemeentelijke Archief Grave

RANB I.300: "Rekeningen, 1671–1674."
RANB I.400: "Resolutieboeken, 1656–1681."
RANB II.400: "Ingekomen stukken, 1670–72, 1673–76."

Gemeentelijke Archief Leiden

Gilden Archieven, No. 350: "'t Boeck van de Mr. Chirurgijns."

Gemeentelijke Archief Zutphen

"Trouwvermeldingen."
"Lidmatenboeken, 1609–1810."
A one-page account of the Groenevelt family in the "Genealogie" folders.

Greater London Record Office

P76/JS1/8: "Marriages, Baptisms, and Burials, 1711–26, St. James Clerkenwell."

London Guildhall

Dutch Church at Austin Friars: 7382, "Register of Baptisms 1602–1874, Marriages 1602–
    1874, and Burials 1671–1853"; 7383, "Register of Burials in the London Dutch
    Church"; 7389, v. 1, "Kerek Rek[ening] Boek van 1658 tot 1705"; 7405, "Lidmaten
    Boek"; 7406, "Register of Members of the London-Dutch Church 1681–1690";
    7401, v. 2, "Register of Members of the Consistory 1666 to 1685"; 7408, "Gen'l
    memoranda book 1594–1714"; 7410, "Deacons Memoranda 1615–1741."
Draft agreement between Fellows and members of R.C.P. to support President and Censors
    of College in their execution of the laws and statutes," 1695.
Society of Apothecaries: 8200, "Court of Assistants, Minute Books, Vol. 4: 1694–1716";
    8202, "Wardens' Account Book, 1692–1718"; 8290, "Papers relating to disputes
    and suits between the Society and the Barber-Surgeon's Company, 1690–1708."

Public Record Office, Chancery Lane

Chancery Proceedings, C7/137/65: Case of Dr. Groenevelt and Dr. Browne.
S.P. 29/311/210: "His Majesty's gracious Declaration for encouraging the subjects of the
    United Provinces of the Netherlands to transport themselves with their estates, and
    to settle in this his Majesty's kingdom of England."
S.P. 44/238/171: "Petition of Dr. William Dawes."
S.P. 44/238/179: "Petitions of Dr. Thomas Burwell, Dr. Richard Torless, and Dr. Thomas
    Gill."

Royal College of Physicians

Annals: "Annales Collegii Medicorum," vols. 3–8 (1608 to after 1716).
SR 108: Dr. Gibbons' report on case of duke of Gloucester.
SR 173: Anon. copybook.
SR 259: Groenevelt, *Dissertatio Lithologica* (1687), with MS notes.
2003/27–28: "Censors petition to the King re their omission to take the oaths of Allegiance and supremacy on taking the Censorial office with Counsel's opinion."
2012/9.
2013/1: "Acts, Ordinances, and Bylaws relating to licentiates."
2022/1: "By what name may the College of Physicians commence any suit at law."
Envelope 235: "Case of Mala Praxis. Declaration of William Withall and his wife Susannah concerning the treatment of Dr. John Groenveldt. Easter Term 9 William III," "Instructions of the Censors to Mr. Richard Swift. 18 May 1697."
Envelope 236: "Objections of Defendants Counsel to the Warrant issued by the Censors Committing Dr. John Groenveldt to Newgate Prison," "Rough notes in hand of Mr. Swift the College Attorney to the Censors return to Dr. Groenveldt's case against them on an action of trespass and false imprisonment," "Declaration by the Censors signed Thomas Burwell, Richard Torlesse, William Dawes, Thomas Gill, 18 May 1697."
Envelope 237: "Brief of Counsel for Complainent."

Royal Society of London

Letter Books: LB.C.8; LB.C.9.
"Classified Papers," vol. 14 (1), "Physick."

University of Leiden

"Archieven van Senaat en Faculteiten der Leidsche Universiteit, Recensielijsten," nos. 38–42.

Worshipful Company of Barbers

"Court Minute Books."

PRINTED PRIMARY SOURCES CITED

Newspapers, Periodicals, and Handbills

"Advertisements, medical." British Library, C.112.f.9.
"Advertisements, medical." British Library, 551.a.32.
Flying Post.
Foreign Post.
London Gazette.
Post Boy.

Post Man.
Protestant Mercury.
Philosophical Transactions.

Books

André, François. *Chemical Disceptations: Or, Discourses upon Acid and Alkali.* Translated by "J.W." London, 1689.

Atkins, William. *A discourse shewing the nature of the gout.* London, 1694.

[Badger, John]. *Doctor Badger's Vindication of Himself, from the Groundless Calumnies and Malicious Slanders, of some London-Apothecaries.* 1701.

Barbette, Paulus. *Opera Omnia et Chirurgicae.* Edited and annotated by Johannes Jacobus Mangeti. Geneva, 1688.

Bartholin, Thomas. *Historiarum anatomicum & medicarum rariorum, centuria V. & VI.* Copenhagen, 1661.

Blankaart, Steven. *Lexicon medium renovatum.* Leiden, 1735.

———. *A Physical Dictionary.* Translated by J.G. London, 1684.

———, ed. *Collectanea medico-physica oft Hollands Jaar-Register der Genees- en Natuurkundige Aanmerkingen van gantsch Europa & Beginnende mett het Jaar MDCLXXX.* Amsterdam, 1680.

———, ed. *Collectanea medico-physica, oft Hollands Jaar-Register: Der Genees- en Natuur-kundige Aanmerkingen van gantsch Europa, etc. Tweede en Derde Deel des Jaars MCDCLXXXI en LXXXII.* Amsterdam, 1683.

[Boerhaave, Herman.] *Boerhaave's Aphorisms: Concerning the Knowledge and Cure of Diseases.* London, 1742.

Boerhaave, Herman. *Prealectiones Academicae de lue venerea.* Leiden, 1762.

———. *Traité des maladies vénériennes.* Paris, 1753.

Bontekoe, Cornelis. *Alle de philosophische, medicinale, en chymische werken.* 2 vols. Amsterdam, 1689.

[Borrichius, Olaus.] *Prosodia Pharmacopaeorum: or the Apothecary's prosody.* [Translated and edited] by Richard Browne. London, 1685.

Boulton, Richard. *A Letter to Dr. Charles Goodall.* London, 1699.

Boyle, Robert. *Experiments, Notes, &c. about the mechanical origin or Production of divers particular Qualities.* Oxford, 1675.

———. *Some Considerations touching the Usefulness of Experimental Naturall Philosophy.* Oxford, 1663.

———. *Works.* Edited by Thomas Birch. 6 vols. 1772. Reprint. Hildesheim: Georg Olms Verlagsbuchhandlung, 1966.

Bracken, Henry. *The Midwife's Companion, or, a Treatise of Midwifery.* London, 1737.

Brown, Tom. *Physick Lies a Bleeding, or the Apothecary turned Doctor.* London, 1697.

[Browne, Richard, ed.?] *Chirurgorum comes: Or the Whole Practice of Chirurgery. Begun by the Learned Dr. Read.* London, 1687.

Busschof, Herman, and Hermann Roonhuis. *Two Treatises, The One Medical, of the Gout, . . . the Other Partly Chirurgical, Partly Medical.* London, 1676.

The Case of the Censors, and other Members of the College of Physitians, London. 1698.

A Catalogue of the Library of the late learned Dr. Francis Bernard . . . which will be sold at auction. 1698.

Catalogue of the several Members of the Society of Apothecaries London: Living in and About the City of London, this present 24th day of August, 1693.

A Catalogue of the several Members of the Society of Apothecaries London: Living in and about the City of London, this present 29th Day of September, 1702.

Cavlier, Petrus. *De Calculo Renum, & Vesicae.* Leiden, 1654.

Celer, Lysiponius [pseud.; poss. Joannes Groenevelt]. *The Late Censors Deservedly Censured; And their Spurious Litter of Libels Against Dr. Greenfield, and Others, justly expos'd to Contempt.* London, 1698.

Clavel, Robert. *The general catalogue of books printed in England since the dreadful fire of London, 1666. To the end of Trinity term, 1674.* London, 1675.

Colbatch, John. *A Physico-Medical Essay Concerning Alkaly and Acid.* London, 1696.

———. *A Treatise of the Gout.* London, 1697.

Cooke, John. *Unum Necessarium: Or, The Poore Mans Case.* London, 1648.

Cotta, John. *A Short Discoverie of the Unobserved Dangers of severall sorts of ignorant and unconsiderate Practicers of Physicke in England.* London, 1612.

Crelle Spinowski, Christophorus. *De calculo renum et vesicae.* Leiden, 1682.

Culpeper, Nicholas. *A Physicall Directory or A Translation of the London Dispensatory.* London, 1649.

Curtius, Alexander Carolus. *De calculo renum et vesicae.* Leiden, 1662.

de Luine, Guillaume. *Relation de tout ce qui s'est passé pendant le siége de Grave en l'année 1674.* Paris, 1753.

Dunk, Eleazer. *The Copy of a Letter written by E.D. Doctour of Physicke to a Gentleman.* London, 1606.

Ettmuller, Michael. *Opera Omnia.* Lyons, 1685.

Garth, Samuel. *The Dispensary: A Poem. In Six Cantos.* London, 1699.

Geyer, Joh. Daniel. *Tractatus physico-medicus de cantharidibus.* Leipzig and Frankfurt, 1687.

Goade, Richard. *Boerhaave's Materia Medica, or the Druggists' Guide, and the Physician and Apothecary's Table-Book.* London, [1755].

Groenevelt, Joannes. *Arthritology: or, A Discourse of the Gout.* London, 1691.

———. *A Compleat Treatise of the Stone and Gravel.* London, 1710.

———. *A compleat treatise of the stone . . . with an ample discourse on lithontriptick, or stone-breaking medicines, etc.,* 2d ed. London, 1712.

———. *De Tuto Cantharidum in Medicina Usu Interno.* London, 1698.

———. *De calculo vesicae.* Utrecht, 1670.

———. *Dissertatio Lithologica, variis observationibus et figuris illustrata.* London, 1684.

———. *Dissertatio Lithologica, variis observationibus et figuris illustrata. Editio secunda, Prior multo Auctior et Emendatior.* London, 1687.

———. *Fundamenta Medicinae Scriptoribus.* London, 1714.

———. *Fundamenta Medicinae Scriptoribus . . . Autore Joanne Groenvelt . . . Secundum Dictata D. Zypaei, Editio Secunda.* London, 1715.

———. *The Grounds of Physick.* London, 1715.

———. Λιθολογια. *A Treatise of the Stone and Gravel.* London, 1677.

————. *The Rudiments of Physick Clearly and Accurately Describ'd and Explain'd.* Sherborne and London, [1753].

————. *A Treatise Of the Safe, Internal Use of Cantharides in the Practice of Physick . . . Translated . . . By John Marten.* London, 1706.

————. *A Treatise Of the Safe, Internal Use of Cantharides in the Practice of Physick . . . Translated . . . By John Marten.* 2d ed. London, 1715.

————. *Tutus Cantharidum In Medicinâ Usus Internus. Editio Secunda, priori locupletior et auctior.* London, 1703.

Groenevelt, Johannes, with Richard Browne, Christopher Crell, Phillipe Guide, and John Pechey. *The Oracle for the Sick.* [1687].

Guide, Philippe. *De la Vertu Singulière du Vin Rouge, Pour guerir La Retention d'Urine. Observations des bons et des mauvais Effets du Quinquina Dans Les Fievres Intermittentes, etc.* London, 1684.

————. *Observations Anatomiques, Faites sur Plusiers Animaux au sortir de la Machine Pneumatique.* Paris, 1674.

————. *Traité de la Nature du Mal Venerien, Tiré de plusieurs expériences Physiques et des Mechaniques.* Paris, 1676.

Harris, Walter. *An Exact Enquiry Into, and Cure of the Acute Diseases of Infants.* Translated by W[illiam] C[ockburn]. London, 1693.

————. *Pharmacologia Anti-Empirica: Or a Rational Discourse of Remedies both Chymical and Galenical.* London, 1683.

[Hildanus], Wilhelm Fabricius. *Lithotomia Vesicae.* Basel, 1628.

————. *Lithotomia Vesicae: That is, An Accurate description of the Stone in the Bladder.* Translated by N.C. London, 1640.

Hulleman, Hermannus. *De Calculo renum & vesicae.* Leiden, 1657.

Hutchinson, Richard. *De calculo.* Utrecht, 1668.

Huyberts, Adrian. *A Corner-Stone Laid towards the Building of a New Colledge (that is to say, a new Body of Physicians) in London.* London, 1675.

Johnson, William. 'Αγυρτο-Μαστιξ, *Or, Some Brief Animadversions Upon two late Treatises.* London, 1665.

Lister, Martin. *Octo Exercitationes Medicinales . . . Altera Editio ab Auctore recondita, & non parum aucta.* London, 1697.

Mandeville, Bernard. *A Treatise of the Hypochondriack and Hysterick Passions.* London, 1711.

Marten, John. *Treatise of all the degrees and symptoms of the venereal disease, in both sexes . . . 6th ed., with Gonosologium Novum: or, a new system of all the secret . . . diseases.* London, [1708].

Maynwaring, Everard. *The frequent, but unsuspected progress of pains, inflammations, tumors . . . and mortifications internal.* London, 1679.

Middegaels, Lambertus. *De calculo vesicae.* Leiden, 1668.

Nedham, Marchamont. *Medela Medicinae: A Plea For the Free Profession, and a Renovation of the Art of Physick.* London, 1665.

The Oath Taken by the Censors, who are the Examiners of the College, before the President of the College, upon the day of their admission into their Office. [1698].

Observations upon the Case of William Rose an Apothecary. London, 1704.

Paré, Ambroise. *Oeuvres.* 4th ed. 1565. Facsimile. Lyons: Editions du Fleuve, 1962.

Pechey, John. *Collections of Acute Diseases, in Five Parts*. London, 1686–91.
———. *The London Dispensatory, Reduced to the Practice of the London Physicians*. London, 1694.
———. *A Plain and Short Treatise of an Apoplexy, Convulsions, Colick, twisting of the Guts, Mother Fits, Bleeding at the Nose, and several other violent diseases that come of a sudden*. London, 1698.
———. *Promptuarium Praxeos Medicae*. London, 1693.
———. *The Store-house of Physical Practice*. London, 1695.
———. *The Whole Works of the Excellent Practical Physician, Dr. Thomas Sydenham*. London, 1696.
Pharmacopoeia Collegii Regalis Londini. London, 1678.
Reasons Humbly Offered to the Right Honourable, the Lords Spiritual and Temporal in Parliament, Assembled, why Dr. Thomas Burwell, Dr. Richard Torlesse, Dr. William Dawes, and Dr. Thomas Gill . . . Should not be excused from the penalty of the Act of 25 Car. II. [1698].
A Reply to the Reasons Against the Censors of the College of Physicians; for not Qualifying themselves according to the Statute of 25 Car. II. [1698].
A Reply to the Remarks upon the Reasons, why the late Censors should not be excus'd from the Penalty of the 25 Car. II. [1697].
Rogers, George. *Oratorio Anniversaria, habita in Theatro Collegii Medicorum Londinensum, Decimo octavo dre Octob. Et divi lucae Festo. 1681*. London, 1682.
Salmon, William. *Pharmacopoeia Londinensis. Or, the New London Dispensatory*. 6th ed. London, 1702.
———. *A Rebuke to the Authors of A Blew-Book; call'd The State of Physick in London*. London, 1698.
Schroeder, Johannes. *Pharmacopoeia Medico-Chymica, Sive Thesaurus Pharmacologicus*. Leiden, 1672.
Securis, Iohn. *A Detection and Querimonie of the daily enormities and abuses committed in physick*. London, 1566.
Sermon, William. *A Friend to the Sick: Or, the Honest English Man's Preservation*. London, 1673.
Sherley, Thomas. *A Philosophical Essay: Declaring The Probable Causes, whence Stones are produced in the Greater World*. London, 1672.
A Short Answer to a Late Book, Entituled Tentamen Medicinale. London, 1705.
Spechtius, Johannes. *De Celebri illo plurimorum tortore calculo*. Leiden, 1657.
Spinke, J. *Quackery Unmask'd: Or, Reflections on the Sixth Edition of Mr. Marten's Treatise of the Venereal Disease, and its Appendix*. London, 1709.
The State of Physick in London. London, 1698.
Straselius, Fransicus. *De Calculo renum & vesicae*. Leiden, 1659.
Stubbe, Henry. *Campanella Revived*. London, 1670.
———. *The Lord Bacons Relation of the Sweating-Sickness Examined . . . Together with a Defense of Phlebotomy . . . in opposition to [George Thomson] and the author of Medela Medicinae, Doctor Whitaker, and Doctor Sydenham*. London, 1671.
Swammerdam, Johannis. *Miraculum naturae sive uteri muliebris fabrica, notis in D. Joh. van Horne prodromum illustrata*. Leiden, 1672.

Sydenham, Thomas. *Tractatus de Podagra et Hydrope*. London, 1683.

————. *A Treatise concerning the Gout lately published in Latine by Dr. Sydenham. Now sett forth in English by John Drake, Med. B.* London, 1685.

Sylvius, François dele Boë. *Idea praxeos medicae, in Tres Libros Divisae*. Frankfurt, 1671.

————. *A New Idea of the Practice of Physic*. Translated by Richard Gower. London, 1675.

————. *Opera Medica*. Amsterdam, 1679.

[Temple, Sir William.] *Miscellanea*. London, 1680.

Ten Rhijne, Willem. *An account of the Cape of Good Hope and the Hottentotes*, in vol. 4 of *A Collection of Voyages and Travels*. London, 1732.

————. *Dissertatio de arthritide: Mantissa schematica: de acupunctura: et orationes tres, I. de chymiae ac botaniae antiquitate et dignitate. II. de physiognomia. III. de monstris*. London, 1683.

————. *Schediasma de Promontorio Bonae Spei, ejusve tractus incolis Hottentottis*. Schaffhausen, 1686.

————. *Verhandelinge van het Podagra en Vliegende Jicht*. Amsterdam, 1684.

Titsingh, Abraham. *Heelkundige Verhandeling over de Steen en het Steensnyden, van Frere Jacques de Beaulieu*. Amsterdam, [1731].

Tolet, François. *Traité de la lithotomie ou de l'extraction de la pierre hors la vessie, avec les figures*. Paris, 1682.

————. *A Treatise of Lithotomy: Or, Of the Extraction of the Stone out of the Bladder*. Translated by A. Lovell. London, 1683.

Tulp, Nicolaes. *Observationes Medicae. Editio Quinta*. Leiden, 1716.

Turquet de Mayerne, Theodore. *Treatise of the Gout*. Translated by T. Sherley. London, 1676.

Tyson, Edward. *Carigueya, seu Marsupiale Americanum; or, the anatomy of an opossum dissected at Gresham College*. London, 1698.

————. *Orang-outang, sive Homo Silvestris: or, the Anatomy of a Pygmie compared with that of a monkey, an ape, and a man. To which is added a Philological Essay. . . .* London, 1699.

————. *Phocaena; or, the anatomy of a Porpess*. London, 1680.

Tyssot de Patot, Simon. *Lettres Choises*. 2 vols. The Hague, 1727.

van Campen, Christophorus. *De calculo renum*. Leiden, 1668.

van der Heyden, Ioachimus. *De Calculo vesicae*. Leiden, 1667.

van Helmont, Joannis Baptista. *Opuscula medica inaudita. I. De lithiasi*. 1644. 2d ed. Amsterdam, 1648.

van Meek'ren, Job. *Heel- en Genees-Konstige Aanmerkkingen*. Amsterdam, 1668.

[Ward, Ned?] *Hell in an Uproar, Occasioned by A Scuffle That Happened between the Lawyers and the Physicians, for Superiority. A Satyr*. [1700].

Yonge, James. *Sidrophel Vapulans: Or, the Quack-Astrologer tossed in a Blanket. . . .* London, 1699.

Zypaeus, Françoise. *Fundamenta medicinae reformatae physico-anatomica. Editio secunda, ex M.S. Authoris aucta, correcta, et emendata*. Brussels, 1687.

————. *Fundamenta medicinae reformatae physico-anatomica. Editio secunda, ex M.S. Authoris aucta, correcta, et emendata*. Lyons, 1692.

REFERENCES, PRINTED MANUSCRIPT SOURCES, AND
MODERN EDITIONS

Album Studiosorum Academiae Lugduno Batavae, 1575–1875. The Hague, 1875.
Album Studiosorum Academiae Rheno-Trajectinae, 1636–1886. Utrecht, 1886.
Arber, Edward, ed. *The Term Catalogues, 1668–1709*. 3 vols. London: Privately printed,
    1903.
Banga, Jelle. *Geschiedenis van de geneeskunde en van hare beoefenaren in Nederland*.
    1868. Introduction by G. A. Lindeboom. Schiedam: Interbook International, 1975.
Bayle, Antoine Laurent Jesse, and Thillaye. *Biographie Médicale par ordre Chronolo-
    gique; D'apres Daniel Leclerc, Éloy, etc*. 2 vols. Paris, 1855.
Bennett, Reginald R. *Medical and Pharmaceutical Latin*. London: J. & A. Churchill,
    1922.
Birch, Thomas. *The History of the Royal Society of London for Improving of Natural
    Knowledge*. 4 vols. 1756–57. Facsimile. Hildesheim: Georg Olms Verlagsbuch-
    handlung, 1968.
Bloom, J. Harvey, and R. Rutson James. *Medical Practitioners in the Diocese of London,
    Licensed Under the Act of 3 Henry VIII, C. 11: An Annotated List 1529–1725*.
    Cambridge: Cambridge University Press, 1935.
Budrys, Stasys, and Valclovas Paprockas, eds. *Alex[ander] Carolus Curtius, Inaugural
    Medical Dissertation on the Kidney and Bladder Stone, Printed in Leiden, 1662*.
    Translated by Anicetas Tamosaitis. Chicago: Lithuanian Medical Association,
    1967.
Callisen, Adolph Carl Peter. *Medicinisches Schriftsteller-Lexicon der Jetzt Leebenden
    Aerzte, Wundarzte, Geburtshelfer, Apotheker, und Naturforscher aller gebildeten
    Volker*. 33 vols. 1830–45. Nieuwkoop: B. de Graaf, 1962–64.
Celsus. *De medicina*. Translated by W. G. Spencer. Cambridge: Harvard University
    Press, 1961.
Cheney, C. R., ed. *Handbook of Dates for Students of English History*. London: Royal
    Historical Society, 1970.
Collection de documents pour servir a l'histoire des hôpitaux de Paris. Paris, 1881.
*A Collection of Ordinances and Regulations for the Government of the Royal Household,
    Made in Divers Reigns. From King Edward III to King William and Queen Mary.
    Also Receipts in Ancient Cookery*. London, 1790.
Dale, Thomas Cyril C., comp. "The Members of the City Companies in 1641 as set forth
    in the return for the poll tax." Society of Genealogists, 1935.
De Beer, E. S., ed. *The Correspondence of John Locke*. 8 vols. Oxford: Clarendon Press,
    1976–89.
————, ed. *The Diary of John Evelyn*. 6 vols. Oxford: Clarendon Press, 1955.
De Smith, S. A. *Judicial Review of Administrative Action*. 3d ed. London: Stevens and
    Sons, 1973.
Dezeimeris, J. E. *Dictionnarie historique de la médecine ancienne et moderne*. 7 vols.
    Paris, 1828–39.
The Diary of Robert Hooke M.A., M.D., F.R.S., 1672–1680. Edited by Henry W.
    Robinson and Walter Adams. London: Taylor and Francis, 1935.

The Diary of Samuel Pepys. Edited by Robert Latham and Williams Matthews. 11 vols. London: G. Bell and Sons, 1970–83.

Dictionary of National Biography. 22 vols. 1890. London: Smith, Elder and Co., 1908.

Dictionnaire de médecine, ou répertoire général des sciences médicales. 2d ed. 30 vols. Paris, 1834.

Dictionnaire des sciences médicales: Biographie médicale. 7 vols. Paris, 1820–25.

Dumbar, Gerhard. *Het Kerkelyk en Wereltlyk Deventer.* 2 vols. Deventer, 1732, 1788.

Elliott, T. H., comp. *State Papers Domestic Concerning the Post Office in the Reign of Charles II.* Introduction by Foster W. Bond. Special Series, no. 20. Postal History Society, 1964.

Eloy, N. F. J. *Dictionnarie historique de la médecine ancienne et moderne: Ou mémoires disposés en ordre alphabétique pour servir a l'histoire de cette science.* 4 vols. Mons, 1778.

English Reports. 178 vols. Edinburgh: William Green and Sons, 1900–1932.

Fockema Andreae, S. J., and Th. J. Meijer. *Album Studiosorum Academiae Franekerensis (1585–1811, 1816–1844).* Franeker: T. Wever, 1969.

Foster, Joseph, comp. and ed. *Alumni Oxonienses, 1500–1714: The Members of the University of Oxford.* 4 vols. Oxford, 1891–92.

Frame, Donald M., ed. *The Complete Works of Montaigne.* Stanford: Stanford University Press, 1943.

Gillispie, C. C., ed. *Dictionary of Scientific Biography.* 18 vols. New York: Scribner's, 1970–90.

The Heidelberg Catechism with Scripture Texts. Grand Rapids: CRC Publications, 1989.

Hessels, Joannes Henricus, ed. *Ecclesiae Londino-Batavae Archivum.* 3 vols. Cambridge, 1887–97.

———, ed. *Register of the Attestations or Certificates of Membership, Confessions of Guilt, Certificates of Marriages, Betrothals, Publication of Banns, Etc. Preserved in the Dutch Reformed Church, Austin Friars, London, 1568 to 1872.* London and Amsterdam, 1892.

Hett, Francis Paget, ed. *The Memoirs of Sir Robert Sibbald (1641–1722).* London: Oxford University Press/Humphrey Milford, 1932.

Hillhouse, James T. *The Grub-Street Journal.* 1928. New York: Benjamin Blom, 1967.

Hippocratic Writings. Edited by G. E. R. Lloyd. Harmondsworth: Penguin, 1978.

Hirsch, August, ed. *Biographisches Lexicon der Hervorragenden Ärzte aller der Zeiten und Völker.* 5 vols. 1884–86. Berlin: Urban & Schwazenberg, 1929–34.

House of Lords Journals. 224 vols. London, HMSO, n.d.

Kennedy, James, W. A. Smith, and A. F. Johnson. *Dictionary of Anonymous and Pseudonymous English Literature, New and Enlarged Edition.* 7 vols. Edinburgh: Oliver and Boyd, 1926–34.

Ketner, F. *Album Promotorum Academiae Rheno-Trajectinae 1636–1815.* Utrecht, 1816.

Keynes, Geoffrey. *The Works of Sir Thomas Browne,* Vol. 4: *Letters.* London: Faber and Faber, 1928.

Knuttel, W. P. C., comp. *Catalogus van de pamfletten-verzameling berustende in de Koninklijke Bibliotheek.* 9 vols. 1890–1920. Utrecht: HES, 1978.

Krivatsy, Peter, comp. *Catalogue of Seventeenth Century Printed Books in the National Library of Medicine*. Bethesda: National Library of Medicine, 1989.

Lindeboom, G. A. *Dutch Medical Biography: A Biographical Dictionary of Dutch Physicians and Surgeons, 1475–1975*. Amsterdam: Rodopi, 1984.

Luttrell, Narcissus. *A Brief Historical Relation of State Affairs from September 1678 to April 1714*. 6 vols. Oxford, 1857.

Mandeville, Bernard. *The Fable of the Bees*. Edited by F. B. Kaye. 2 vols. Oxford: Clarendon Press, 1924.

Mangeti, Joannis Jacobi. *Bibliotheca scriptorum medicorum, veterum et recentiorem*. 2 vols. Geneva, 1731.

Meertens, P. J., ed. *Nederlands repertorium van familienamen*. Vol. 6, *Overijssel*. Assen: Van Gorcum, 1968.

Meynell, G. G. *Materials for a Biography of Dr. Thomas Sydenham*. Folkestone: Winterdown Books, 1988.

Moens, William J. C., ed. *The Marriage, Baptismal, and Burial Registers, 1571 to 1874 . . . of the Dutch Reformed Church, Austin Friars, London*. Lymington, 1884.

Molhuysen, P. C. *Bronnen tot de geschiedenis der Leidsche Universiteit*. 4 vols. The Hague: Martinus Nijhoff, 1913–20.

Munk, W. R. *The Roll of the Royal College of Physicians*. 2 vols. London, 1861.

Nieuw nederlandsch biographisch woordenboek. 10 vols. Leiden: Sijthoff's 1911–37.

Nouvelle biographie générale. 46 vols. Paris, 1855–66.

Opuscula selecta neerlandicorum De Arte Medica. 19 vols. Amsterdam: Sumptibus Societatis, 1907–48.

Ovid. *Ibis*. Edited by Frideric Walther Lenz. Turin: G. B. Paravia, 1956.

Palmer, George Herbert, ed. *The English Works of George Herbert*. Boston and New York: Houghton Mifflin, 1905.

Pharmacopoea Ultrajectina. 1656. Facsimile with introduction by D. A. Wittop Koning. Ghent: Christian de Backer, 1974.

Plomer, H. R. *A Dictionary of the Printers and Booksellers Who Were at Work in England, Scotland, and Ireland from 1668 to 1725*. Bibliographical Society, 1922.

Ploucquet, Guilielmus Godofredus, ed. *Literatura medica digesta*. 4 vols. Tübingen, 1808.

Postma, Coenraad, comp. *Nederland in vroeger tijd: 18e eeuwse beschrijving van steden en dorpen in Nederland*. Vol. 29: *Overijssel*. Zaltbommel: Europese Bibliotheek, 1966.

Poynter, F. N. L., ed. *The Journal of James Yonge*. [1647–1721]. London: Longmans, 1963.

Rijksarchief in Overijssel: Repertorium op de leenregisters van de leen- en hofhorige goederen van de proosdij van St. Lebuinis te Deventer, 1408–1809. 3 Vols. Compiled by Albertus Jans Mensema. Zwolle: 1981.

Schillings, A. *Matricule de L'Université de Louvain*. Brussels: Palais Des Académies, 1963.

Schutte, O. *De Wapenboeken der Gelders-Overijsselse studentenverenigingen*. The Hague: Koninklijk Nederlandsch Genootschap voor Geslacht- en Wapenkunde, 1975.

Shaw, William A., ed. *Letters of Denization and Acts of Naturalization for Aliens in*

England and Ireland, 1603–1700. Publications of the Huguenot Society of London, vol. 18. 1911.

Smit, W. A. P., ed. *Jacobus Revius, Over-Ysselsche sangen en dichten*. 2 vols. Amsterdam: Uitgeversmaatschappij Holland, 1930.

Statutes of the Realm. 9 vols. London, 1810–22.

Stow, John. *Survey of the Cities of London and Westminster*. Edited and augmented by John Strype. 2 vols. London, 1720.

ten Harmsel, Henrietta, ed. and transl. *Jabocus Revius, Dutch Metaphysical Poet: A Parallel Dutch/English Edition; Selected Poems*. Detroit: Wayne State University Press, 1968.

A Transcription of the Registers of the Worshipful Company of Stationers: From 1640–1708 A.D. 3 vols. London: Privately printed, 1913–14.

van Beresteyn, E. A. *Genealogisch repertorium*. The Hague: Centraal Bureau voor Genealogie, 1972.

van der Aa, A. J., ed. *Biographisch woordenboek der Nederlanden*. 12 vols. Haarlem, 1858–78.

Venn, John, and J. A. Venn. *Alumni Cantabrigienses: A Biographical List of All Known Students, Graduates, and Holders of Office at the University of Cambridge, from the Earliest Times to 1900*. 2 vols. Cambridge: Cambridge University Press, 1924–54.

Vigilius von Creutzenfeld, Stephani Hieronymi de. *Bibliotheca chirurgica*. 2 vols. Vienna, 1781.

von Haller, Albertus. *Bibliotheca anatomia: Qua scripta ad anatomen et physiologiam facientia a rerum initiis recensentur*. 2 vols. Zurich, 1774.

———. *Bibliotheca chirurgica: Qua scripta ad artem chirurgicam facientia a rerum initiis recensentur*. 2 vols. Basel and Bern, 1774.

———. *Bibliotheca medicinae practicae qua scripta ad partem medicinae practicam facientia a rerum initiis recensentur*. 4 vols. Bern and Basel, 1779.

Wallis, P. J., and R. V. Wallis, comp. Assisted by T. D. Whittet. *Eighteenth-Century Medics (Subscriptions, Licenses, Apprenticeships)*. Newcastle upon Tyne: Project for Historical Biobibliography, 1985.

Ward, G. R. M., transl. and ed. *Oxford University Statutes*. London, 1845.

Wrop, J. A., ed. *De Briefwisseling van Constantijn Huygens*. Vol. 6, *1663–1687*. The Hague: Martinus Nijhoff, 1917.

SECONDARY SOURCES CITED

Allen, Phyllis. "Medical Education in Seventeenth Century England." *Journal of the History of Medicine* 1 (1946): 115–43.

Appleby, Joyce Oldham. *Economic Thought and Ideology in Seventeenth-Century England*. Princeton, N.J.: Princeton University Press, 1980.

Ashcraft, Richard. *Revolutionary Politics and Locke's "Two Treatises on Government."* Princeton, N.J.: Princeton University Press, 1986.

Ashley, Maurice. *John Wildman, Plotter and Postmaster: A Study of the English Republican Movement in the Seventeenth Century*. London: Jonathan Cape, 1947.

Ashley Montague, M. F. *Edward Tyson, M.D., F.R.S., 1650–1708, and the Rise of Human and Comparative Anatomy in England: A Study in the History of Science.* American Philosophical Society, Memoirs, no. 20. Philadelphia: American Philosophical Society, 1943.

Avalon, J. "Une auto-opération au XVIIe siècle." *Bulletin Société Française d'Histoire de la Médecine* 16 (1922): 309–11.

Aveling, James H. *The Chamberlens and the Midwifery Forceps: Memorials of the Family and an Essay on the Invention of the Instrument.* 1882. New York: Arno Press, 1977.

Bahlman, Dudley W. R. *The Moral Revolution of 1688.* The Wallace Notestein Essays. New Haven: Yale University Press, 1957.

Barlow, Frank. "The King's Evil." *English Historical Review* 95 (1980): 3–27.

Barrett, C. R. B. *The History of the Society of Apothecaries of London.* London: Elliot Stock, 1905.

Bates, Donald G. "Thomas Sydenham: The Development of His Thought, 1666–1676." Ph.D. diss., Johns Hopkins University, 1975.

Batty Shaw, A. "East Anglian Bladder Stone." *Journal of the Royal Society of Medicine* 72 (1979): 222–28.

Baumann, E. D. *François Dele Boe Sylvius.* Leiden: E. J. Brill, 1949.

———. "Job van Meekren." *Nederlandsch tijdschrift voor geneeskunde* 67, no. 5 (1923): 456–79.

Beukers, H. "Clinical Teaching in Leiden from Its Beginning until the End of the Eighteenth Century." *Clio Medica* 21 (1987–88): 139–52.

———. "Het laboratorium van Sylvius." *Tijdschrift voor de geschiedenis der geneeskunde, natuurwetenschappen, wiskunde, en techniek* 3 (1980): 28–36.

———. "Mechanistiche principes bij Franciscus dele Boë, Sylvius." *Tijdschrift voor de geschiedenis der geneeskunde, natuurwetenschappen, wiskunde en techniek* 5 (1982): 6–15.

Birken, William. "Dr. John King (1614–1681) and Dr. Assuerus Regimorter (1615–1650)." *Medical History* 20 (1976): 276–95.

Bitter, H. "Stadsoperateurs en steensnijders in de 17de en 18de Eeuw, te Haarlem." *Nederlands Tijdschrift voor Geneeskunde* 58, no. 2 (1914): 568–76.

Bloch, Marc. *The Royal Touch: Sacred Monarchy and Scrofula in England and France.* French ed. 1961. Translated by J. E. Anderson. London: Routledge and Kegan Paul, 1973.

Blockmans, Wim. "Corruptie, patronage, makelaardij, en venaliteit als symptomen van een ontluikende staatsvorming in de Bourgondisch-Habsburgse Nederlanden." *Tijdschrift voor sociale geschiedenis* 11 (1985): 231–47.

Boerma, N. J. A. F. "Wondergeval van Jan de Dood, een smit t' Amsterdam 1651." *Nederlandsch tijdschrift voor geneeskunde* 85, no. 3 (1941): 3631.

Boulton, Jeremy. *Neighbourhood and Society: A London Suburb in the Seventeenth Century.* Cambridge: Cambridge University Press, 1987.

Boxer, Chalres R. *The Dutch Seaborne Empire, 1600–1800.* London: Hutchinson, 1965.

Boys, Richard C. *Sir Richard Blackmore and the Wits: A Study of "Commendatory Verses on the Author of the Two Arthurs" and the "Satyr against Wit" (1700).* University of Michigan Contributions in Modern Philology. Ann Arbor: University of Michigan Press, 1949.

Brewer, John. *The Sinews of Power: War, Money, and the English State, 1688–1783*. London: Unwin Hyman, 1989.

Brockliss, L. W. B. "The Development of the Spa in Seventeenth-Century France." In *The Medical History of Waters and Spas*, edited by Roy Porter, 23–47. Medical History Supplements, no. 10. London: Wellcome Institute for the History of Medicine, 1990.

Brugmans, H., ed. *Gedenkboek van het Athenaeum en de Universiteit van Amsterdam, 1632–1932*. Amsterdam: Stadsdrukerij, 1932.

Bussemaker, Cavel Hendrik Theodoor. *Geschiedenis van Overijssel gedurende het eerste stadhouderlooze tijdperk*. The Hague, 1888–89.

Bylebyl, Jerome J. "Galen on the Non-Natural Causes of Variation in the Pulse." *Bulletin of the History of Medicine* 45 (1971): 482–85.

Cameron, James K. "Humanism in the Low Countries." In *The Impact of Humanism on Western Europe*, edited by Anthony Goodman and Angus MacKay, 137–63. London: Longman, 1990.

Carrubba, Robert W., and John W. Bowers. "The Western World's First Detailed Treatise on Acupuncture: Willem Ten Rhijne's *De Acupunctura*." *Journal of the History of Medicine* 29 (1974): 371–97.

Carter, Richard B. *Descartes' Medical Philosophy: The Organic Solution to the Mind-Body Problem*. Baltimore: Johns Hopkins University Press, 1983.

Clark, George N. *A History of the Royal College of Physicians of London*. 2 vols. Oxford: Clarendon Press, 1964–66.

Colie, Rosalie L. *Light and Enlightenment: A Study of the Cambridge Platonists and the Dutch Arminians*. Cambridge: Cambridge University Press, 1957.

Cook, Harold J. " 'Against Common Right and Reason': The College of Physicians against Dr. Thomas Bonham." *American Journal of Legal History* 29 (1985): 301–22.

———. *The Decline of the Old Medical Regime in Stuart London*. Ithaca, N.Y.: Cornell University Press, 1986.

———. "Good Advice and Little Medicine: The Professional Authority of Early Modern English Physicians." *Journal of British Studies* 33 (1994): 1–31.

———. "Living in Revolutionary Times: Medical Change under William and Mary." In *Patronage and Institutions: Science, Technology, and Medicine at the European Court, 1500–1750*, edited by Bruce T. Moran, 111–35. Woodbridge: Boydell, 1991.

———. "Medical Innovation or Medical Malpractice? Or, a Dutch Physician in London: The Case of Joannes Groenevelt, 1694–1700." *Tractrix* 2 (1990): 63–91.

———. "The New Philosophy and Medicine in Seventeenth-Century England." In *Reappraisals of the Scientific Revolution*, edited by David C. Lindberg and Robert S. Westman, 397–436. Cambridge: Cambridge University Press, 1990.

———. "Physicians and the New Philosophy: Henry Stubbe and the Virtuosi-Physicians." In *Medical Revolution in the Seventeenth Century*, edited by Roger French and Andrew Wear, 246–71. Cambridge: Cambridge University Press, 1989.

————. "Physick and Natural History in Seventeenth-Century England." In *Revolution and Continuity: Essays in the History and Philosophy of Early Modern Science,* edited by Peter Barker and Roger Ariew, 63–80. Studies in Philosophy and the History of Philosophy, vol. 24. Washington, D.C.: Catholic University Press of America, 1991.

————. "Policing the Health of London: The College of Physicians and the Early Stuart Monarchy." *Social History of Medicine* 2 (1989): 1–33.

————. "Practical Medicine and the British Armed Forces after the 'Glorious Revolution.' " *Medical History* 34 (1990): 1–26.

————. "The Rose Case Reconsidered: Physic and the Law in Augustan England." *Journal of the History of Medicine* 45 (1990): 527–55.

————. "Sir John Colbatch and Augustan Medicine: Experimentalism, Character, and Entrepreneurialism." *Annals of Science* 47 (1990): 475–505.

————. "The Troubles of Adriaan Huyberts in London: A Clash of Medical Ideas and Medical Values" (forthcoming).

Cook, Richard I. *Bernard Mandeville.* New York: Twayne Publishers, 1974.

Cope, Zachary. *William Cheselden, 1688–1752.* Edinburgh and London: E. & S. Livingstone, 1953.

Cranston, Maurice. *John Locke: A Biography.* 1957. London: Longmans, 1966.

Crosse, John Green. *A Treatise of the Formation, Constituents, and Extraction of the Urinary Calculus.* London, 1841.

Cummins, S. Lyle. "Some Early British Phthisiologists." *Proceedings of the Royal Society of Medicine* 37 (1944): 517–24.

Cunningham, Andrew. "Sir Robert Sibbald and Medical Education, Edinburgh, 1706." *Clio Medica* 13 (1978): 135–61.

————. "Thomas Sydenham: Epidemics, Experiment, and the 'Good Old Cause.' " In *The Medical Revolution of the Seventeenth Century,* edited by Roger French and Andrew Wear, 164–90. Cambridge: Cambridge University Press, 1989.

Dankmeijer, J. "De biologische studies van René Descartes." *Leidse voordrachten,* no. 9. Leiden: Universitaire Pers, 1951.

Darnton, Robert. *The Great Cat Massacre and Other Episodes in French Cultural History.* New York: Basic Books, 1984.

Davis, Natalie Zemon. *The Return of Martin Guerre.* Cambridge: Harvard University Press, 1983.

De Beer, E. S. "The English Newspapers from 1695 to 1702." In *William III and Louis XIV: Essays 1680–1720 by and for Mark A. Thomson,* edited by R. Hatton and J. S. Bromley, 117–29. Liverpool: Liverpool University Press, 1968.

De Booy, Engelina Petronella. *De weldaet der scholen: Het plattelandsonderwijs in de Provincie Utrecht van 1580 tot het begin der 19de eeuw.* Stichtse Historische Reeks, no. 3. 1977.

————. *Kweekhoven der wijshied: Basis- en vervolgonderwijs in de steden van de provincie Utrecht van 1580 tot het begin der 19e eeuw.* Stichtse Historische Reeks, no. 5. Zutphen: De Walburg Pers, 1980.

de Hoog, Adriaan Cornelius. *Some Currents of Thought in Dutch Natural Philosophy: 1675–1720.* D.Phil. thesis, Oxford University, 1974.

De Hullu. "Bijdrage tot de kerkelijke geschiedenis van Deventer, 1578–1587." *Archief voor de geschiedenis van het Aartsbisdom van het Utrecht* 41 (1915): 1–51.

de Jong, Henk J. "The Study of the New Testament in the Dutch Universities, 1575–1700." *History of Universities* 1 (1981): 113–29.

De Krey, Gary Stuart. *A Fractured Society: The Politics of London in the First Age of Party, 1688–1715.* Oxford: Clarendon Press, 1985.

de Lint, J. "Comment Jan De Doot, Forgeron, S'Opéra D'un Calcul de la Vessie." *Asculape* 18 (1928): 50–53.

de Moulin, Daniel. "Paul Barbette, M.D.: A Seventeenth-Century Amsterdam Author of Bestselling Textbooks." *Bulletin of the History of Medicine* 59 (1985): 506–14.

De Vries, Jan. *Barges and Capitalism: Passenger Transportation in the Dutch Economy (1632–1839).* Utrecht: H&S, 1981.

———. *The Dutch Rural Economy in the Golden Age, 1500–1700.* New Haven: Yale University Press, 1974.

———. *European Urbanization, 1500–1800.* Harvard Studies in Urban History. Cambridge: Harvard University Press, 1984.

———. "On the Modernity of the Dutch Republic." *Journal of Economic History* 32 (1973): 191–202.

Dewhurst, Kenneth. "Dr. Robert Pitt's Letters to John Locke." *Saint Bartholomew's Hospital Journal*, no. 11 (1962): 258–67.

———. *Dr. Thomas Sydenham (1624–1689): His Life and Original Writings.* Berkeley and Los Angeles: University of California Press, 1966.

———. *John Locke (1632–1704), Physician and Philosopher: A Medical Biography, with an Edition of the Medical Notes in His Journals.* London: Wellcome Historical Medical Library, 1963.

Dibon, Paul. *La philosophie néerlandaise au siècle d'or.* Paris: Elsevier, 1954.

Dijkstra, Jan Gerard. *Een epidemiologische beschowing van de Nederlandsche pest-epidemieën der XVIIde eeuw.* Amsterdam: Volharding, 1921.

Dollinger, Phillippe. *The German Hansa.* Translated and edited by D. S. Ault and S. H. Steinberg. Stanford: Stanford University Press, 1970.

Duffy, Eamon. "Valentine Greatrakes, the Irish Stroker: Miracle, Science, and Othodoxy in Restoration England." *Studies in Church History* 17 (1981): 251–73.

Ekberg, Carl J. *The Failure of Louis XIV's Dutch War.* Chapel Hill: University of North Carolina Press, 1979.

Ellis, Frank H. "The Background to the London Dispensary." *Journal of the History of Medicine* 20 (1965): 197–212.

———. "Garth's Harveian Oration." *Journal of the History of Medicine* 18 (1963): 8–19.

Ellis, Harold. *A History of Bladder Stone.* Oxford and Edinburgh: Blackwell, 1969.

Fisher, F. J. *London and the English Economy, 1500–1700.* Edited by P. J. Corfield and N. B. Harte. London: Hambledon, 1991.

Fix, Andrew C. *Prophecy and Reason: The Dutch Collegiants in the Early Enlightenment.* Princeton, N.J.: Princeton University Press, 1991.

Formsma, W. J. "De nieuwe geschiedenis, staatkundig beschouwd." In *Geschiedenis van Overijssel*, edited by B. H. Slicher van Bath, 119–35. Deventer: Kluwer, 1970.

Fortgens, H. W. *Schola Latina: uit het verleden van ons voorbereidend hoger onderwijs.* Zwolle: Mij. W. E. J. Tjeenk Willink, 1958.

Foxon, D. F. "Libertine Literature in England, 1660–1745." *Book Collector* 12 (1963): 21–36.

Frank, Robert G., Jr. "The Image of Harvey in Commonwealth and Restoration England." In *William Harvey and His Age,* edited by J. J. Bylebyl, 103–43. Baltimore: Johns Hopkins University Press, 1979.

French, Roger. "Harvey in Holland: Circulation and the Calvinists." In *The Medical Revolution of the Seventeenth Century.* Edited by Roger French and Andrew Wear, 46–86. Cambridge: Cambridge University Press, 1989.

Frijhoff, Willem Th. M. "Deventer en zijn gemiste universiteit: Het Athenaeum in de sociaal-culturele geschiedenis van Overijssel." *Overijsselse Historische Bijdragen* 97 (1982): 45–79.

———. *La Société Néerlandaise et ses gradués, 1575–1814: Une Recherche sérielle sur le statut des intellectuels à pertir des registres universitaires.* Amsterdam: APA–Holland University Press, 1981.

———. " 'Non satis dignitatis . . .': Over de maatschappelijke status van geneeskundigen tijdens de Republiek." *Tijdschrift voor geschiedenis* 96 (1983): 379–406.

———. "Wetenschap, beroep en status ten tijde van de Republiek: De intellectueel." *Tijdschrift voor de geschiedenis der geneeskunde, natuurwetenschappen, wiskunde, en techniek* 6 (1983): 18–30.

Frijhoff, W. Th. M., B. Looper, J. van der Kluit, C. E. M. Reinders, R. C. C. de Savornin Lohman, F. W. J. Scholten, and R. Wartena, eds. *Geschiedenis van Zutphen.* Zutphen: De Walburg Pers, 1989.

Fruin, R. *The Siege and Relief of Leyden in 1574.* Translated by Elizabeth Trevelyn. With an introduction by George Macaulay Trevelyan. The Hague: Martinus Nijhoff, 1927.

Geertz, Clifford. *The Interpretation of Cultures: Selected Essays.* New York: Basic Books, 1973.

Geyl, A. *De geschiedenis van het Roonhuysiaansch geheim.* Rotterdam: Meidert Boogaerdt, 1905.

Geyl, Pieter. *The Netherlands in the Seventeenth Century: Part Two, 1648–1715.* New York: Barnes and Noble, 1964.

———. *Orange and Stuart, 1641–1672.* Translated by Arnold Pomerans. New York: Scribner's, 1969.

———. *The Revolt of the Netherlands, 1555–1609.* 1932. New York: Barnes and Noble, 1958.

Gijswijt-Hofstra, Marijke, and Willem Frijhoff, eds. *Witchcraft in the Netherlands, Fourteenth to Twentieth Centuries.* Rotterdam: Universitaire Pers Rotterdam, 1990.

Ginzburg, Carlo. *The Cheese and the Worms: The Cosmos of a Sixteenth-Century Miller.* Translated by John Tedeschi and Anne Tedeschi. Baltimore: Johns Hopkins University Press, 1982.

Goldsmith, M. M. *Private Vices, Public Benefits: Bernard Mandeville's Social and Political Thought.* Cambridge: Cambridge University Press, 1985.

———. "Regulating Anew the Moral and Political Sentiments of Mankind: Bernard

Mandeville and the Scottish Enlightenment." *Journal of the History of Ideas* 49 (1988): 587–606.

Gottlieb, Paula. "Aristotle and Protagoras: The Good Human Being as a Measure of Goods." *Aperion* 24 (1991): 25–45.

Grafton, Anthony. "Civic Humanism and Scientific Scholarship at Leiden." In *The University and the City: From Medieval Origins to the Present,* edited by Thomas Bender, 59–78. New York: Oxford University Press, 1989.

———. *Joseph Scaliger: A Study in the History of Classical Scholarship.* Vol. 1: *Textual Criticism and Exegesis.* Oxford: Clarendon Press, 1983.

Grafton, A., and L. Jardine. *From Humanism to the Humanities: Education and the Liberal Arts in Fifteenth- and Sixteenth-Century Europe.* Cambridge: Cambridge University Press, 1986.

Grell, Ole Peter. *Dutch Calvinists in Early Stuart London: The Dutch Church in Austin Friars, 1603–1642.* Leiden: E. J. Brill, 1989.

Groenhuis, Gerrit. *De Predikanten: De sociale positie van de gereformeerde predikanten in de Republiek der Verenigde Nederlanden voor + − 1700.* Groningen: Wolters-Noordhoff, 1977.

Habermas, Jürgen. *The Structural Transformation of the Public Sphere: An Inquiry into a Category of Bourgeois Society.* 1962. Translated by Thomas Burger. Assisted by Frederick Lawrence. Cambridge: MIT Press, 1989.

Haley, K. H. D. *The British and the Dutch: Political and Cultural Relations through the Ages.* London: George Philip, 1988.

———. *An English Diplomat in the Low Countries: Sir William Temple and John De Witt, 1665–1672.* Oxford: Clarendon Press, 1986.

Hall, A. Rupert, and Marie Boas Hall, eds. *The Correspondence of Henry Oldenburg.* 13 vols. Madison: University of Wisconsin Press; London: Mansell, and Taylor and Francis, 1965–86.

Hall, Marie Boas. "Acid and Alkali in Seventeenth Century Chemistry." *Archives internationales d'histoire des sciences* 34 (1956): 13–28.

Harris, Michael. *London Newspapers in the Age of Walpole: A Study in the Origins of the Modern English Press.* Cranbury, N.J.: Associated University Presses, 1987.

Hart, Simon. *Geschrift en Getal: Een keuze uit de demografisch-, economisch- en sociaal-historische studiën op grond van Amsterdamse en Zaanse archivalia, 1600–1800.* Dordrecht: Historische Vereninging Holland, 1976.

Haver Droeze, J. J. *Het Collegium Medicum Amstelaedamense, 1637–1798.* Haarlem: De Erven F. Bohn, 1921.

Hofman, J. H., ed. "Deventer in de tweede helft der 16e eeuw en daarna." *Archief voor de geschiedenis van het Aartsbisdom Utrecht* 19 (1892): 337–419.

Hoppen, K. Theodore. *The Common Scientist in the Seventeenth Century: A Study of the Dublin Philosophical Society, 1683–1708.* Charlottesville: University Press of Virginia, 1970.

Houck, M. E., and Ch. Dixon. *Deventer onder de Stadhouders uit het Huis van Oranje.* Deventer, 1898.

Howell, Wilbur S. *Logic and Rhetoric in England, 1500–1700.* 1956. New York: Russell and Russell, 1961.

Huizinga, Johan. *Erasmus and the Age of Reformation.* 1924. Translated by F. Hopman. New York: Harper Torchbook, 1957.

Hunter, Michael. *Establishing the New Science: The Experience of the Early Royal Society.* Woodbridge: Boydell, 1989.

―――. *The Royal Society and Its Fellows, 1660–1700: The Morphology of an Early Scientific Institution.* Chalfont St. Giles: British Society for the History of Science, 1982.

Imhof, Arthur E. "From the Old Mortality Pattern to the New: Implications of a Radical Change from the Sixteenth to the Twentieth Century." *Bulletin of the History of Medicine* 59 (1985): 1–29.

Israel, Jonathan I. *The Anglo-Dutch Moment: Essays on the Glorious Revolution and Its World Impact.* Cambridge: Cambridge University Press, 1991.

―――. *European Jewry in the Age of Merchantilism, 1550–1750.* Oxford: Clarendon Press, 1985.

Jaffe, Louis L., and Edith G. Henderson, "Judicial Review and the Rule of Law: Historical Origins." *Law Quarterly Review* 72 (1956): 345–64.

Jappe Alberts, W. *De Nederlandse Hanzesteden.* Bussum: Fibula-Van Dishoeck, 1969.

Jellicoe, Sidney. *The Septuagint and Modern Study.* Oxford: Clarendon Press, 1968.

Jensma, G. Th., F. R. H. Smit, and F. Westra, eds. *Universiteit te Franeker, 1585–1811: Bijdragen tot de geschiedenis van de Friese Hogeschool.* Leeuwarden: Fryske Akademy, 1985.

Jones, Ellis. "The Life and Works of Guilhelmus Fabricius Hildanus (1560–1634)." *Medical History* 4 (1960): 112–34, 196–209.

Jones, Peter Murray. "Thomas Lorkyn's Dissections, 1564/5 and 1566/7." *Transactions of the Cambridge Bibliographical Society* 9 (1988): 209–29.

Jurriaanse, M. W. *The Founding of Leyden University.* Translated by J. Brotherhood. Leiden: E. J. Brill, 1965.

Justin-Godart, M. "L'Opération de la taille mise en musique par un compositeur du dix-huitième siècle: Marin Marais (1656–1728)." *Histoire de la médecine* 4 (December 1954): 27–35.

Karstens, W. K. H., and Herman Kleibrink. *De Leidse Hortus: Een botanische erfenis.* Uitgeverij Waanders, 1984.

Keevil, John J. *Hamey the Stranger.* London: G. Bles, 1952.

―――. *The Stranger's Son.* London: G. Bles, 1953.

Kerkhoff, A. H. M. *Over de geneeskundige vergorging in het staatse leger.* Nijmegen: R. Tissen et al., 1976.

Keuning, H. J. *Kaleidoscoop der Nederlandse landschappen: De regionale verscheidenheid van Nederland in historisch-geographisch perspectief.* The Hague: Martinus Nijhoff, 1979.

King, Lester S. *The Road to Medical Enlightenment, 1650–1695.* New York: American Elsevier, 1970.

Koch, A. C. F. "The Reformation in Deventer in 1579–1580: Size and Social Structure of the Catholic Section of the Population during the Religious Peace." *Acta Historiae Neerlandicae* 6 (1976): 27–66.

Laguette, J. A. Ph. "Beleg en herovering van Grave in 1674." *Militaire spectator* 143 (1974): 547–56.

Landes, David S. *Revolution in Time: Clocks and the Making of the Modern World.* Cambridge: Harvard University Press, Belknap Press, 1983.

Latour, Bruno. *Science in Action: How to Follow Scientists and Engineers through Society.* Cambridge: Harvard University Press, 1987.

Lawler, John. *Book Auctions in England in the Seventeenth Century (1676–1700).* London, 1898.

Lewis, Gillian. "The Faculty of Medicine." In *History of the University of Oxford,* vol. 3: *The Collegiate University,* edited by J. K. McConica, 213–56. Oxford: Clarendon Press, 1986.

Lindeboom, G. A. *Descartes and Medicine.* Amsterdam: Rodopi, 1979.

———. "Dog and Frog: Physiological Experiments." In *Leiden University in the Seventeenth Century: An Exchange of Learning,* edited by Th. H. Lunsingh Scheurleer and G. H. M. Posthumus Meyjes, 279–93. Leiden: Universitaire Pers, E. J. Brill, 1975.

———. *Florentius Schuyl (1619–1669) en zijn betekenis voor het Cartesianisme in de geneeskunde.* The Hague: Martinus Nijhoff, 1974.

———. *Herman Boerhaave: The Man and His Work.* Forward by E. Ashworth Underwood. London: Methuen, 1968.

———. "Jan Swammerdam als microscopist." *Tijdschrift voor de geschiedenis der geneeskunde, natuurwetenschappen, wiskunde en techniek* 4 (1981): 87–110.

———. "Medical Education in the Netherlands, 1575–1750." In *The History of Medical Education,* edited by C. D. O'Malley, 201–16. Berkeley and Los Angeles: University of California Press, 1970.

———, ed. and comp. *Ontmoeting met Jan Swammerdam.* Ontmoetingen met Mystici, no. 3. Kampen: Uitgeversmaatschappij J. H. Kok, 1980.

Lindeboom, Johannes. *Austin Friars: History of the Dutch Reformed Church in London, 1550–1950.* Translated by B. D. De Iongh. The Hague: Martinus Nijhoff, 1950.

Lloyd, G. E. R. *Science, Folklore and Ideology.* Cambridge: Cambridge University Press, 1983.

———, ed. *Hippocratic Writings.* Harmondsworth: Penguin, 1978.

Longfield-Jones, G. M. "Buccaneering Doctors." *Medical History* 36 (1992): 187–206.

Lonie, Ian M. "The 'Paris Hippocrates': Teaching and Research in Paris in the Second Half of the Sixteenth Century." In *The Medical Renaissance of the Sixteenth Century,* edited by Andrew Wear, Roger K. French, and Ian M. Lonie, 155–74, 318–26. Cambridge: Cambridge University Press, 1985.

Lovejoy, Arthur O. *The Great Chain of Being: A Study of the History of an Idea.* Cambridge: Harvard University Press, 1942.

Lunsingh Scheurleer, Th. H., and G. H. M. Posthumus Meyjes, eds. *Leiden University in the Seventeenth Century: An Exchange of Learning.* Leiden: Universitaire Pers, E. J. Brill, 1975.

Luyendijk-Elshout, Antonie M. "Death Enlightened: A Study of Frederik Ruysch." *Journal of the American Medical Association* 212, no. 1 (1970): 121–26.

McAdoo, H. R. *The Structure of Caroline Moral Theology.* London: Longmans, Green, 1949.

MacFarlane, A. D. J. *Witchcraft in Tudor and Stuart England.* London: Routledge and Kegan Paul, 1970.

McGahagan, T. A. "Cartesianism in the Netherlands, 1639–1675: The New Science and the Calvinist Counter-reformation." Ph.D. diss., University of Pennsylvania, 1976.

McInnes, E. M. St. Thomas' Hospital. London: George Allen and Unwin, 1963.

McLaren, Angus. A History of Contraception: From Antiquity to the Present Day. Oxford: Blackwell, 1990.

Matthews, Leslie G. "Philip Guide, Huguenot Refugee Doctor of Medicine (c. 1640–1716)." Proceedings of the Huguenot Society of London 22 (1974): 345–52.

Mayhew, Henry, and John Binny. The Criminal Prisons of London and Scenes of Prison Life. 1862. London: Frank Cass, 1968.

Mayr, Otto. Authority, Liberty, and Automatic Machinery in Early Modern Europe. Baltimore: Johns Hopkins University Press, 1986.

Metzger, Hélène. Les doctrines chimiques en France du début du XVIIe à fin du XVIIIe siècle. Paris: Libraire Scientifique et Technique, 1969.

Meynell, G. G. Materials for a Biography of Dr. Thomas Sydenham. Folkestone: Winterdown Books, 1988.

Monro, Hector. The Ambivalence of Bernard Mandeville. Oxford: Clarendon Press, 1975.

Moore, Norman. The History of St. Bartholomew's Hospital. 2 vols. London: C. Arthur Pearson, 1918.

Moran, Bruce T. The Alchemical World of the German Court: Occult Philosophy and Chemical Medicine in the Circle of Moritz of Hessen (1572–1632). Sudhoffs Archiv, Beiheft 29. Stuttgart: Franz Steiner Verlag, 1991.

Muir, Edward, and Guido Ruggiero. Microhistory and the Lost Peoples of Europe. Translated by Eren Branch. Baltimore: Johns Hopkins University Press, 1991.

Murray, John J. Flanders and England: A Cultural Bridge; the Influence of the Low Countries on Tudor-Stuart England. Antwerp: Fonds Mercator, 1985.

Napjus, J. W. De hoogleeraren in de geneeskunde aan de hogeschool en het athenaeum te Franeker. Edited by G. A. Lindeboom. Nieuwe Nederlandse Bijdragen tot de Geschiedenis der Geneeskunde en der Natuurwetenschappen, no. 15. Amsterdam: Rodopi, 1985.

Neibyl, P. H. "The Non-Naturals." Bulletin of the History of Medicine 45 (1971): 486–92.

Nijenhuis, W. "Variants within Dutch Calvinism in the Sixteenth Century." Low Countries History Yearbook 12 (1979): 48–64.

Noorthouck, John. A New History of London, including Westminster and Southwark. London, 1773.

Nöske, Hans-Dieter. Lithotomia Vesicae. Munich: Zuckeschwerdt, 1982.

Nutton, Vivian. "Hippocrates in the Renaissance." In Die Hippokratischen Epidemien: Theorie—praxis—tradition, edited by Gerhard Baader and Rolf Winau, 420–39. Sudhoffs Archiv, Beiheft. Stuttgart: Franz Steiner Verlag, 1990.

Oberman, Heiko A. Devotio Moderna: Basic Writings. Translated by John van Engen. New York: Paulist Press, 1988.

O'Malley, Charles D., ed. The History of Medical Education. Berkeley and Los Angeles: University of California Press, 1970.

Ong, Walter J. Ramus: Method, and the Decay of Dialogue: From the Art of Discourse to the Art of Reason. 1958. Cambridge: Harvard University Press, 1983.

———. Ramus and Talon Inventory. Cambridge: Harvard University Press, 1958.

Ottley, Richard R. *A Handbook to the Septuagint*. London: Methuen, 1920.

————. *An Introduction to the Old Testament in Greek*. 2d ed. Cambridge: Cambridge University Press, 1914.

Pagel, Walter. *Paracelsus: An Introduction to Philosophical Medicine in the Era of the Renaissance*. New York: S. Karger, 1958.

Palm, L. C. "Italian Influences on Antoni van Leeuwenhoek." In *Italian Scientists in the Low Countries in the Seventeenth and Eighteenth Centuries*, edited by C. S. Maffioli and L. C. Palm, 147–63. Amsterdam: Rodopi, 1989.

Parker, Geoffrey. *The Dutch Revolt*. 1977. Harmondsworth: Penguin, 1985.

Parsons, F. G. *The History of St. Thomas's Hospital*. 3 vols. London: Methuen, 1932–36.

Patist, C. R. *Het beleg van de stad Grave in 1674*. Nijmegen: U.H.N., 1974.

Peachey, G. C. "The Two John Peacheys, Seventeenth Century Physicians: Their Lives and Times." *Janus* 23 (1918): 121–41.

Pettegree, Andrew. *Foreign Protestant Communities in Sixteenth-Century London*. Oxford: Clarendon Press, 1986.

Phelps Brown, E. H., and S. V. Hopkins, "Seven Centuries of Building Wages." In *Essays in Economic History*, edited by E. M. Carus-Wilson, 2:168–78. London, 1954–62.

————. "Seven Centuries of the Prices of Consumables Compared with Builders' Wage Rates." In *Essays in Economic History*, edited by E. M. Carus-Wilson, 2:179–96. London, 1954–62.

Pinto, John D., and Richard B. Selander. *The Bionomics of Blister Beetles of the Genus "Meloe" and a Classification of the New World Species*. Illinois Biological Monographs, no. 4. Urbana: University of Illinois Press, 1970.

Porter, Dorothy, and Roy Porter. *Patient's Progress: Doctors and Doctoring in Eighteenth-Century England*. Stanford: Stanford University Press, 1989.

Porter, Roy. *Health for Sale: Quackery in England, 1650–1850*. Manchester: Manchester University Press, 1989.

————. "The Patient's View: Doing Medical History from Below." *Theory and Society* 14 (1985): 175–98.

————, ed. *The Medical History of Waters and Spas*. Medical History Supplements, no. 10. London: Wellcome Institute for the History of Medicine, 1990.

————, ed. *Patients and Practitioners: Lay Perceptions of Medicine in Pre-industrial Society*. Cambridge: Cambridge University Press, 1985.

Post, Regnerus Richardus. *The Modern Devotion: Confrontation with Reformation and Humanism*. Leiden: E. J. Brill, 1968.

Posthumus, N. W. *Inquiry into the History of Prices in Holland*. 2 vols. Leiden: E. J. Brill, 1946–64.

Posthumus Meijes, E. J. W. *Jacobus Revius, zijn leven en werken*. 2 vols. Amsterdam, 1895.

Postma, F. "Nieuw licht op een oude zaak: De oprichting van de nieuwe bisdommen in 1559." *Tijdschrift voor geschiedenis* 103 (1990): 10–27.

Power, D'Arcy. *A Short History of Surgery*. London: John Bale and Sons, 1933.

Poynter, F. N. L., ed. *The Evolution of Medical Education in Britain*. London: Pitman, 1966.

Prest, John. *The Garden of Eden: The Botanic Garden and the Re-creation of Paradise.*
New Haven: Yale University Press, 1981.

Purver, Margery. *The Royal Society: Concept and Creation.* London: Routledge and
Kegan Paul, 1967.

Rather, L. J. "The 'Six Things Non-Natural': A Note on the Origin and Fate of a Doctrine
and a Phrase." *Clio Medica* 3 (1968): 337–47.

Rattansi, P. M. "Paracelsus and the Puritan Revolution." *Ambix* 11 (1963): 24–32.

Raymond, Georges. "La lithotomie musciale ou le théâtre de l'opération de la taille de
Marin Marais." *Histoire des sciences médicales* 22 (1988): 141–49.

Regin, Deric. *Traders, Artists, Burghers: A Cultural History of Amsterdam in the Seventeenth Century.* Assen and Amsterdam: Van Gorcum, 1976.

Reitsma, Rients. *Centrifugal and Centripetal Forces in the Early Dutch Republic: The
States of Overijssel, 1566–1600.* Amsterdam: Rodopi, 1982.

Risse, Guenter B. *Hospital Life in Enlightenment Scotland: Care and Teaching at the
Royal Infirmary of Edinburgh.* Cambridge: Cambridge University Press, 1986.

Robb-Smith, A. H. T. "Cambridge Medicine." In *Medicine in Seventeenth-Century England,* edited by Allen G. Debus, 327–69. Berkeley and Los Angeles: University
of California Press, 1974.

Robinson, Howard. *Britain's Post Office: A History of Development from the Beginnings
to the Present Day.* London: Oxford University Press, 1953.

Rodríguez-Salgado, M. J. *The Changing Face of Empire: Charles V, Philip II, and
Habsburg Authority, 1551–1559.* Cambridge: Cambridge University Press, 1988.

Rogers, Pat. *Grub Street: Studies in a Subculture.* London: Methuen, 1972.

Rook, Arthur. "Medical Education at Cambridge, 1600–1800." In *Cambridge and Its
Contribution to Medicine,* edited by Arthur Rook, 49–64. London: Wellcome
Institute for the History of Medicine, 1971.

Rosen, George. "Sir William Temple and the Therapeutic Use of Moxa for Gout in
England." *Bulletin of the History of Medicine* 44 (1970): 31–39.

Rosenberg, Albert. "The London Dispensary for the Sick-poor." *Journal of the History
of Medicine* 14 (1959): 41–56.

Rosenberg, Aubrey. *Tyssot de Patot and His Work, 1655–1738.* The Hague: Martinus
Nijhoff, 1972.

Rowen, Herbert H. *John de Witt, Grand Pensionary of Holland, 1625–1672.* Princeton,
N.J.: Princeton University Press, 1978.

———. *The Princes of Orange: The Stadholders in the Dutch Republic.* Cambridge:
Cambridge University Press, 1988.

Ruestow, Edward Grant. *Physics at Seventeenth and Eighteenth Century Leiden.* The
Hague: Martinus Nijhoff, 1973.

———. "The Rise of the Doctrine of Vascular Secretion in the Netherlands." *Journal
of the History of Medicine* 35 (1980): 265–87.

Russell, Andrew W., ed. *The Town and State Physician in Europe from the Middle Ages
to the Enlightenment.* Wolfenbütteler Forschungen. Wolfenbüttel: Herzog August
Bibliothek, 1981.

Russell, K. F. "A Seventeenth Century Surgeon, Anatomist, and Plagiarist." *Bulletin of
the History of Medicine* 33 (1959): 393–414, 503–25.

Schama, Simon. *An Embarrassment of Riches: An Interpretation of Dutch Culture in the Golden Age.* New York: Knopf, 1987.

Schenkeveld, Maria A. *Dutch Literature in the Age of Rembrandt: Themes and Ideas.* Amsterdam and Philadelphia: John Benjamins, 1991.

Schöffer, I., H. Van der Wee, and J. A. Bornewasser, eds. *De lage landen van 1500 tot 1780.* Amsterdam: Elsevier, 1983.

Schokkaert, E., and H. Van der Wee. "A Quantitative Study of Food Consumption in the Low Countries during the Sixteenth Century." *Journal of European Economic History* 17 (1988): 131–58.

Seaver, Paul. *Wallington's World: A Puritan Artisan in Seventeenth-Century London.* Stanford: Stanford University Press, 1985.

Sharp, Buchanan. "Popular Political Opinion in England, 1660–1685." *History of European Ideas* 10 (1989): 13–29.

Sherman, Nancy. *The Fabric of Character: Aristotle's Theory of Virtue.* Oxford: Clarendon Press, 1989.

Sigerist, Henry E. "Alexandre Ricord's Dissertation of 1824." *Bulletin of the History of Medicine* 9 (1941): 468–74.

Singer, Charles. "Benjamen Marten, a Neglected Predecessor of Louis Pasteur." *Janus* 16 (1911): 81–98.

Slicher van Bath, B. H., G. D. Van der Heide, C. C. W. J. Hijszelere, A. C. F. Koch, E. C. Maschewski, and E. Vroom, eds. *Geschiedenis van Overijssel.* Deventer: Kluwer, 1970.

Smith, Wesley D. *The Hippocratic Tradition.* Ithaca, N.Y.: Cornell University Press, 1979.

Solomon, Harry M. *Sir Richard Blackmore.* Boston: Twayne, 1980.

Sondervost, F.-A. *Geschiedenis van de geneeskunde in België.* Brussels: Elsevier, 1981.

———. *Histoire de la médicine belge.* Zeventem: Sequoia, 1981.

Sonnino, Paul. *Louis XIV and the Origins of the Dutch War.* Cambridge: Cambridge University Press, 1988.

Southgate, B. C. " 'Forgotten and Lost': Some Reactions to Autonomous Science in the Seventeenth Century." *Journal of the History of Ideas* 50 (1989): 249–68.

Spence, Jonathan D. *The Question of Hu.* New York: Random House, 1988.

Spufford, Margaret. *The Great Reclothing of Rural England: Petty Chapmen and Their Wares in the Seventeenth Century.* London: Hambledon Press, 1984.

Staff, Frank. *The Penny Post, 1680–1918.* London: Lutterworth Press, 1964.

Steneck, Nicholas. "Greatrakes the Stroker: The Interpretations of Historians." *Isis* 73 (1982): 161–71.

Szczeniak, Boleslaw. "John Floyer and Chinese Medicine." *Osiris* 11 (1954): 137–56.

Talbot, C. H. *The Anglo-Saxon Missionaries in Germany.* New York: Sheed and Ward, 1954.

TeBrake, Wayne Ph. *Regents and Rebels: The Revolutionary World of an Eighteenth-Century Dutch City.* Studies in Social Discontinuity. Cambridge, Mass.: Basil Blackwell, 1989.

TeBrake, William H. *Medieval Frontier: Culture and Ecology in Rijnland.* College Station: Texas A&M University Press, 1985.

Temkin, Owsei. "The Role of Surgery in the Rise of Modern Medical Thought." *Bulletin of the History of Medicine* 25 (1951): 248–59.

Thijssen-Schoute, C. Louise. "De Nederlandse vriendenkring van John Locke." In *Uit de republiek der letteren*, 90–103. The Hague: Martinus Nijhoff, 1967.

———. "Le cartésianisme aux pays-bas." In *Descartes et le cartésianisme hollandais: Etudes et documents*, 183–260. Amsterdam: Editions Françaises D'Amsterdam, 1950.

———. *Nederlands Cartesianisme*. 1954. Utrecht: Hes Uitgevers, 1989.

Thomas, Donald, ed. *State Trials*. 2 vols. London: Routledge and Kegan Paul, 1972.

Thoren, Victor E. *The Lord of Uraniborg: A Biography of Tycho Brahe*. Cambridge: Cambridge University Press, 1990.

Todd, T. *William Dockwra and the Rest of the Undertakers: The Story of the London Penny Post, 1680–1682*. Edinburgh: C. J. Cousland and Sons, 1952.

Torlesse, Francis Harriet. *Bygone Days*. London: Harrison and Sons, 1914.

Toulmin, Stephen, and June Goodfield. *The Discovery of Time*. New York: Harper and Row, Harper Torchbooks/Science Library, 1966.

Tracy, James D. *A Financial Revolution in the Habsburg Netherlands: Renten and Renteniers in the County of Holland, 1515–1565*. Berkeley and Los Angeles: University of California Press, 1985.

———. *Holland under Habsburg Rule, 1506–1566: The Formation of a Body Politic*. Berkeley and Los Angeles: University of California Press, 1990.

Trevor-Roper, Hugh. "The Paracelsian Movement." In *Renaissance Essays*, 149–99. London: Fontana Press, 1986.

Troyer, Howard William. *Ned Ward of Grubstreet: A Study of Sub-literary London in the Eighteenth Century*. Cambridge: Harvard University Press, 1946.

Ulrich, Laurel. *A Midwife's Tale: The Life of Martha Ballard, Based on Her Diary, 1785–1812*. New York: Knopf, 1990.

van Andel, M. A. "Geneesmiddelen tegen den steen der nieren en der blase." *Nederlandsch Tijdschrift voor Geneeskunde* 79, no. 3 (1935): 3307–12.

———. "Plague Regulations in the Netherlands." *Janus* 21 (1916): 410–41.

van Berkel, K. "Descartes in debat met Voetius: De mislukte introductie van het Cartesianisme aan de Utrechtse Universiteit (1639–1645)." *Tijdschrift voor de geschiedenis der geneeskunde, natuurwetenschappen, wiskunde, en techniek* 7 (1984): 4–18.

———. *In het voetspoor van Stevin: Geschiedenis van de natuurwetenschap in Nederland 1580–1940*. Amsterdam: Boom Meppel, 1985.

———. *Isaac Beeckman (1588–1637) en de mechanisering van het wereldbeeld*. Amsterdam: Rodopi, 1983.

van der Hoeven, J. "Het Chirurgijn-gilde te Deventer." *Nederlandsch tijdschrift voor geneeskunde* 78, no. 2 (1934): 1547–59.

van der Pas, Peter W. "The Earliest European Descriptions of Japan's Flora." *Janus* 61 (1974): 281–95.

van der Stigchel, J. W. B. "Geneesmiddelen tegen den steen der nieren en der blaas." *Nederlandsch tijdschrift voor geneeskunde* 79, no. 4 (1935): 4658–59.

van der Wall, E. G. E. *De mystieke chiliast Petrus Serrarius (1600–1669) en zijn wereld*. Leiden, 1987.

van der Wee, H. "Antwoord op een industriël uitaging: De Nederlandse steden tijdens de late middeleeuwen en nieuwe tijd." *Tijdschrift voor geschiedenis* 100 (1987): 169–84.

van der Woude, A. M. "Demografische ontwikkeling van de Noordelijke Nederlanden, 1550–1800." In *Algemene geschiedenis der nederlanden*. Haarlem: Fibula-Van Dishoeck, 1980, Vol. 5.

van Deursen, A. T. *Plain Lives in a Golden Age: Popular Culture, Religion, and Society in Seventeenth-Century Holland*. Translated by Maarten Ultee. Cambridge: Cambridge University Press, 1991.

van de Velde, A. J. J. "Bijdrage tot de studie der werken van der geneeskundige Cornelis Bontkoe." *Koninklijke Vlaamsche Academie voor Taal en Letterkunde, verslagen en mededeelingen* (1925): 3–48.

———. "Bijdrage tot de studie der werken van Stephanus Blankaart." *Koninklijke Vlaamsche Academie voor Taal en Letterkunde, verslagen en mededeelingen* (1924): 453–94.

van de Ven, A. J. "Een steensnijding in 1653." *Nederlandsch tijdschrift voor geneeskunde* 79, no. 3 (1935): 3300–3307; 3750–60.

van Dorssen, J. M. H. "Willem ten Rhijne." *Geneeskunde tijdschrift voor Nederlands Indië* 51 (1911): 134–228.

van Dorsten, J. A. *The Anglo-Dutch Renaissance: Seven Essays*. Leiden: E. J. Brill, 1988.

———. *Poets, Patrons, and Professors: Sir Philip Sidney, Daniel Rogers, and the Leiden Humanists*. Leiden: Leiden University Press, 1962.

van Engen, John, trans. *Devotio Moderna: Basic Writings*. New York: Paulist Press, 1988.

van Gelder, J. B., E. Grendel, and D. A. Wittop Koning. "Deventer en de farmacie." *Pharmaceutisch Weekblad* 101, no. 42 (1966): 940–52.

van Gils, J. B. F. "Spaansche vlieg." *Nederlandsch tijdschrift voor geneeskunde* 90, no. 1 (1946): 377–80.

van Houtte, J. A. *An Economic History of the Low Countries, 800–1800*. London: Wedenfeld and Nicholson, 1977.

van Lieburg, M. J. "Isaac Beeckman and His Diary-Notes on William Harvey's Theory on Bloodcirculation." *Janus* 69 (1982): 161–83.

———. "Pieter van Foreest en de rol van de stadsmedicus in de Noord-Nederlandse steden van de 16e eeuw." In *Pieter van Foreest: Een Hollands medicus in de zestiende eeuw*, edited by H. L. Houtzager, 41–72. Amsterdam: Rodopi, 1989.

———. "Zacharias Sylvius (1608–1664), Author of the 'Praefatio' to the First Rotterdam Edition (1648) of Harvey's *De Motu Cordis*." *Janus* 65 (1978): 241–57.

van Slee, Jacob Cornelius. *De Illustre School te Deventer, 1630–1878*. The Hague: Martinus Nijhoff, 1916.

van Stuijvenberg, J. H. " 'The' Weber Thesis: An Attempt at Interpretation." *Acta Historiae Neerlandicae* 8 (1975): 50–66.

van Thiel, P. H. *Anopheles en malaria in Leiden en naaste omgeving*. Leiden: Eduardo Ijdo, 1922.

van Zanden, J. L. "Op zoek naar de 'missing link': Hypothesen over de opkomst van Holland in de late Middeleeuwen en de vroeg-moderne tijd." *Tijdschrift voor social geschiedenis* 14 (1988): 359–86.

Veendorp, H., and L. G. M. Baas Becking. *Hortus Academicus Lugduno Batavus, 1587–1937: The Development of the Gardens of Leyden University.* Haarlem: Enschedaiana, 1938.

Verbeek, Theo. *Descartes and the Dutch: Early Reactions to Cartesian Philosophy, 1637–1650.* Carbondale: Southern Illinois University Press, 1992.

———, ed. and trans. *La Querelle D'Utrecht: René Descartes et Martin Schoock.* Paris: Les Impressions Nouvelles, 1988.

Verhulst, Adriaan. "The Origins of Towns in the Low Countries and the Pirenne Thesis." *Past and Present,* no. 122 (1989): 3–35.

Viseltear, Arthur J. "Joanna Stephens and Eighteenth Century Lithontriptics: A Misplaced Chapter in the History of Therapeutics." *Bulletin of the History of Medicine* 42 (1968): 199–220.

Walker, R. B. "Advertising in London Newspapers, 1650–1750." *Business History* 15 (1973): 112–30.

Wangensteen, Owen H., and Sarah D. Wangensteen. *The Rise of Surgery.* Minneapolis: University of Minnesota Press, 1978.

Ward, H. Gordon. "An Unnoted Poem by Mandeville." *Review of English Studies* 7 (1931): 73–76.

Weber, Max. *The Protestant Ethic and the Spirit of Capitalism.* Translated by Talcott Parsons. With a foreword by R. H. Tawney. New York: Scribner's, 1958.

Webster, Charles. "English Medical Reformers of the Puritan Revolution: A Background to the 'Society of Chymical Physitians'." *Ambix* 14 (1967): 16–41.

———. *The Great Instauration: Science, Medicine, and Reform, 1625–1660.* New York: Holmes and Meyer, 1975.

Westfall, Richard S. *Never at Rest: A Biography of Isaac Newton.* Cambridge: Cambridge University Press, 1980.

Willcock, John W. *The Laws Relating to the Medical Profession.* London, 1830.

Williamson, Raymond. "The Germ Theory of Disease: Neglected Precursors of Louis Pasteur (Richard Bradley, Benjamin Martin, Jean-Baptiste Goiffon)." *Annals of Science* 11 (1955): 44–57.

———. "John Martyn and the *Grub-Street Journal,* with Particular Reference to His Attacks on Richard Bentley, Richard Bradley, and William Cheselden." *Medical History* 5 (1961): 361–74.

Wilson, Charles. *Holland and Britain.* London: Collins, n.d.

———. *Profit and Power: A Study of England and the Dutch Wars.* London: Longmans, Green, 1957.

Winn, James Anderson. *John Dryden and His World.* New Haven: Yale University Press, 1987.

Wittop Koning, D. A. "De oorsprong van de Amsterdamse Pharmacopee." *Pharmeceutisch Weekblad* 85 (1950): 801–3.

———. "De voorgeschiedenis van het Collegium Medicum te Amsterdam." *Jaarboek Amstelodamum* (1947): 1–16.

———. Introduction to *Fascimile of the First Amsterdam Pharmacopoeia, 1636.* Nieuwkoop: B. de Graaf, 1961.

Wood, Thomas. *English Casuistical Divinity during the Seventeenth Century: With Special Reference to Jeremy Taylor.* London: SPCK, 1952.

Wrigley, E. A. "A Simple Model of London's Importance in Changing English Society and Economy, 1650–1750." *Past and Present,* no. 37 (1967): 44–70.

Wrigley, E. A., and Roger S. Schofield. *The Population History of England, 1541–1871: A Reconstruction.* Cambridge: Harvard University Press, 1981.

Yates, Frances A. *The Rosicrucian Enlightenment.* London: Routledge and Kegan Paul, 1972.

Index

Library of Congress Cataloging-in-Publication Data

Cook, Harold John.
   Trials of an ordinary doctor : Joannes Groenevelt in seventeenth-century London /
Harold J. Cook.
     p.   cm.
   Includes bibliographical references and index.
   ISBN 0-8018-4778-8 (acid-free)
    1. Groeneveld, Joannes, 1647–1710?   2. Physicians—Netherlands—Biography.
3. Physicians—England—Biography.   4. Dutch—England.   5. Medicine—Europe—
History—17th century.   I. Title.
R489.G79C66   1994
610′.92—dc20   93-39733
[B]